The History of Veterinary Education in Edinburgh

Dedicated with thanks to
the late John Clewlow and his widow Ailsa
of the Veterinary History Society
and
the Archivists and Research Services Team
at the Centre for Research Collections, Main University Library,
The University of Edinburgh

The History of Veterinary Education in Edinburgh

ALASTAIR A. MACDONALD AND
COLIN M. WARWICK

WITH CHAPTER 8 BY
ALASTAIR A. MACDONALD,
MARIA DŁUGOŁĘCKA-GRAHAM
AND COLIN M. WARWICK

EDINBURGH
University Press

Edinburgh University Press is one of the leading university presses in the UK. We publish academic books and journals in our selected subject areas across the humanities and social sciences, combining cutting-edge scholarship with high editorial and production values to produce academic works of lasting importance. For more information visit our website: edinburghuniversitypress.com

Edinburgh University Press Ltd
The Tun – Holyrood Road
12 (2f) Jackson's Entry
Edinburgh EH8 8PJ

Typeset in 11/13 Adobe Garamond by
Cheshire Typesetting Ltd, Cuddington, Cheshire, and
printed and bound in Great Britain

A CIP record for this book is available from the British Library

ISBN 978 1 3995 2558 9 (hardback)
ISBN 978 1 3995 2559 6 (paperback)
ISBN 978 1 3995 2560 2 (webready PDF)
ISBN 978 1 3995 2561 9 (epub)

Contents

Figures

Plates

Tables

Preface

We began the research that underpins this book some twenty years ago (Warwick and Macdonald 2003). Our aim then, as now, was to seek out and uncover the various stories of veterinary education in Edinburgh (Macdonald, Warwick and Johnston 2005). We have therefore published our findings in the Edinburgh Research Archive (ERA) as a series of detailed articles that focused on particular aspects of that development. The initial core of the research material lay, sometimes openly, sometimes well hidden, on the shelves of the libraries in the Royal (Dick) School of Veterinary Studies, in the archives of the Royal Highland and Agricultural Society of Scotland and within the National Library of Scotland. The unfolding evidence soon led us to the Centre for Research Collections (CRC) in the Edinburgh University Library, to the Edinburgh Room of the City Library, to the Archives of the City of Edinburgh and beyond.

It was quickly clear that the evolution of the teaching of veterinary medicine and surgery in Edinburgh was not the province of one school or college alone. It was also obvious that there had been secure anatomical and medical foundations in Edinburgh upon which to build this academic and clinical discipline. But why had it not happened sooner? What caused the delay? As the data was gathered and sorted, the various timelines of veterinary education in Edinburgh became visible. The personality and family background to the institution in 1823 of the William Dick Veterinary School, once known, were obvious. The establishment of separate Colleges of Veterinary Medicine, established in 1857 by John Gamgee and in 1873 by William Williams, were understandably distinctive entities when it was clear why they had budded off from William Dick's College. The perhaps unexpected establishment of the wartime Polish Veterinary Faculty, from its beginnings in 1943, to become another largely self-contained entity, but associated with the Royal (Dick) Veterinary College, raised a plethora of questions and a wholly unexpected new finding. During the nineteenth century there was a curious dichotomy in the constant, sometimes ambivalent institutional arm's-length, 'veterinary presence' of the University of Edinburgh, when compared with the many critical, indeed essential, individual medical contributions of teaching, examining and research support to veterinary education provided over those decades by medical staff at Edinburgh University. This made a comprehensive and cohesive description of these contributions awkward.

The involvement of the university with the veterinary college was progressively resolved during the twentieth century. It followed the establishment of veterinary degrees in the University of Edinburgh in 1911 and the later embodiment of the Royal (Dick) Veterinary College within the University of Edinburgh in 1952. One offshoot of the veterinary college's long association with the university was the development of the postgraduate Centre for Tropical Veterinary Medicine in 1970. Thereby, yet another centre of veterinary education came into being, embedded within, yet quite distinctly different from, the Veterinary School; how did such an organisation dealing with tropical animal diseases come to be located in temperate Scotland?

We have been pragmatic in dividing the remaining time periods into largely chronological chapters. These partitions are associated with important changes in the teaching accommodation, adjustments in internal administration and finally with an all-too-brief summary of two hundred years of veterinary student life in Edinburgh. Who were these men and women and where did they come from? What was it that brought them from all over the world to the veterinary schools and colleges of Edinburgh? What did they do and how did they live when they were here? And where did they go to after they received their veterinary education? The whole student topic is clearly worthy of detailed analysis and presentation in a book on its own.

We have taken care to accurately source all the information presented in the book and have presented references to assist the reader's access to further information. We have been assisted in the compilation and analysis of information by many people in libraries, universities, museums, archives and veterinary institutions in this country and abroad, as well as by the alumni of the Royal (Dick) School of Veterinary Studies. However, we take responsibility for any errors that may have crept in.

References

ERA. https://era.ed.ac.uk/handle/1842/898/discover (accessed 4 August 2022).

Macdonald, A. A., Warwick, C. M. and Johnston, W. T. 2005. Locating veterinary education in Edinburgh in the nineteenth century. *Book of the Old Edinburgh Club*, New Series, 6, 41–71. https://era.ed.ac.uk/handle/1842/2199 (accessed 4 August 2022).

Warwick, C. M. and Macdonald, A. A. 2003. The New Veterinary College, Edinburgh, 1873 to 1904. *The Veterinary Record*, 153, 380–6. https://era.ed.ac.uk/handle/1842/2198 (accessed 4 August 2022).

Acknowledgements

We gratefully acknowledge the provision, by all the Deans and Heads of School at the Royal (Dick) School of Veterinary Studies, of the research environment which has enabled us to carry out our veterinary historical investigations. These span a combined total of seventy-four years of employment in the university and a combined 102 years of association as staff and honorary fellows of the Dick Vet. The professional assistance given to us by administrative members of staff at the Dick Vet over this period, including Bruce Nelson, Janet Hackel, Marianne Watson and Lindsay Dalziel, was fundamental to our research and much appreciated. The library staff, including Fiona Brown, Doreen Graham, Bogusia McRoberts and Gail Gray of the Lady Smith of Kelvin Library and Eileen Burdekin and Anne Kennett at the Summerhall library of the Royal (Dick) School of Veterinary Studies, have always been most helpful to us. The late Dr 'Bean' Phillips fully deserves very special mention for having routinely and carefully collected together and guarded the bulk of the early archives of material relating to the Dick Vet. In a host of different ways, the research assistance of the Centre for Research Collections in the University of Edinburgh Library, into which that archive was carefully transferred, has had a very direct impact on our book. We thank the earlier staff, Arnott Wilson, Joe Marshall, Tricia Boyd, Sally Pagan, Denise Anderson, Hazel Robertson and Ann Henderson and the current archivists Grant Buttars, Rachel Hosker, Aline Brodin, Fiona Menzies, and the Research Services Team of Francesca Baseby, Scott Docking, Paul Fleming, Elliot Holmes, Danielle Howarth, Lauren McKay, Louise Scollay, Danielle Spittle, Daisy Stafford and Stephen Willis. The work of Marshall Dozier in opening our internet access to libraries and newspapers (such as the Scotsman Historical Archive) nationally and worldwide had a hugely beneficial effect on our historical research, for which we are profoundly grateful. Similarly, we thank Theo Andrew for enabling us to put our research information online, and thereby widely available, in the Edinburgh Research Archive (https://www.era.lib.ed.ac.uk/).

For many years the historical knowledge and archival assistance of the late Willie Johnston, the librarian of the Royal Highland and Agricultural Society of Scotland, was of great benefit to our studies. We also deeply appreciate the professional assistance given to us by the librarians of the National Library of Scotland, the Edinburgh Room of the City of Edinburgh main Library, the Edinburgh City Archives, the General Register House, the Royal Botanic Gardens of Edinburgh, Queen Margaret University College, Edinburgh, the Royal Commission on the Ancient and Historical Monuments of Scotland (RCAHMS), now part of Historic Environment Scotland (HES), the National Archives of Scotland, the Royal College of Veterinary Surgeons, the Royal Veterinary College in London, the British Library, Jonathan Farmer, Librarian at the National Archives based at Kew, the Wellcome Trust and the American Veterinary Medical Association. Our thanks too to James Hamilton, Research Principal of the WS Society at the Signet Library, Edinburgh and to Craig Statham and staff in the Reading Room, National Library of Scotland. The information and assistance provided to us by Jacqueline Williams, Adrian Allan, Thomas Chisholm and the staff of the special collections and archives of the University of Liverpool Library was much valued.

We thank Mandy Wise and Dan Mitchell in the University College London, Library Services, Special Collections for their assistance in gaining access to the John Barclay manuscript, O. Charnock Bradley's grandniece, Mrs Frances Harrison, for access to his personal diaries, Captain G. E. Locker and the staff at Home Headquarters The Light Dragoons for historical military information, Michael Knott and Cynthia Hendrickx for information and photos relating to chapter 8, the Hogarth-Scott Family for the unique Dick Vet blazer and tie, and Sian Lexmond, Vivian Yu, Joey Luxmore, Lorna Linfield and the other students for assistance with the contents of chapter 14.

The assistance of Janina Kowalska, Deputy Archivist, and reading room assistants Klaudia Kierepka, Paulina Gabryszak-Stevens and Katarzyna Pobideł at the Polish Institute and Sikorski Museum in London was much appreciated, as was the assistance of Grzegorz Pisarski, the Deputy Chief Librarian of the Polish Library POSK in London. We are also indebted to Dr Agnieszka Zawiejska, mgr. Maria Jankowska, emeritus Vice-Head of Poznań's Saint Adalbert Publishing House (Wydawnictwo Św. Wojciecha) and an emeritus Chief Redactor of Poznań Adam Mickiewicz University Publishing House. Lindsay Dalziel, Leslie Harrison, Tony Smith, Darren

Shaw and Kate Ainsworth graciously provided assistance with postgraduate data. Acknowledgement is happily given to Sandie Howie, Joe Rock, Trenton Boyd and to Andrew Gardiner, Paul Watkins, Clare Boulton and other members of the Veterinary History Society for helpful conversations, discussions and assistance. We extend our thanks to the many photographers who gave us permission to reproduce their work: Paul Dodds, Fiona Manson, Ali Humphreys, Brian Mather and Alex Hennessey of Ron Taylor. We are also grateful for the contributions made by Mary Packer, John Frace (Travelling Tabby), Valentin Jonathan Hunzinger and Ketan Lad, and Diane Fagen of the American Veterinary Medical Association.

Penultimately, but certainly by no means least, we are grateful to all the students and alumni of the Dick Vet with whom we have had personal conversations, email and letter correspondence for all their stories, recollections, photographs and medals shared with us. Similarly, we thank all those from the Dick Vet and the other veterinary institutions based in Edinburgh who have gone before and left manuscript notes, letters, printed journal articles, books of recollections, lecture notes, records of session attendance, places of residence, fees paid, photographs, newspaper stories, College publications and other veterinary ephemera.

Thanks to the team at Edinburgh University Press: Tom Dark, Isobel Birks and Eddie Clark, with particular thanks to Michelle Houston for her careful guidance of us when we were compiling our work in 'book proposal' form and then guiding this through its first few steps in 2021 and 2022. Thanks too to copy-editor Ian Brooke.

We gratefully acknowledge the financial assistance to our research from the University of Edinburgh Development Trust, the University of Edinburgh, Mhaoin leabhar and the Balloch Trust.

Chapter 1

Foundations of Veterinary Education in Scotland (1696–1817)

Eighteenth-century Edinburgh experienced significant changes in thought patterns, education and the resulting ways of living following the transfer of the Scottish Royal Court to London in 1603, the removal of the Scottish Parliament to London in 1707, the Jacobite Rebellion in 1745 and the blossoming of the Scottish Enlightenment (Houston 1994). The town had also felt the political and social impacts of the French Revolution, the war in Europe (1789–99) and the Napoleonic Wars (1803–15). Scattered in the archives of national, city and university libraries in Edinburgh there are many traces of these events. Among them can be found fragments of evidence of enlightened eighteenth-century publications, lectures, proposals and discussions indicating that the topic of veterinary education (in its broadest sense) had been debated in Edinburgh. It is also evident that these conversations had begun more than one hundred years before the 1820s, when the first groups of students were enrolled in William Dick's Veterinary School. This chapter draws specific attention to the contributions made by William Hope, Alexander Monro and his son and grandson, the new School of Medicine in the University of Edinburgh, James Clark and his family, James Jeffray, the Frenchman John Feron, Jeremiah Kirby, Edward Harrison, the Highland Society of Scotland and John Barclay. The 1784 map of Edinburgh by Kincaid (Figure 1.1) has been labelled to indicate the locations discussed in the narrative.

The beginnings

Formal veterinary education in Edinburgh can be said to have stemmed from lessons learned in France. Sir William Hope of Kirkliston

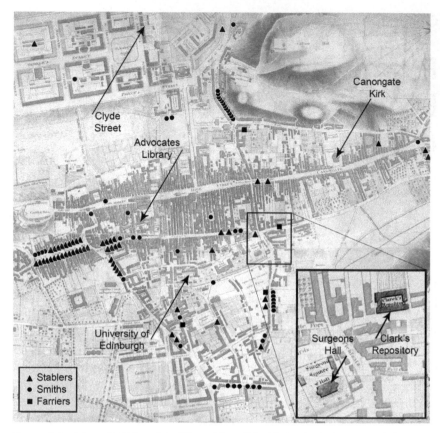

Figure 1.1 Map of Edinburgh by Kincaid (1784) highlighting the locations of places mentioned in the text. With permission of the WS Society, The Signet Library.

(1660–1724), a skilled horseman who served in the army, travelled widely in Europe. He met Jacques de Solleysel (1617–80) in Paris and became his pupil for two years (Smith 1919). Back in Edinburgh, during his time as Deputy Governor of Edinburgh Castle, Hope translated into English the 1691 edition of Solleysel's famous book, *Le Parfait Maréchal* (Solleysel 1691). This was printed in Edinburgh in 1696 as a splendid folio edition of six hundred pages. Hope supplemented the translation with the works of William Cavendish (1592–1676) and others and expressed his wish that farriers could somehow receive a more formal education (Solleysel 1696). He deplored the absence of skilled veterinary practitioners in Britain (Smith 1919). In 1707 the Scots anatomist James Douglas (1675–1742), who was based in London, published his book on the detailed comparative anatomy of the human and the dog (Douglas 1707). He is considered to have been one of the most important anatomists of the eighteenth century for having introduced meticulous and scientific methods for studying human anatomy (Koutsouflianiotis et al. 2019). It was also at about this time that the teaching of anatomy in Edinburgh entered a new period (Struthers 1867). The College of Surgeons reported to Edinburgh Town Council in 1697 that it had completed an Anatomical Theatre in Surgeons' Hall (Figure 1.1), where dissections of the human body could be carried out with access restricted to the regular apprentices and pupils of Surgeons. The title Professor of Anatomy was conferred by the Town Council on the surgeon selected to carry out the dissection. The fourth surgeon appointed as Professor of Anatomy was Alexander Monro, a student of James Douglas (Struthers 1867).

Alexander Monro *primus* (1697–1767)

Alexander Monro (Figure 1.2) had already studied anatomy during his teenage years in Edinburgh. In 1717 he travelled first to London and then on to Paris and Leiden as part of his two-year study tour to further develop his anatomical knowledge and teaching techniques. During his time as a student in Leiden in 1719 he used animal dissections and the knowledge gained from Douglas to explain to his fellow students the differences in muscular structure between animals and man (Bower 1817; Erlam 1954). Following his return to Edinburgh in the autumn of 1719, Monro was examined by the College of Surgeons and admitted as a member (Bower 1817; Struthers 1867). The subsequent year he was proposed to the Town Council as the next Special Teacher in Anatomy. In 1722, at the age of twenty-five, he was formally appointed Professor of Anatomy in the University of Edinburgh (Figure 1.1). Monro initially gave lectures in the anatomy theatre in the basement of Surgeons' Hall. Thereafter he moved into the 'townis college' (University of Edinburgh) in 1725, where a new dissection theatre had been built for him. His anatomical investigations led him to dissect dogs, cows, domestic fowl and fish. The results of these studies were fed into his detailed comparative anatomy lectures, and the dissected specimens went into his anatomical museum (Monro 1775, 1797, 1798). Within ten years the numbers of medical students and surgical scholars and apprentices attending his classes doubled in size, to over a hundred young men (Bower 1817; Struthers 1867). One of the scholars in his 1737–8 class of 123 students was James Robertson, an apprentice to the surgeon-apothecary John Kennedy (Macdonald et al. 2011). Robertson later became the father-in-law of James Clark (1732–1808), the next significant character in the development of veterinary education in Scotland. Monro's interest in animals extended beyond his study of comparative anatomy, as he made clear in a manuscript autobiography

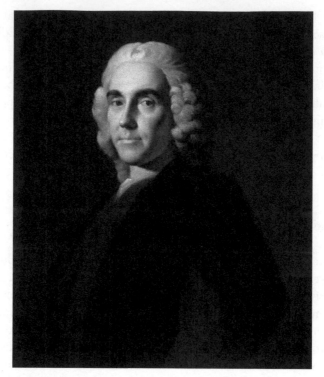

Figure 1.2 Alexander Monro of Auchenbowie *primus* (1697–1767) by Allan Ramsay (1713–84). National Galleries of Scotland. Purchased 1990.

(Erlam 1954; Macdonald et al. 2011). In the 1760s Monro wrote that he had a small estate near Stirling, called Auchinbowie, where he had planned to retire when he reached sixty years of age (1757), and to set aside one day of the week

> for the Cure of diseased Cattle, of whom the Farrier's son was to take Care as also directed by the old Gentleman [Monro himself] – The young Doctors for the human and brute Patients, were to dissect both sound and morbid Bodies of Animals, and were afterwards to be sent to the proper Schools to complete their Education.

Sadly he fell ill that year, and then 'some Circumstances of his Family Affairs put a Stop to it' (his retirement plan).

James Clark (1732–1808)

James Clark was a well-educated, enterprising and highly experienced farrier living in Edinburgh. Long regarded as the most significant British contributor to the veterinary literature of the period, he was further characterised as the 'father of Veterinary Hygiene, not only in this country but in Europe' (Smith 1924).

Almost nothing is known of the first thirty years of Clark's life other than that he was born about 1732 (Greig 1948). This was the same year that William Burdon published in Edinburgh:

> A Farrier is as useful a Trade as any other in His Majesty's Dominions; we commonly call him Doctor, because he professes Physick and Surgery among Horses; and some are good sensible Men; but People who are able to give their Sons Learning, seldom bind 'em to that Trade; so that Farriers are oblig'd to take such Apprentices as they can get without Regard to their Education ... Thus many are illiterate, and some totally incapable of Improvement. I have great Compassion for that noble and serviceable Creature a Horse, when I consider how precarious his Life is in the Hands of such Men. (Burdon 1732)

We know that in 1758, aged twenty-six, Clark travelled south to London and spent about eleven months working at his trade there (Greig 1948; Macdonald et al. 2011). On 9 December 1764, in the Trinity College Kirk, Edinburgh, he married Jean Robertson, a milliner from the Tolbooth Parish of Edinburgh. She was the daughter of the aforementioned James Robertson, the medical surgeon at Torryburn, Fife, and his wife Elizabeth née Langlands. Although no records of conversations within the Clark family have come to light, it is highly likely that James and his father-in-law shared discussions of a farriery/veterinary nature. Dr Robertson had studied anatomy under Alexander Monro, who presented to him detailed lectures on the comparative anatomy of the organs in the abdomen, thorax and neck of the dog and cow (Macdonald et al. 2011). In 1765 Clark in his turn enrolled to attend the equivalent set of anatomy classes given by Monro's son, referred to as Alexander Monro *secundus* (Monro 1765). He may also have had some lectures from his father, Monro *primus*, in the newly built (1764) anatomy theatre, which could now hold three hundred students. Clark matriculated in the University of Edinburgh in 1765 and 1766 (Album 1762). As a student, he would have had access to the books in the university's library as well as those of various other libraries in the town. For example, he may well have had access, via friends and colleagues, to the very well-stocked Advocates Library (Figure 1.1); its 1776 catalogue listed books of 'farriery interest' by H. Bracken, G. L. Le Clerc (Count de Buffon), R. Berenger and S. Hales, as well as Sir W. Hope's translation of Jacques de Solleysel, among others (Wellburn 1989).

Clark published his first veterinary textbook in 1770, three years after undertaking his university studies of human and comparative animal anatomy (Clark 1770). Within five years a much-expanded edition of this book was published (the number of pages had increased from 62 to 203). This gave a detailed account of the diseases of the horse's foot; Clark donated a copy to Edinburgh University Library (Clark 1775). Both books entered the catalogue of the Advocates Library between 1776 and 1787 (Macdonald et al. 2011). The text of the expanded edition was republished in 1782 as the third edition (Clark 1782).

In 1771 Clark established a 'Livery Stables and Repository for Horses' at the head of the South Back of Canongate (Figure 1.1) (Macdonald et al. 2005). It was situated outside the city wall, due north-east of Surgeons' Hall. The number of 'stablers' listed in the 1775 Edinburgh *Directory* (fifty-two, with two stablers in Leith) gives some measure of the population of horses coming into the town at that time (Williamson 1775). The same *Directory* listed James Clark as a ferrier [farrier] in the South Back of the Canongate, Peter Clark as a farrier in Toderick's Wynd in the Cowgate and James Thomson as a farrier in Broughton. Although George Christie at the Pleasance was the only listed Blacksmith, an additional sixty-one men were included as 'smiths' (with eight in Leith). There is good evidence from other sources, such as the Register of Marriages, that a number of these and other younger men were also considered farriers or blacksmiths (Macdonald et al. 2011). Clark's good reputation was such that on 31 January 1776 he was appointed, and on 25 September that year registered, as Farrier to His Majesty in Scotland (George III) (Greig 1948; Macdonald et al. 2005).

Alexander Monro *secundus* (1733–1817)

During this period in Clark's life there had been a substantial increase in the reputation of the University of Edinburgh's Medical School and Monro *primus* had been succeeded to the Chair in Anatomy in 1754 by his son, Alexander Monro *secundus* (Struthers 1867). Like his father, Monro *secundus* (Figure 1.3) first spent time abroad, in London, Leiden, Paris and Berlin, furthering his anatomical knowledge and research skills, before returning to Edinburgh in 1758 to teach (Struthers 1867). He continued the development of his father's lectures on human and comparative anatomy and presented these to ever-increasing numbers of students (Macdonald et al. 2011). In 1775 Douglas's book on comparative anatomy (human and dog) was republished in Edinburgh (Douglas 1775). Six years later, Monro *secundus* published the *Treatise on Comparative Anatomy* as part of his father's complete works, and two years thereafter published an extended and revised version of this *Comparative Anatomy* (Monro 1783). Perhaps in part inspired by Douglas's book, this revised

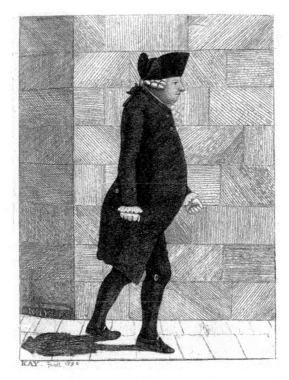

Figure 1.3   Drawing [1790] of Alexander Monro *secundus* (1733–1817) by John Kay (1742–1826). Courtesy of Sheila Szatkowski, Edinburgh.

version now contained, in addition to the previous twenty-nine pages on dog anatomy, a detailed eighteen-page description of the musculature of the dog. There was also the following explanation in a footnote to the Introduction:

> the myology of animals seems exceedingly necessary for young anatomists, who generally begin with dissecting them before they have access to human bodies. For this reason, we have added, not indeed a complete myology, but an account of the particulars wherein the muscles of a dog differ from those of man; this being the animal most frequently chosen for dissections, and one of those whose structure bears no small resemblance to that of the human species.

It was therefore clearly stated that in the University of Edinburgh most of the practical medical and surgical instruction on muscular anatomy was being learned from the dissection of the dog. In 1781 James Clark's eldest son, James, matriculated in the University of Edinburgh and enrolled in the anatomy classes given by Monro *secundus*. He enrolled for classes again during the 1782–3 session (Macdonald et al. 2011).

James Jeffray (1759–1848)

James Jeffray (Figure 1.4) was another of the 328 students who enrolled in the 1782–3 Anatomy classes by Monro *secundus* (Macdonald et al. 2011). He had gone to Glasgow University in 1772 and after the five-year course obtained his MA degree in 1778 (Macdonald et al. 2011). He then came to Edinburgh to study Medicine at the university in 1782 and was listed as attending the 1783–4 classes in Natural History given by John Walker and the 1784–5 lectures in Botany by John Hope (Macdonald et al. 2011). Other Medical School teachers also taught in the vernacular and these included William Cullen on the Practice of Medicine, Joseph Black on Chemistry and Medicine, Francis Home on Dietetics, Materia Medica and Pharmacy, James Gregory on the Institutions of Medicine and Alexander Hamilton on Obstetrics and Midwifery. On 30 November 1782, Jeffray was accepted as a member of the Medical Society of Edinburgh. This student society was established in 1737 and not only had an active programme of lectures and debates but also had its own library (Macdonald et al. 2011). Jeffray was elected one of the four annual presidents of the Society for 1784–5. On 13 February 1783, he joined the newly formed Natural History Society of Edinburgh (Macdonald et al. 2011). Jeffray presented two essays to this society: 'Observations on the Placenta' on 22 May 1783 and 'On the analogy that subsists between animals and vegetables' on 11 March 1784. These titles are indicative of the range of subjects selected by the medical students for presentation. In 1786 (aged twenty-seven) he submitted his thesis and graduated MD (Macdonald et al. 2011).

That same year Jeffray released his first publication, *An address to the public, on the present state of farriery* (Jeffray 1786). This document is interesting and pertinent from several points of view. Firstly, it reveals how politically well-connected Jeffray appears to have been; he described himself as 'Farrier to his Royal Highness the Prince of Wales for Scotland' (Prince George Augustus Frederick, the future George IV). This link may have been achieved through his connections with Andrew Duncan, the editor of *Medical Commentaries*, then the only medical journal in Britain, who had recently been appointed Physician to the Prince of Wales for Scotland (Macdonald et al. 2011). Secondly, Jeffray seems to have been directing his writing to the Prince, and thereafter to a horse-owning readership based more in England than in Scotland. Thirdly, he stated that he had gained experience of horse dissection during the preceding three years and had had access to books on farriery by Snape, Gibson, Bourgelat and De la Fosse, as well as those from the European veterinary schools (Jeffray 1786). He wrote:

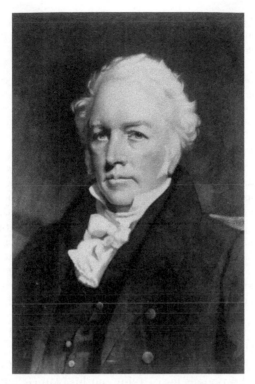

Figure 1.4 James Jeffray (1759–1848) from the photograph by Thomas Annan (1829–87) of a portrait by John Graham-Gilbert (1794–1866). © CSG CIC Glasgow Museums and Libraries Collection: The Mitchell Library, Special Collections.

Farriery must be studied, not as a system of empyricism, consisting of complex, inelegant recipes, and jarring contradictory facts; but as a branch of Medicine, and on a Scientific plan . . . A scientific knowledge of Anatomy, of the phaenomena and causes of diseases, together with an accurate acquaintance with the operation of remedies, so essentially necessary in Medicine, is equally useful and necessary in Farriery; and, that acquaintance with the structure, diseases, and remedies of other animals, particularly of man, added to the stock of knowledge to be acquired in a stable, will make a blacksmith, or a groom, a better farrier, however qualified he might have been.

He went on to argue:

At present everyone who wishes to acquire a superior knowledge of this art, must either dissect alone, and read over the innumerable and voluminous authors, who have written on the subject, without having any one to assist him in clearing away the rubbish, and condensing their scattered facts; or, he must go to Paris or Lyons, and study in the Veterinary Schools. In these seminaries, founded and endowed by the Crown, Professors are appointed to lecture on the anatomy and physiology of horses; on their diseases, and the medicines employed in their cure. And there are extensive stables for horses labouring under every kind of disease, where the student has it in his power to see the truth or fallacy of what he reads, or hears, fully established or overthrown, by an immediate and candid appeal to practice. Pupils have been sent almost from every court in Europe: **that of Britain as yet has sent none** [our emphasis].

Jeffray went on to explain that:

> This can only be done by the institution of an Academy, on a plan somewhat similar to that of the [French] Veterinary Schools . . . There the first object must be, To demonstrate the structure of the Horse, and to point out the nature, the causes, and the seat of his various disorders; the second, To ascertain the effects of medicines on him, and the peculiarities of his constitution . . . To accomplish the first of these ends, a proper place must be fitted up for dissection, demonstration, and preserving preparations, to shew the structure of his different parts in health, and their derangement in disease. As for the last, it is impossible it can be effected, except the horses be continually under the eye of the Mareschall, and entrusted to his people alone; which renders the erection of Stables, or an Infirmary, absolutely necessary.

Jeffray did not hide his opinion that 'a considerable expense must be incurred before this plan can be executed in its full extent'.

Later that year Jeffray followed up his published *Address* with the publication of a set of proposals for carrying out his plan (Jeffray 1786). This document emphasised that in addition to having studied the subject for the last three years,

> he has studied and compared most of the publications on it; he has examined the structure of the horses, by careful dissection; he has improved [that is, learned from] every opportunity that offered, of observing the diseases of Horses, with the effects produced on them by Medical remedies and operations.

His farriery studies in Edinburgh had been unassisted and so he indicated that he intended to spend the 'two following years in attending the Veterinary Academies on the Continent'. Before embarking on this scheme, he invested time into looking for sponsors willing to take the risk of supporting him. Interestingly, the spendthrift Prince George was not persuaded to provide the necessary funding to his 'Farrier in Scotland'. Local Scottish financiers were similarly not attracted to sponsor him. Perhaps the reticence of the latter was because of his statement that following his studies in France, he planned to establish the Veterinary School in London. In 1787 he set off for the continent for other reasons (Jeffray 1787).

Further proposals for veterinary education

It should be understood that in the 1780s hundreds of young men were coming to Edinburgh each year for a medical education. In Edinburgh they were receiving lectures and dissection experience of comparative anatomy as well as participating in discussions of comparative biology as part of their training. Books on these and related medical subjects were being published regularly in the town (Douglas 1775; Monro 1783). James Clark's new book on veterinary hygiene was published in 1788 (Clark 1788). In the preface he regrets that:

> A regular mode of education [in farriery] is not to be attained on any terms, at least in this country. In France, a regular academy [Lyon in 1761 and Alfort in 1765] for the instruction of young farriers has been instituted. The attempt is laudable, and worthy of imitation.

He also goes on to say that:

> Professors of Anatomy, Materia Medica and the Practice of Physic should be available for those anxious to study the diseases of animals; nothing is at present available to them but reading [and this] is not sufficient to qualify a man either for the profession of physician or farrier.

These thoughts and ideas must have been circulating in Edinburgh. They were clearly being discussed within the Clark household. In January 1790 his second son, John, during his interview to be accepted as a pupil at the School of Design in Edinburgh, put forward the proposal 'to institute a Veterinarian School in Scotland' (Macdonald et al. 2005). On 5 October of that year, James Clark wrote to the Odiham Agricultural Society (approximately 60 km south-east of London) with 'a proposal for establishing a veterinarian School in Edinburgh'. However, this application arrived too late. A detailed proposal to establish a veterinary school in London had already been submitted to the Odiham Agricultural Society by Vial de Saint Bel and had been accepted by the Society. Clark's proposal was unsuccessful. The London Veterinary College was established in 1791 with Benoît Charles Marie Vial (also known as Vial de Saint Bel) as the College's first Principal (Veterinary College 1793; Cotchin 1990).

Clark pressed on. In 1793 and 1794 he prepared lectures 'on the prospect of a Veterinary School being established at Edinburgh, under the direction of the Author.' He wrote:

> This school was to have been patronized by some of the first noblemen and gentlemen of the country; and, at the same time, the Author had the fullest assurance of the countenance of Government for its aid and support. For

which reason, he declined the offer then made to him by the Directors of the Veterinary College at London, of standing as a candidate for the vacant Professorship, following the death of M. St Bel their first Professor. (Clark 1806)

It is possible that Clark's comments may have referred in part to Sir John Sinclair (1754–1835), who between 1791 and 1799 published the twenty-one-volume *Statistical Account of Scotland* and who in 1793 had been made President of the newly formed British Board or Society for the Encouragement of Agriculture and Internal improvement (Sinclair) (Figure 1.5). Clark's preference for Scotland was because he

anticipated the many advantages that would be derived from an institution of this kind in Edinburgh, from its vicinity to an University so justly famed for the celebrity of its medical and surgical Professors, and attended by a numerous concourse of Medical Students from all parts of Europe; that whilst many of them were attending other branches of medical education, some might be induced to attend the Veterinary Class. The many advantages arising to the science from this circumstance alone, of being studied by men who had the advantage of a liberal education, would have been the surest means of improving the art, and of disseminating veterinary knowledge throughout the kingdom in a highly improved state. Another circumstance of equal importance attending a Veterinary School at Edinburgh is, that young men who propose to follow the operative branch of shoeing horses, and indeed mechanics in general, get a better or more liberal education in this country, than their more southern brethren of the same professions in England. (Clark 1806)

Clark was a wealthy man by this time, and for the preceding twenty years had been a bold entrepreneur in Edinburgh (Macdonald et al. 2005). He may have considered creating the veterinary college from his own resources. However, various circumstances militated against this course of action. Firstly, he was now over sixty years old. Without doubt, he was aware of the 1778 attempt by Edward Snape, Farrier to George III in England, to establish a Hippiatric Infirmary for the instruction of pupils in Knightsbridge, London; and of its collapse when backers failed to shoulder some of the financial burden (Smith 1924). He was also well aware of the troubled early years experienced by the new London College (Veterinary College 1793). The political situation in Britain due to the 1789 revolution in France and the Napoleonic Wars must also have played a role (Clark 1806).

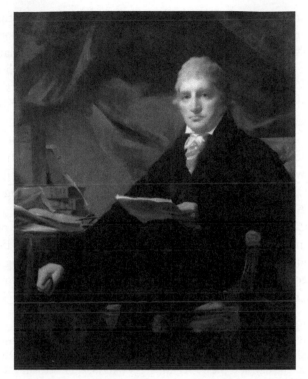

Figure 1.5   Sir John Sinclair (1754–1835) by Sir Henry Raeburn (1756–1823).
© National Portrait Gallery, London.

John Feron (c. 1754–1824)

It was the French Revolution that brought into town the next contributor to the Edinburgh discussion of veterinary education, in the form of a
French Royalist refugee. John Feron (Jean Féron) was born about 1754,
and according to his own account was a military man first (Regiment
of Carabineers) before becoming 'equerrer' and public demonstrator of
equine anatomy in Nantes, Brittany from 1779 to 1789 (Feron 1796). He
said that he had been encouraged by 'Monsieur de S. Bell' to go with him
to England 'to second him in his undertaking of a Veterinary College in
London, which I could not refuse, on account of the long friendship that
had subsisted between us'. Interestingly, Feron's claim that he 'had the
honour of being named Second Professor [of the London School], charged
with the general care of the Infirmary, &c' is not evident in the histories of
the London Veterinary College (Veterinary College 1793; Cotchin 1990).

Feron said that three months after the death of Vial de Saint Bel (on
21 August 1793) he left London and came to Edinburgh via Dublin.

Sometime in 1794 or 1795 Feron reportedly gave a public lecture on the veterinary art to an audience in Edinburgh (Feron 1796). It is possible that James Clark attended this lecture. The event may have stimulated Clark to continue with his writing. The account of the lecture, which was published in 1796, contained a list of thirty subscribers to Feron's proposed veterinary institution (Feron 1796). How many of these may have been the same people that had supported Clark is not clear. At about this time (1794) the *Directory* listed seven 'ferriers' for Edinburgh, and an additional one for Leith; James Clark was listed as a 'coach hyrer'. In the same lists there were fifty-three 'smiths' and sixty-one 'stablers' in Edinburgh (Figure 1.1), with eight smiths and five stablers in neighbouring Leith.

On 28 April 1796 Feron advertised that he had 'Fitted up a FORGE and Opened an INFIRMARY for the reception of SICK or LAME HORSES' in former stable premises under the North Bridge in Edinburgh (Anonymous 1796a). In June he advertised that he was going to give a course of lectures on farriery in July (Anonymous 1796b), and these were specified in a further advertisement on 16 July (Anonymous 1796c):

FARRIERY
M. FERON, Professor of VETERINARY MEDICINE, respectfully informs the Nobility and Gentry, That his proposed COURSE of LECTURES will begin on Tuesday next the 19th curt. at Two o'clock, in Bernard's Rooms, Thistle-street; when he will deliver his First Lecture, containing a General Description of the Horse; with various Remarks on the Geometrical Proportions of the Race and other kinds of Horses.
LECTURE 2d, on Wednesday,
Containing a particular description of the Horse's Foot, externally and internally, &c.
LECTURE 3d, on Thursday,
Of the Position of the Foot upon the Ground, and of the Concave Form of the Lower Surface of the Foot, considered in respect to Shoeing.
LECTURE 4th, on Friday the 22d,
On Paring the Hoof, Accidents resulting from the unskilful performance of that operation, and on Shoeing the Good, the Flat, and the Convex Foot.
Admittance to the whole Course, One Guinea – to a Single Lecture, Seven Shillings.
Tickets may be had of Mr FERON, at his INFIRMARY, under the North Bridge, where he continues to admit LAME or SICK HORSES, not affected with any contagious [sic] disorder, using the most effectual means for their speedy and perfect cure.
EDINR. July 14, 1796.

During the summer of 1796 Feron worked as a farrier with the cavalry at West Barns, East Lothian, under the command of Major General Sir James Stewart (Stewart 1797?; Feron 1797?). He gave his course of farriery lectures to the troops there, the first such series of lectures in Scotland. The next we know of his movements is that he went to London on business in the autumn, and on his return to Edinburgh in 1797 published the prospectus for his Edinburgh Veterinary School entitled *Veterinary Institution* (Feron 1797; Macdonald et al. 2011). In this he indicated that he was now 'ready to receive Pupils, in order to teach the Anatomy of the Horse, and the Veterinary Medicine'. He set his fees and outlined a programme of study, with the study of the horse beginning in May and ending in October, and the study of anatomy and the 'animal economy' beginning in November and ending in April of the following year. In addition, a series of fourteen public lectures on the anatomy and diseases of the horse were offered at the cost of 1 guinea, with tickets to be obtained from him in Edinburgh. However, nothing seems to have come of this. He returned to London and in 1799 attended the short three- to four-month-long course at the same London Veterinary College in which he said he had taught some eight years earlier; he obtained his Diploma on 12 October 1799 (Macdonald et al. 2011). Within days, on 24 October 1799, at the age of forty-five, he enlisted as a veterinary surgeon with the 13th Regiment of the Light Dragoons (Macdonald et al. 2011). Meanwhile, James Clark continued writing his lectures on veterinary physiology in Edinburgh. He lived out the last years of his life in his home near Comely Gardens at the east end of London Road. He died there, aged seventy-six, on 29 July 1808 and was buried in the Canongate cemetery, Edinburgh (Greig 1948; Macdonald et al. 2005) (Figure 1.1).

Jeremiah Kirby (1774–1827)

Jeremiah Kirby qualified MD from the Edinburgh Medical School in 1802. He made a significant contribution to veterinary education with his reviews of Farriery in the *Encyclopaedia Britannica* (Kirby 1810) and of Veterinary Medicine in the *Encyclopaedia Edinensis* (Kirby 1827). His authorship of the former was hidden from sight until the prefaces of the 5th (1815) and 6th (1823) editions were published (Molony and Warwick 2013). Although his reviews relied heavily on his choice of direct quotations from the works of others, he had an outstanding ability to assimilate, analyse and present a breadth of knowledge and depth of understanding superior to any of those from whom he sourced material (Molony and Warwick 2013).

Edward Harrison (1766–1838)

The discussion of veterinary education in Edinburgh appears to have been somewhat muted during the Napoleonic Wars years. Nevertheless, thought was being given to post-war improvements in animal (and human) medical care. Edward Harrison (1766–1838) had been trained in Edinburgh University's Medical School at the same time that James Clark junior and James Jeffray were students there. In 1810 he published in Edinburgh copies of his sketch of a bill 'for the improvements of the medical and surgical and veterinary sciences and for regulating the practice thereof'; copies were also circulating in England (Harrison 1810). This was a proposal to regulate the medical and veterinary professions; it was a long way ahead of its time. He wrote

> that it is expedient that provision should be made, as well for regulating the practice of the medical and surgical and veterinary sciences, as for promoting the due education of practitioners in the different branches . . . a register to be kept for that purpose, [recording] his **or her** [our emphasis] Christian and surname and place of abode . . . and . . . a certificate shall be given to every person so registered of the capacity or capacities to practice. Every person practicing as a . . . veterinary practitioner . . . shall annually . . . take out a certificate and that . . . all sums of money so to be raised for such registering and certificates . . . shall go and be applied . . . to promote the improvement of the medical and surgical and veterinary sciences, and the education of the practitioners.

It would be over thirty years before these ideas matured to fruition with regard to veterinary education and the registration of its practitioners, and somewhat later for human medicine. Nevertheless, these thoughts kept the topic alive in Edinburgh. The specific forum of the influential in Scotland, that was critical to the future development of these considerations, was the Highland Society of Scotland.

The Highland Society of Scotland (1784–present)

The Highland Society of Edinburgh had been established in 1784. Three years later it received its first Royal Charter as 'The Highland Society of Scotland at Edinburgh'. It had been formed by the 'great and the good', with the 5th Duke of Argyll as its first President and Sir John Sinclair (1754–1835) a founding and very active member in its early years. Monro *secundus* was another founding member (Ramsay 1879; Davidson 1984). The original objects of the Society included: the improvement of

the Highlands and Islands of Scotland and the conditions of their inhab-
itants; an enquiry into the means of their improvement by establishing
towns and villages – facilitating communications by roads and bridges
– advancing agriculture – extending fisheries – introducing useful trades
and manufactures; and the preservation of the language, poetry and music
of the Highlands. The Society's agricultural interests dated from 1785,
when medals for essays on agricultural subjects were first offered. In 1790
the Chair of Agriculture in the University of Edinburgh was founded on
the Society's initiative. Sir John Sinclair's *Statistical Account of Scotland*
established the bases for the Society's considerations of further development throughout Scotland. In 1803 two essays on the diseases of black
cattle were published by the Society (MacNab 1803; Stewart 1803). As
a direct result of these, the Society established a prize essay competition
to gather comparable information on the diseases of sheep. The thirteen
essays submitted were synthesised into a 196-page treatise on the subject
(Duncan 1807).

On 28 August 1816 the Lord Provost of Edinburgh, Sir William
Arbuthnot (also a member of the Highland Society), moved in the Town
Council of Edinburgh

> that in order to maintain the high reputation and consequence of the
> University of Edinburgh, a committee be appointed to consider the pro-
> priety and necessity of the Patrons instituting a Chair for Comparative
> Anatomy and Veterinary Physic and Surgery on a scale similar to that of the
> celebrated Cuvier at Paris.

The Magistrates and Council approved. A report was prepared the following day (Macdonald et al. 2011). The discussions that then took place
within the University and between the University and the Town Council
have been examined in some detail (Gardiner 2007). John Barclay
(1758–1826) (Figure 1.6), who had been tipped for the post, was a man
of brilliance, vision and charm (Kaufman 2007). He taught anatomy pri-
vately and very successfully outside the University, at 10 Surgeon Square
(Macdonald et al. 2011). Professor Alexander Monro *tertius* (1773–1859),
the Anatomy Professor inside the university, was much less successful as
a teacher of anatomy. Both he and other professors were very apprehen-
sive about the impact that this new professorship would have on their
subject 'territories' and future income (Gardiner 2007; Kaufman 2007).
The unfortunate timing of the suggestion may also have contributed to
the outcome. It arrived just as the members of the Senatus were preoc-
cupied with the last stages of their judging of the competition for the
design of the College buildings. It is not easy to see where accommodation
for Veterinary Physic and Surgery might have been fitted into Playfair's

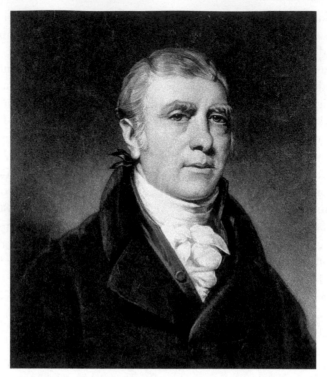

Figure 1.6   John Barclay (1758–1826). Mezzotint by T. Hodgetts, 1820, after J. S. C. Syme, 1818. Wellcome Collection. Public Domain Mark.

plan for the college site (Fraser 1989). On 11 December 1816, the Chair Committee of Edinburgh Town Council, although it argued fluently against the report from the University, also stated that 'we will conceive it our duty at all times to endeavour as far as we are able to promote the establishment . . . [of] . . . a separate School of veterinary medicine connecting it with an hospital for sick animals and a Forge' (Edinburgh Council 1816). The chair was not established. John Barclay, although denied the opportunity to become the first Professor of Comparative Anatomy and Veterinary Physic and Surgery in the University of Edinburgh, contributed significantly to the next steps in the establishment of veterinary education in Edinburgh.

References

Album, 1762. Album Academiae Jacobi VI Regis Scotorum quae est Edinburgi 1762–1786 & 1786–1803. Edinburgh University Library Da34; *Index to Matriculations in Medicine 1762–63 – 1860–61.* Manuscript. Edinburgh University Library.

Anonymous, 1796a. *Caledonian Mercury*, Thursday, 28 April 1796, p. 1, col. 4; Saturday, 7 May 1796, p. 1, col. 4.

Anonymous, 1796b. *Caledonian Mercury*, Thursday, 23 June 1796, p. 1, col. 2.

Anonymous, 1796c. *Caledonian Mercury*, Saturday, 16 July 1796, p. 1, col. 4.

Bower, A. 1817. *The History of the University of Edinburgh.* Vol. 2. Edinburgh: A. Smellie.

Burdon, W. 1732. *The gentleman's pocket-farrier; shewing how to use your horse on a journey: and what remedies are proper for common misfortunes that may befal him on the road.* Edinburgh: [s.n.].

Clark, J. 1770. *Observations upon the Shoeing of Horses: with an anatomical description of the bones in the foot of the horse.* Edinburgh: A. Donaldson.

Clark, J. 1775. *Observations upon the Shoeing of Horses: together with a new inquiry into the causes of diseases in the feet of horses, in two parts. Part I. Upon the shoeing of horses. Part II. Upon the diseases of the feet.* Edinburgh: J. Balfour, and London: T. Cadell.

Clark, J. 1782. *Observations upon the Shoeing of Horses: together with a new inquiry into the causes of diseases in the feet of horses, in two parts. Part I. Upon the shoeing of horses. Part II. Upon the diseases of the feet.* 3rd edition. Edinburgh: William Creech.

Clark, J. 1788. *A treatise on the prevention of diseases incidental to horses from bad management in regard to stables, food, water, air, and exercise. To which are subjoined observations on some of the surgical and medical branches of farriery.* Edinburgh: printed for the author by W. Smellie.

Clark, J. 1806. *First lines of veterinary physiology and pathology.* Vol. 1. Edinburgh: [s.n.].

Cotchin, E. 1990. *The Royal Veterinary College London: A Bicentenary History.* Buckingham: Barracuda.

Davidson, J. D. G. (ed.) 1984. *The Royal Highland and Agricultural Society of Scotland. A Short History: 1784–1984.* Edinburgh: Blackwood Pillans & Wilson.

Douglas, J. 1707. *Myographiae comparatae specimen: or, a comparative description of all the muscles in a man, and in a quadruped.* London: G. Strachan.

Douglas, J. 1775. *Myographiæ comparatæ specimen: or, a comparative description of all the muscles in a man, and in a quadruped. A new edition, with improvements. To which is now added, An account of the blood-vessels and nerves.* Edinburgh: J. Bell.

Duncan, A. (ed.) 1807. A treatise on the diseases of sheep; drawn up from [thirteen] original communications presented to the Highland Society of Scotland. *Prize Essays and Transactions of the Highland Society of Scotland*, 3, 339–535.

Edinburgh Council, 1816. Edinburgh City Council Records, 11 December 1816, TCM, 172, 322–36.

Erlam, H. D. (ed.) 1954. Alexander Monro *primus. University of Edinburgh Journal*, 17, 77–105. [An autobiography.]

Feron [Féron], J. 1796. *An address most humbly dedicated to the subscribers of the veterinary institution in the City of Edinburgh.* Edinburgh: J. Moir.

Feron [J. 1797?] *Veterinary Institution.* Edinburgh: [s.n.] n.d.

Fraser, A. G. 1989. *The Building of Old College: Adam, Playfair & The University of Edinburgh.* Edinburgh: Edinburgh University Press.

Gardiner, A. 2007. Elephants and exclusivity: An episode from the 'pre-Dick' history of veterinary education in Edinburgh. *Veterinary History*, 13, 299–309.

Greig, J. R. 1948. James Clark: A great and forgotten veterinarian, *Veterinary Record*, 60, 662–3.

Harrison, E. 1810. *Copies of communications relative to Dr Harrison's plan for a medical reform, and the sketch of a bill for the improvements of the medical and surgical and veterinary sciences and for regulating the practice thereof.* Edinburgh: D. Schaw and Son.

Houston, R. A. 1994. *Social Change in the Age of Enlightenment: Edinburgh, 1660–1760.* Oxford: Clarendon Press.

Jeffray, J. [1786?] *Proposals for carrying into effect, the plan contained in an Address to the Public, on the present state of farriery.* [Edinburgh?]; [s.n.].

Jeffray, J. 1786. *An address to the public, on the present state of farriery.* Edinburgh: [s.n.].

Jeffray, J. 1787. Letters to William Hamilton, Professor of Anatomy and Botany, Glasgow University, from: Genoa, 19 February 1787; Rome, 6 April 1787; Turin, 9 April 1787; Bologna, 24 April 1787; Geneva, 27 May 1787. Manuscripts. Glasgow University Library: MS Gen 1356/54-58. (In 1790, following William Hamilton's early death that year, Jeffray moved to Glasgow University, where he was appointed Regius Professor of Anatomy and Botany. He retained the Chair in Anatomy until his death in 1848, a separate Chair in Botany having been founded in 1818.)

Kaufman, M. H. 2007. *Dr John Barclay (1758–1826): Extra-mural teacher of human and comparative anatomy in Edinburgh*. Edinburgh: The Royal College of Surgeons of Edinburgh.

[Kirby, J.] 1806–10. Farriery. In J. Millar (ed.), *Encyclopaedia Britannica*, 4th edition. 8 (2). Edinburgh: Archibald Constable and Co.

Kirby, J. 1827. Medicine veterinary. In J. Millar, J. Kirby and R. Poole (eds), *Encyclopaedia Edinensis*, 5, 84–103. Edinburgh: J. Anderson.

Koutsouflianiotis, K. N., Paraskevas, G. K., Kalitsa, N., Iliou, K. and Noussios, G. 2019. The anatomist James Douglas (1675–1742: his life and scientific work. Cureus 2019 Jan; 11 (1): e3919. Doi: 10.7759/cureus.3919.

Macdonald, A. A., Warwick, C. M. and Johnston, W. T. 2005. Locating veterinary education in Edinburgh in the nineteenth century. *Book of the Old Edinburgh Club*, New Series, 41–71. <http://www.era.lib.ed.ac.uk/handle/1842/2199>

Macdonald, A. A., Warwick, C. M. and Johnston, W. T. 2011. Early contributions to the development of veterinary education in Scotland. *Veterinary History*, 16 (1), 11–40.

Macnab, A. 1803. Observations on the economy of black cattle farms, under a breeding stock. *Prize Essays and Transactions of the Highland Society of Scotland*, 2, 204–11.

Molony, V. and Warwick, C. M. 2013. Jeremiah Kirby Author of 'Farriery' in the 1806–1823 Editions of the *Encyclopaedia Britannica*. *Veterinary History*, 16(4), 353–60. <era.ed.ac.uk/handle/1842/6681> (accessed 11 September 2022).

[Monro, A.] 1765. List of Anatomy Students 1720–74. Manuscript. Edinburgh University Library: Da.50.1; ['1765, paid. [No.]129 James Clark, S[cottish], a Ferrier. £3.3.-.'].

[Monro, A.] 1775. *An essay on comparative anatomy*. London: John Nourse. (A second edition was published in 1775.)

Monro, A. 1783. *A treatise on Comparative Anatomy published by his son, Alexander Monro. A new edition with considerable improvements and additions by other hands*. Edinburgh: Charles Elliot.

[Monro, A.] 1797. Catalogue of Anatomical Preparations presented to the University of Edinburgh by Dr Alexr Monro Senr in the year 1797 [Manuscript]. Edinburgh University Library: Da.50.902.

[Monro, A.] 1798. Catalogue of Anatomical Preparations presented to the University of Edinburgh by Dr Alexr Monro Senr in the year 1798 [Manuscript]. Edinburgh University Library: Da.50.903.

Ramsay, A. 1879. *History of the Highland and Agricultural Society of Scotland: With notices of anterior societies for the promotion of agriculture in Scotland*. Edinburgh: W. Blackwood.

Sinclair, J. Significant Scots; Sir John Sinclair. <electricscotland.com/history/other/sincla ir_john.htm> (accessed 11 September 2022).

Smith, F. 1919. *The Early History of Veterinary Literature and its British Development, I. From the earliest period to A.D. 1700*. London: Baillière, Tindall & Cox.

Smith, F. 1924. *The Early History of Veterinary Literature and its British Development, II. The Eighteenth Century*. London: Baillière, Tindall & Cox.

Solleysel, J. de 1691. *Le parfait maréschal, qui enseigne à connoistre la beauté, la bonté, & les defauts des chevaux. . . . Revue avec exactitude & augmenté methodiquement*. 8th edition. Paris: A. La Haye, chez Henry van Bulderen.

Solleysel, J. de 1696. *The parfait maréschal, or compleat farrier: Which teacheth, I. To know the shapes and goodness, as well as faults and imperfections of horses . . . / written originally in French by the Sieur de Solleysel Escuyer . . . and translated from the last Paris impression, by Sir William Hope of Kirkliston. Edinburgh: Printed by George Mosman.

Stewart, A. 1803. Observations on the economy of black cattle farms, under a breeding stock. *Prize Essays and Transactions of the Highland Society of Scotland*, 2, 212–19.

Stewart, J. 1797? Letter in: Feron, *Veterinary Institution* [1797?]. National Archives of Scotland: GD 45/24/106.

Struthers, J. 1867. *Historical sketch of the Edinburgh Anatomical School.* Edinburgh: Maclachlan and Stewart.

Veterinary College. 1793. *An account of the veterinary college, from its institution in 1791.* London: James Phillips.

Wellburn, P. 1989. The living library. In P. Cadell and A. Matheson (eds), *For the encouragement of learning: Scotland's national library 1689–1989.* Edinburgh: Her Majesty's Stationary Office, pp. 186–214. ('From about 1770 the curators of the Advocates' Library begin to record a considerable rise in the number of applications from non-members of the library.')

Williamson, P. 1775. *Williamson's Directory for the city of Edinburgh, Canongate, Leith, and suburbs, from June 1775 to June 1776.* Edinburgh: Peter Williamson.

Chapter 2

The Establishment of William Dick's Veterinary School (1817–57)

Early veterinary education of William Dick

Around the time that there were discussions in Edinburgh about the possible creation of a school of veterinary medicine (1787), a young farrier, John Dick, moved south from Aberdeenshire to Edinburgh with his wife, Jean Anderson (Bradley 1923). They took up lodgings at the foot of the Canongate, probably in White Horse Close, where they lived for over a decade (Figure 2.1). Although it is not known precisely where this bright and ambitious farrier found employment, his relatively close geographical proximity to James Clark's business premises is likely to have led to a sharing of views between the two men. The Dicks's first child, Mary, was born at White Horse Close on 1 June 1791, as was their son William two years later, on 6 May 1793 (Bradley 1923). The early years of their family life in the old and new towns of Edinburgh have been described in detail elsewhere (Macdonald and Warwick 2019). However, it is important to point out that the formative period from 1800 to 1814 for these two youngsters was when they lived in the small cluster of five houses on Mud Island below Calton Hill at the south-west end of Leith Walk (Figure 2.2). James Burt, the only veterinarian in Edinburgh at that time, had based his practice beside their home there. In that way, Mary and William got to see all sorts of different animal health problems, with their father and James Burt able to explain and demonstrate how they were being dealt with clinically. Farriery with John Dick and veterinary surgery with James Burt became core parts of the children's every-day lives as they grew into and went through their teenage years (Macdonald and Warwick 2019). Further foundations were being laid.

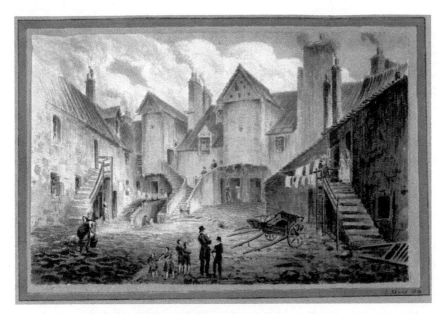

Figure 2.1 White Horse Close, Old White Horse Inn, Canongate by J. Skene, c. 1818. Permission granted by Central Library, George IV Bridge, Edinburgh.

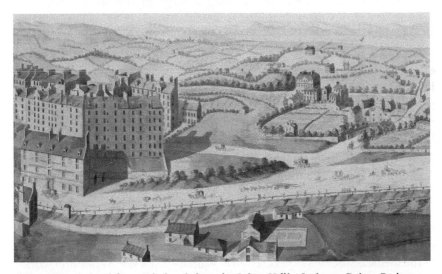

Figure 2.2 A detail from *Edinburgh from the Calton Hill* by Irishman Robert Barker (1739–1806), who invented the word 'Panorama'. It was painted in 1792 from the (recently completed) roof of the old observatory on Calton Hill. Mud Island is in the foreground and is where John Dick and his family lived before moving to Clyde Street. Behind Mud Island is Leith Street (running from left to right). University of Edinburgh (Coll-1709). Permission granted by CRC, The University of Edinburgh.

In 1811 the census had recorded 120,000 people in Edinburgh, of whom 11,000 were spinsters. Mary was now twenty years old, and never did marry. Some years later, William fell in love with the daughter of one of the local bankers, but her father did not agree to the match: 'we weren't good enough for her'. She married someone else. William and the woman remained very good friends for the rest of their lives (Bradley,1923). He never cared for another woman like that ever again (Macdonald and Warwick 2019). In March 1811 the famous singer, Miss Elizabeth Feron, came to perform in Edinburgh (Macdonald, Warwick and Johnston 2011). She was the daughter of John Feron, and her presence would likely have prompted family discussions about the various attempts having been made by her father to establish a veterinary school in Edinburgh (Macdonald and Warwick 2019). In the autumn of 1811, Alex Grey, the twenty-four-year-old son of Alexander Grey, one of the senior farriers in Edinburgh, set off for London to study at the Veterinary College there. This was something that the eighteen-year-old William Dick would have been very well aware of.

By 1815 John Dick and his family had moved from Edinburgh's New Town to live in their recently built house at 15 Clyde Street (Figure 2.3). The ambitious John Dick had secured a forge in the stable courtyard behind 10 Clyde Street. It was conveniently situated diagonally across the road from his home (Macdonald and Warwick 2019). The family noticed in the April 1815 issue of *The Farmers Magazine* that a three-month course of classes on comparative anatomy for farriers was to be run from May by Dr Barclay at Surgeon Square (Macdonald and Warwick 2012). Doubtless there were family discussions about this and perhaps big-sister encouragement for William to attend. Certainly, the timing, three days after William Dick's twenty-second birthday, supports the speculation that he responded to these advertisements by going to this inaugural course of Comparative Anatomy lectures. The timing also implies that it was William Dick who took his young friend and neighbour, William Dumbreck, to these lectures. What is clear is that Barclay rapidly recognised, and was greatly impressed by, the intellectual capability of William Dick, and 'lavished his commendations' on him (Bradley 1923). For example, when told by one of the medical students in his class that William Dick was a common working blacksmith, Barclay, who knew nothing of him at that time, retorted, 'Well, well. All I can say is, that whether he be blacksmith or whitesmith, he's the cleverest chap among you.' Once so identified, Barclay probably encouraged Dick to attend the lectures on chemistry and the practice of healing disease in Edinburgh University (Bradley 1923). The content of the lectures given by Barclay has been described in some detail elsewhere, as have the likely benefits to William Dick of them and the accompanying

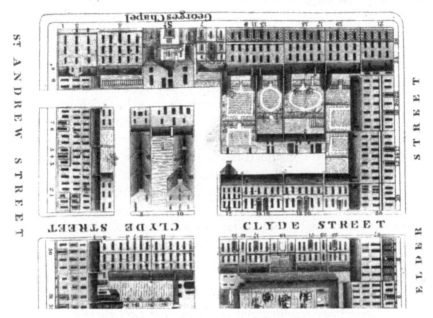

Figure 2.3 The Clyde Street courtyard; an extract from Kirkwood's 1819 city plan of Edinburgh, which shows the front elevations of buildings. The farrier's forge and the upstairs dissection room used by John and William Dick were located on the right (east) side behind number 10. With permission of the WS Society, The Signet Library.

practical classes in comparative anatomy (Macdonald and Warwick 2014). In 1816 *The Farmers Magazine* continued to press for the establishment of veterinary education in Edinburgh (Macdonald and Warwick 2012). As indicated in chapter 1, the University of Edinburgh Senatus had declined to accept this proposal from the Edinburgh Town Council (Jacyna 1994; Gardiner 2007; Macdonald and Warwick 2012).

An indication that veterinary discussion within the Dick family had continued was the reported statement from Mary Dick to Mrs Burt, the veterinary surgeon's wife, 'oor Willum's gawn tae be a graun' veet'nar tae. He's saved enough siller noo tae tak the lang road coach for London' [Our William's going to be a grand veterinarian too. He has saved enough money now to take the long road coach to London] (Bradley 1923). Mary's life-long association with the Dick family's business finance and accountancy may even be suggested by this long-remembered comment.

William Dick begins teaching

In the autumn of 1817, further encouraged by Dr Barclay, William Dick, now aged twenty-four, took the coach to London, to its Veterinary College. There, like other students over the previous fifteen or more years, he received three months of veterinary instruction. His notes record ninety lectures of varying length, the early ones dealing with the blood and blood vessels, the last being on the external conformation of the horse (Dick 1817–18). At the end of January 1818 he applied for his examination and obtained his Diploma (Bradley 1923).

As soon as William got back home his desire to start a veterinary school in Edinburgh sought expression (Bradley 1923; Macdonald and Warwick 2012). He was recommended by Dr Barclay to a Mr Scott of Parton, who was establishing an academical institution in Edinburgh in which, among other sciences, veterinary surgery was intended to be taught. No students enrolled that year (1818), but the following year four students attended, although only one came regularly to hear Dick's daily lecture. The 1820s were filled with the growth and development of William's veterinary teaching and veterinary practice. In 1820–1 Dick had nine students at the one-month-long series of free lectures which he gave in the largest side room of the Calton Convening Rooms (now part of Howie's Restaurant), Waterloo Place (Figure 2.4). In 1821–2 seventeen farriers attended the twenty-four lectures he gave, without payment, at the School of Arts, Niddry Street; the building is known today as St Cecilia's Hall. In 1822–3 the School of Arts again hosted his one-hour-long lectures, which were freely given every Saturday evening from 12 October for the following seven or eight months (Macdonald and Warwick 2012).

In the spring of 1823 John Barclay once again stepped in to assist William. On 21 May 1823, at a meeting of the Directors of the Highland Society of Scotland (of which Barclay was one), the importance of having a professorship or a public lecturer giving instruction in veterinary surgery was discussed. At the General Meeting of the Highland Society one week later a sum not exceeding £50 was placed at the disposal of the Directors to promote 'public instruction in the ensuing season, in the veterinary art and the diseases of livestock'. The Directors and the Committee identified in William Dick

> a practical man, a graduate of the Veterinary College of London, ready to undertake the duty of delivering suitable lectures, and to provide the necessary accommodation, on receiving the countenance and patronage of the Society. (Macdonald and Warwick 2012)

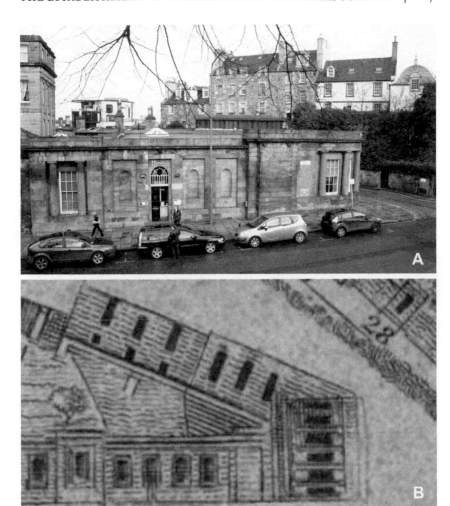

Figure 2.4 A. The Calton Convening Rooms, Waterloo Place, built in 1818–19, now Howies Restaurant. Photo credit: Colin M. Warwick; B. The Calton Convening Rooms as depicted by Kirkwood in 1819. With permission of the WS Society, The Signet Library.

The first Veterinary School in Edinburgh

William Dick (Figure 2.5), now thirty years old, was appointed to the post for a trial period of one year. Once again, he rented the side room of the Calton Convening Rooms (Figures 2.4 and 2.6) and delivered the first lecture in the evening of Monday, 24 November 1823, the recognised date of the founding of his Veterinary School. Twenty-five practical or professional students attended (farriers and smiths; new

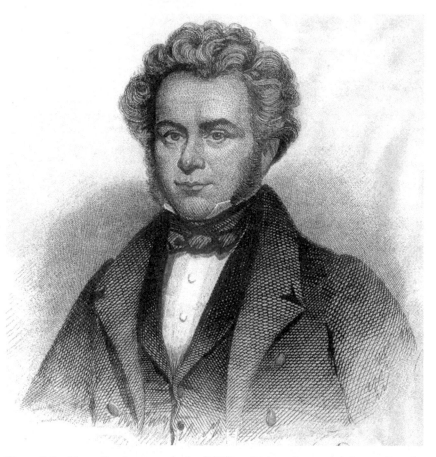

Figure 2.5 The earliest known portrait of William Dick, perhaps in his thirties. Detail from a Diploma awarded by the Edinburgh Veterinary Medical Society. Photographer: Colin M. Warwick.

students paying 2 guineas, former students being charged 1 guinea), as well as various interested general or so-called amateur students (medical men and members of the Highland Society's Committee). A series of forty-six lectures were given in the Calton Convening Rooms, on Monday and Thursday evenings at 7pm, spread over the following twenty-three weeks, concluding in April 1824 (Macdonald and Warwick 2012). The material covered the anatomy and diseases of horses, cattle, sheep, pigs and dogs, a range far wider than that covered by the London School, and one which better fitted the requirements of the Scottish economy. Dick gave practical instruction at his father's forge in the Clyde Street court-yard (Figure 2.3). At the end of this course, three of these men, William Carrick from Cupar in Fife, William Stewart from Aberdeenshire and George Tait from Meigle in Perthshire, were accredited by the Highland

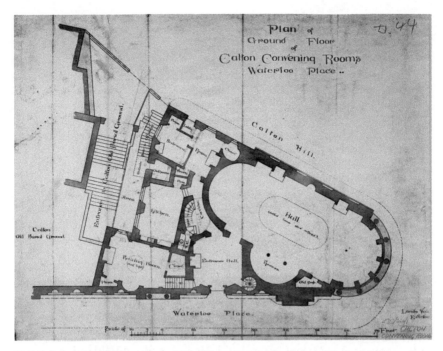

Figure 2.6 Ground-floor plan of the Calton Convening Rooms. The 'retiring room' was for six years the site of the Highland Society's Veterinary School in Edinburgh. Image: Edinburgh City Archives.

Society as Veterinary Surgeons (Pringle 1869; Macdonald and Warwick 2023).

Dr Barclay reported positively to the Directors of the Highland Society and the Committee recommended that the lectures should be continued the following year, with 30 guineas suggested as the appropriate fee to be given to William Dick for 1824–5. In 1825 a circular was sent by the Highland Society to members of the Society, noblemen, landowners and farmers, recommending the school of veterinary surgery established by William Dick in Edinburgh under their patronage and support; for a long time, it was referred to as the Highland Society's Veterinary School in Edinburgh (Macdonald 2013). The time of the classes during the second session in the Calton Convening Rooms was adjusted to enable students of agriculture at the University to attend. In 1827 William also gave a popular course of lectures there in the morning which was attended by a large number of country gentlemen, members of the Highland Society and others. It was not until the end of the fifth session, on 23 April 1828, that the first public examination of students, by six eminent medical practitioners, took place (Bradley 1923; Macdonald and Warwick 2012). A certificate was given to each of the seven students who passed that examination:

Veterinary School under the Patronage of the Highland Society of Scotland.

Edinburgh, 23d April 1828.

Having been requested by the Directors of the Highland Society of Scotland to assist in the examination of the students of Mr Dick, Lecturer upon Veterinary Science under the Society's patronage, we attended accordingly, and do hereby certify that [name of student], who has studied at the Veterinary School for [length of time], having been this day examined by us, we consider him qualified to practise the Veterinary Art.

[signed] Dr [George] Ballingall, Professor of Military Surgery
      Dr [Robert] Graham, Professor of Botany
      Dr [George Augustus] Borthwick, [physician and surgeon]
      Mr William Wood, [Royal College of Surgeons, Edinburgh]
      Mr William Newbigging, [Royal College of Surgeons, Edinburgh]
      Dr [Robert] Knox, Lecturer on Comparative Anatomy

It was at the end of the sixth session, in April 1829, that the Highland Society's Directors decided that the period of study should be extended to a minimum of two years before students were examined for the Society's veterinary certificate. The first thirty-one veterinary surgeons to have been trained by William Dick and accredited as such (Pringle 1869; Macdonald and Warwick 2023) had attended lectures at the Highland Society's Veterinary School in Edinburgh in the Calton Convening Rooms. Later that month Dick went to the Continent, where he inspected several veterinary colleges in France and the Low Countries.

The Clyde Street Veterinary School

In the autumn of 1829 William transferred his course of lectures from the Calton Convening Rooms to Clyde Street, in all likelihood to the old building at number 8, diagonally across the road and to the west of the Dick family home at 15 Clyde Street (Figure 2.3). The building at number 8 was subsequently purchased by William and his father from Alexander Munro (*tertius*) on 12 November 1831. The number of lectures he gave that session was extended to seventy, and the addition of a stable to the available facilities was noted (Macdonald and Warwick 2012). The name 'Edinburgh Veterinary School' now became more widely used.

An important consequence of the students in Edinburgh receiving instruction on the anatomy and diseases of all domesticated animals was that there was soon hardly a dairy or distillery in Scotland (where many cattle were fattened) which was not now being superintended by an adequately trained veterinary surgeon. The same was not true south of the border at this time (Clark 1833).

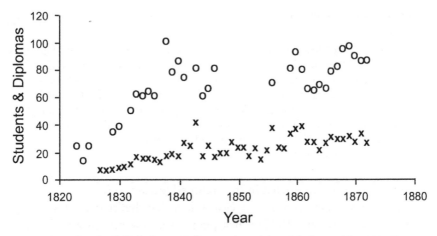

Figure 2.7 Graph of Clyde Street College students (o) and diplomas (x), 1820–70.

The number of students attending the course continued to increase (Figure 2.7), such that in June 1831 the veterinary committee complained that the lecture room at Clyde Street was not comfortable, the museum was small and there was no infirmary stable available for the students (Bradley 1923; Macdonald and Warwick 2012). Indeed, two accounts of these facilities give us contemporary insight. The first, by James Castley in 1830, reports:

> One could wish to see Mr. Dick's lecture-room look somewhat less like the appendage of a forge; but then he never has to lecture to 'empty benches'. You may fancy to yourself a room of no very great dimensions in an old and apparently long untenanted house in Clyde Street. You enter it from the street door, and are immediately struck with the delightful confusion which seems to reign within. Skeletons of all descriptions, 'from a child's shoe to a jack boot' – from a horse to an ape, not ranged in 'regular order all of a row', but standing higglety pigglety, their ranks having been broken by the professor's table, and their heads looking in all directions, as if thrown together by chance. Over the professor's 'devoted head' is seen suspended a portion of inflated and injected intestine, with its mesenteric expansion dangling in the air, something like a lure for flies; whilst all around the room, and especially in the corners, are heaped together vast quantities of diseased bones, and other preparations, seemingly without order, and without arrangement. Here we see no numbered specimens – no classification of morbid anatomy – no description book – all of which would tend to give the collection a pretty effect. Yet the lecturer has not only sufficient, but abundance for his purpose: his table is always covered with choice preparations. That portion of the house which is set apart for the audience . . . is fitted up with rough deal planks, set upon as rough props; the seats rising tier above tier, until your head touches the top of a very dark coloured ceiling.

In the second account, in 1834, John Stewart writes:

> Above the forge, there was, indeed, what had once been an old hay-loft, but which in my time, had been economically converted into a dissecting-room, and a receptacle for lumber . . . The fees at Mr Dick's school are all comprised in ten guineas of entrance money, upon payment of which, the pupil has the privilege of attending the lectures as long as he pleases; of witnessing Mr Dick's practice, which is pretty extensive; of attending the lectures of several eminent medical men in town; and there is no additional expense incurred for the diploma.

Examinations were conducted in the cramped lecture room.

This accommodation was now clearly less than befitted Dick's growing reputation (Bradley 1923). Dick planned a new building to replace 8 Clyde Street. The architecture was designed by Richard and Robert Dickson and the building was constructed by Messrs. Smith and Watson. It was completed in 1833, Dick's fortieth year, at the then substantial cost of £2,500 paid largely by Dick himself (Figure 2.8). The Highland Society contributed the modest sum of £50 towards fitting out the lecture theatre and the museum (Bradley 1923; Macdonald and Warwick 2012).

The classical façade consisted of three storeys, each with three windows, those of the second storey being decorated with pediments (Figure 2.8). Two simple columns between two pilasters supported a frieze comprising a carved row of animal heads, of stallion, dog, bull, and ram on both sides of the central stag's head, set into the building above the second-floor windows (Figure 2.9). These icons powerfully represented the breadth of animal material being taught by William Dick. They were also consistent with the desire of the Highland Society to have veterinary surgeons trained to treat all domestic farm livestock in Scotland and reflected the comparative anatomical training provided to William Dick by his mentor John Barclay (Macdonald and Warwick 2014a). The sculpture of a rising horse was placed on the plinth at the top of the façade (see Figure 4.2). It was by A. Wallace, a partner in the firm Wallace and White.

The Dick family home and the space for the domestic staff occupied the rooms in the top two floors of this new building (Macdonald 2020). The classroom was on the first floor (about 32 m^2 in floor area) and was large enough to hold about fifty students and their lecturer (Figure 2.10). This was comparable to the lecture-room seating density experienced by William Dick when he was a student under Barclay (Macdonald and Warwick 2014). The classroom was well lit by two west-facing and two east-facing windows. Access to the museum (about 17 m^2 in floor area) was via the classroom. Shelving for the museum specimens was arranged along the north wall.

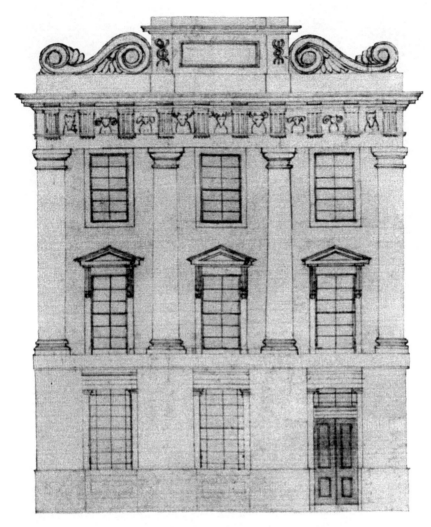

Figure 2.8 Cleaned copy of the 1833 architect's drawing of the 'Elevation to Clyde Street' façade of the new Veterinary School 'proposed to be erected on Clyde Street by Mr Dick'. Image: Royal Commission of Ancient and Historic Monuments of Scotland.

The Veterinary School office was on the ground floor and had a floor area of about 17.5 m². Access to it was from the lobby on the left, once inside the front entrance (Macdonald 2020). The drug room and dispensary was also on the ground floor with access to it via the passageway on the east side of the building. Horse box and stable accommodation was constructed under the students' classroom and museum. The ground-level plan of the Clyde Street veterinary courtyard remained modest (Figure 2.11).

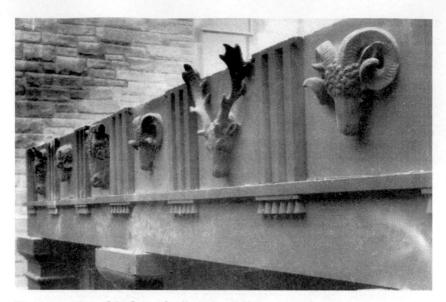

Figure 2.9 Part of the frieze of stallion, dog, bull, ram and stag stone heads on the façade of the Veterinary College in Clyde Street, c. 1952. Photographer: Colin McWilliam, retouched by Colin M. Warwick.

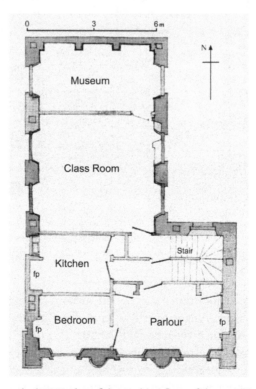

Figure 2.10 Retouched 1833 plan of the teaching floor of the new Veterinary School on Clyde Street. fp = fireplace. Image: Royal Commission of Ancient and Historic Monuments of Scotland.

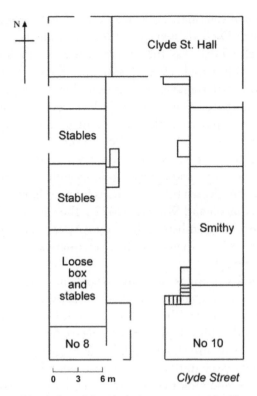

Figure 2.11   Ground-level plan of the Clyde Street courtyard buildings, 1833.

The Edinburgh teaching and living environment

In the 1830s, the teaching environment of the Veterinary School in Clyde Street comprised many different components for each of the students who attended. Clearly the physical environment was an essential element, as was the structural layout of the neighbourhood and indeed of the town of Edinburgh itself (Macdonald 2020). Briefly stated, Edinburgh and its dependencies in 1833 were said to have the following: a population of 187,000 people; one university; two theatres; 60 churches and chapels; 122 mail and stage coaches; seven London steamships; 100 hackney coaches; 300 physicians, surgeons and dentists; 560 teachers of various branches of education; 500 grocers; 470 spirit dealers; 170 taverns and eating houses; 64 livery stables; 270 bakers; 270 fleshers; 350 booksellers, binders, stationers and engravers. Its main manufacturing industry was said to be shawl-weaving. The town was also busy with baking, brewing, distilling, book printing, wire-drawing, coach-building and the manufacture of machinery for paper mills (Macdonald 2020).

There were two veterinary surgeons on the Clyde Street teaching staff in 1833; William Dick assisted by his former student, Josiah Cheetham (Table 2.1). John Dick was the senior farrier. In addition to the farriery expertise within each class of students, there was probably additional blacksmith staff available each session; this is borne out by the 1841 census, which suggested that Thomas Milke, Andrew Steel and William Vanderman were employed as blacksmiths. In addition to this, and by way of personal agreement with William Dick, the classes of the whole medical curriculum in Edinburgh University were open to the veterinary students (Macdonald 2020). This had a major guiding influence on the published material soon to be selected by the students for their library in Clyde Street (Macdonald, Johnston and Warwick 2022). The students also had practical access to the other members of the veterinary community in Edinburgh and beyond. In 1832–3 there were five veterinary surgeons practising in Edinburgh (Table 2.1).

William Dick's lectures initially began in mid-November, after the potato harvest in October. By 1840 they were starting earlier, on Wednesday, 4 November. The lectures ran until the Diploma examination time during the third week of April. The student-teaching session was therefore about six months long. Dick began by giving evening lectures at 7pm, three times a week until mid-January. From mid-January he lectured four times a week, and after the middle of February, increased his lectures to five times a week. Every Saturday he carried out a one-and-a-half- to two-hour-long careful examination lecture period with the students (Macdonald 2020). The end-of-session Diploma examination was largely carried out by senior medical men.

A comprehensive collection of skeletal and other anatomical specimens had been accumulated by Dick and placed in the museum. Sir George Ballingall was invited by the Highland Society to compile a catalogue of this material (Ballingall 1834; Johnston 2002). His inventory of 348 preparations included the complete skeletons of a thoroughbred mare, a horse with curvature of the spine, a cow, a ram, a greyhound, a pug dog and a Lapland reindeer, as well as those of a baboon and a human. There were numerous specimens of diseased and fractured bones, as well as anatomical preparations with blood vessels injected and demonstrated. A large assortment of horses' hooves, shod with a wide variety of different shoes, was also present in the collection, as were examples of healthy and diseased abdominal organs, such as heart, spleen, reproductive tract, stomach and intestine. The students were also entitled to visit the large collection of comparative anatomy specimens that had been compiled by John Barclay, subsequently added to by Robert Knox, that were held in the newly constructed museum of the College of Surgeons (Macdonald and Warwick

Table 2.1 Veterinary surgeons in Edinburgh 1832–41, farriers in 1839–40, the number of veterinary students and practical men and the number of Diploma examination passes from 1832 to 1841.

Veterinary Surgeons	Address in Edinburgh 1839	1832–33	1833–34	1834–35	1835–36	1836–37	1837–38	1838–39	1839–40	1840–41
Aitken, John	142 Causewayside								Y	Y
Cheetham, J.P. g1828	8 Clyde Street	Y					Y	Y		
Dick, William	8 Clyde Street	Y	Y	Y	Y	Y	Y	Y	Y	Y
Gray, Alex	31 Pleasance & 119 Rose St	Y	Y	Y	Y	Y	Y	Y	Y	Y
Gray, Alexander g1836	31 Pleasance							Y	Y	Y
Henderson, William	[100 Rose Street]	Y	Y	Y	Y	Y	Y			
Kennedy, John	[23 Rose Lane]				Y	Y				
Medd, George	1 Windsor Street							Y	Y	
Ritchie, Thomas g1830	35 Rose Street					Y	Y	Y	Y	Y
Seton, Henry g1835	129 Rose Street Lane								Y	Y
Watt, James	[6 St James Place]	Y	Y	Y	Y	Y	Y			
Watt, Alexander g1837	6 St James Place						Y	Y	Y	Y
Worthington, William g1840	10 Clyde Street								Y	Y
Farriers										
Aitkens, James	14 Potterrow								Y	
Aitkens, T.	45 Charlotte Street								Y	
Dick, John	8 Clyde Street								Y	
Mather, T.	6 Nottingham Place								Y	
Smilbert, James	91 St Andrew Street								Y	
Number of students		50	62	>60	64	>60	?	101	78	86
Practical men		30	16	15	20	14			48	
Passed diploma examination		11	16	15	15	14	12	17	18	17

2013, 2014b; Macdonald 2020). Material for student dissection and anatomical study probably came largely from the animals that had presented
for clinical examination and treatment but had either died or had had to
be destroyed. Students were encouraged to prepare illustrative dissections,
and in 1837 a silver medal was presented to James Moore by Dick for the
best anatomical preparation. The benefits of this practice were discussed,
and in 1839 it was decided that from then on no student should be
allowed to become a candidate for the Highland and Agricultural Society
Diploma unless he produced an anatomical preparation executed by his
own hand (Macdonald 2020).

Student and staff cohesion around the new Clyde Street Veterinary
School building resulted in the 1834 establishment of the Edinburgh
Veterinary Medical Society (Macdonald, Warwick and Johnston 2005;
Macdonald 2020; Macdonald, Johnston and Warwick 2022). This was an
association of veterinary surgeons and veterinary students, who met weekly
in the Clyde Street lecture theatre for the advancement and diffusion of
veterinary knowledge. As indicated above, the Society began to accumu-
late a collection of books. These were probably housed in cupboards in
the Clyde Street classroom. Diplomas were issued as a matter of course to
veterinary surgeons when they became members, as well as to students, but
only after the latter had attended regularly for six months, conformed to
the rules of the Society, presented an essay to the Society, and had defended
the same (Macdonald, Warwick and Johnston 2005). Among the twenty
practical men who attended the 1835–6 session (the total student number
was sixty-four) was the first student from North America. In 1838–9 there
were 101 students, and in subsequent years students began to arrive from
Australia (1839–40), Russia (1844–5), Norway (1845–6) and South Africa
(1846–7) (Macdonald, Warwick and Johnston 2005). In January 1838
Dick drew up a memorial requesting recognition of the eligibility of graduates from the Edinburgh Veterinary School for commissions as veterinary
surgeons in the army and in the Honorary East India Company's service.
The Highland Society approved this. It was forwarded by the Society's
President to the 'proper quarters' and by April of that year the Government
had agreed to the Highland Society's request (Anonymous 1879).

William Dick was a highly experienced and very successful veterinary
practitioner. He gathered many clients (Bradley 1923). As a result, his students had lots of opportunities to see examples of the diseases and injuries
that he described to them in lectures. They were able to learn how to practise and perform their treatment in the courtyard. William applied a medical teaching idea (from John Thomson [Jacyna 1994]) to his own clinical
practice and treated the animals of the poor for no payment. This brought
into the Clyde Street Veterinary School many examples of animals that

needed urgent surgery or medical care, which were of great benefit to his students' education (Macdonald and Warwick 2019). The students also had access to the animals in the Royal Edinburgh Zoological Gardens, located relatively close by, to the north-east of the veterinary college. These had opened to the public in 1839. Dick was an ordinary director of the association which managed the Zoological Gardens, and his veterinary opinion was sought when animals showed signs of illness or died. An overview of additional details of the teaching and learning environment experienced by the Clyde Street Veterinary School students between 1833 and 1841 has been presented elsewhere (Macdonald 2020).

Mary Dick

Mary Dick was a businesswoman. She looked after the book-keeping side of the family's veterinary and farriery work. She also took a great interest in the welfare of every student and was always anxious to care for the real good within each one of them (Dollar 1894; Macdonald and Warwick 2019). She made it part of her business to be fully acquainted with all their outgoings and incomings. She was not slow to note minor offences (Bradley 1923). Part of her role was to be the general censor of the students' manners and morals. All the idle, noisy or dissipated delinquents had to appear before her, much to their embarrassment. There were very few misdemeanours that escaped her detection. No discovered culprits escaped reproof. However, she could tell that they all held her in sincere respect and with affectionate regard (Dollar 1894; Bradley 1923): 'I may have been a bit despotic, but my rule was kindly and helpful when they were in sickness or trouble' (Macdonald and Warwick 2019). Former students were constant and regular correspondents. They frequently sent her newspapers that contained personal paragraphs; these she declined to have destroyed (Macdonald and Warwick 2019). It was also about this time that Mary had her portrait painted by Thomas Fraser, who had a studio round the corner in North St Andrew Street. Mary was very fond of this piece of art, called perhaps 'portrait of a lady', and kept it close by her for the rest of her life. It was willed to a friend, Janet Inglis. Its whereabouts thereafter remains a mystery (Macdonald and Warwick 2019).

The Queen's College

In 1839 William Dick joined a number of the other 'extra-academical' lecturers in Edinburgh, a private group made up largely, though not exclusively, of Fellows of the Royal Colleges of Physicians and Surgeons, in the formation of the Queen's College. One intention was to combine and concentrate the exertions of individual, non-university lecturers who had hitherto taught without any mutual co-operation (Macdonald, Warwick and Johnston 2005). The Edinburgh Veterinary School participated in the 1839–40 session and the following two sessions (Macdonald 2013). In April 1840 the Highland Society examiners awarded medals for general excellence to one more veterinary student than the Queen's College rules proposed; John Wright Charles was rewarded for his efforts (Figure 2.12). The closeness of William Dick's association with the Queen's College may be gauged from the number of extra-mural lecturers who attended the annual dinner held by the Veterinary School for its students, examiners and friends at the London Hotel, St Andrew Square, on the evening of the prize-giving ceremonies. However, the very success of the Queen's College stimulated anxiety within some of the professors at the University, and the resulting political controversy in the town led to the demise of this co-operative venture within a few years (Macdonald, Warwick and Johnston 2005).

Nevertheless, the significance of the short-lived Queen's College for veterinary education in Edinburgh lay in the benefits derived from the codified aims and aspirations of this group of extra-mural lecturers. These provided a framework of support for efforts which William Dick had already begun to put into practice over the previous decade. Two days after the Queen's College prize-giving, on 24 April 1840, the Directors of the Highland Society approved a petition from forty-five students at the Clyde Street School requesting that in future it should bear the name

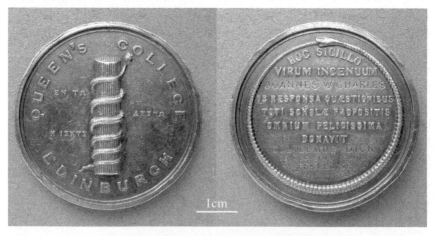

Figure 2.12 Queen's College medal awarded to John Wright Charles. Courtesy of Miss E. K. Charles. Photographer: Colin M. Warwick.

'Veterinary College', and that their teacher, William Dick, should be given the title 'Professor'. Both suggestions were approved (HASS 1840). Dick had encouraged each student to have a library of reference of his own and suggested eleven books that would usefully form the core of their collection (Dick 1839). In 1840 the Edinburgh Veterinary Medical Society established its library of books and journals, which grew to over four hundred volumes within two decades (Macdonald 2022). In 1837 Dick was appointed Veterinary Surgeon to Queen Victoria and proudly displayed her royal crest on the north wall of the college courtyard (Plate 2.1). The lozenge (diamond shape) on the crest indicated the arms of an unmarried woman, before her marriage to Albert on 10 February 1840 (Macdonald 2013).

Clyde Street Veterinary College developments

Increasingly in the 1830s, William had become involved with Edinburgh Town Council through his elected role as Deacon-Convenor of the Trades of Edinburgh (Macdonald, Warwick and Johnston 2005; Macdonald and Warwick 2019). The political situation within the Edinburgh city government and the academic environment which it had largely controlled made this a very sensible move (Jacyna 1994). Dick became *ex officio* General Commissioner of Police, and in that position, on Saturday, 4 September 1842, he was in charge of the detachment of High Constables at the Mercat Cross guarding the keys of Edinburgh town. These were to be symbolically presented to Queen Victoria. A miniature replica of Dick's High Constable's ceremonial baton (Figure 2.13) was presented to him. In 1852 'his friends thought of putting him up as a Liberal parliamentary candidate for Edinburgh. He never entered very heartily into the idea' (Dixon 1870).

During this period a number of properties in the Clyde Street courtyard came onto the market and were purchased by Dick. These were structurally modified and adapted to the needs of the Veterinary College over the following fifteen years. In this way the College was able to expand and better accommodate the eighty or so students now being enrolled each year (Figure 2.7).

In 1844 John Dick died aged about seventy-five, his wife Jean having died seven years earlier due to the influenza epidemic. In 1844 the Royal College of Veterinary Surgeons (RCVS) was granted its Royal Charter and established offices in London – veterinary practice was now legally recognised as a profession – and Dick was elected to its Council (Macdonald, Warwick and Johnston 2005). Also in 1844, Dick took on additional teaching staff. William Worthington (1803–75) had been his clinical

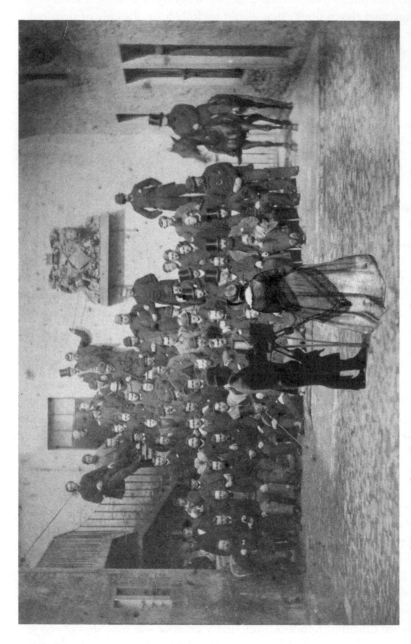

Plate 2.1   Photo montage of the interior of the Clyde Street courtyard with staff, students, Mary Dick and photographer (c. 1864). Montage photographer: Brian Mather.

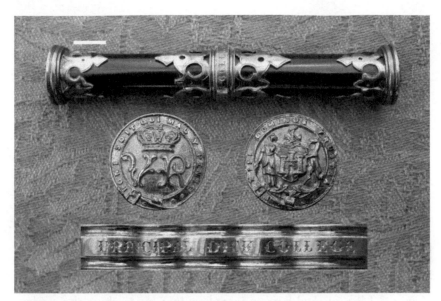

Figure 2.13 Small Ornamental High Constable's Baton, scale 1 cm. The two enlarged end pieces show the monogram of Queen Victoria and the City of Edinburgh Coat of Arms. The enlarged central band reads 'Principal Dick College'. Photographer: Colin M. Warwick.

assistant since 1840, and now George Wilson (1818–59), one of the extra-mural lecturers in Edinburgh, came to teach the students Chemistry (Bradley 1923). John Barlow (1815–56), from Cheshire, who obtained his Diploma from Clyde Street in April 1844, joined the staff to lecture on the anatomy and physiology of the domestic animals and later to give a systematic course of lectures on pathology and the diseases of cattle (Warwick and Macdonald 2006). The examinations that month were carried out by Highland Society and RCVS examiners.

In June 1844 Sir John Graham Dalyell suggested to the Highland Society's Veterinary Committee that the Veterinary College should join the University. However, the Committee considered it premature to consider any of these suggestions further (Macdonald, Warwick and Johnston 2005). Redesigned membership certificates of the Edinburgh Veterinary Medical Society, signed by William Dick and inscribed 'Medica Societas Collegii Regii Veterinarii Civitatis Edinensis', were awarded from April 1844. These represented one of the earliest contemporary pieces of evidence of the application of the title 'Royal' to the name of the College (Macdonald 2013).

The RCVS in London took over the examination of students in April 1845, 1846 and 1847, and the Highland Society suspended its examinations during those years (Bradley 1923). However, following great dissatisfaction with the arrangements of the RCVS examinations, the Highland Society reinstated its exams in April 1848. The Society deliberately scheduled them to take place a few days before the RCVS examinations, to enable students to attend both if they wished (Macdonald, Warwick and Johnston 2005).

By 1844 nearly eight hundred men had attended the Edinburgh Veterinary College as students, of whom just over one-third had obtained diplomas (Figure 2.7; HASS 1844). Many students, since as early as 1827, had been attending the session of lectures on more than one occasion, and had also been coming back for parts of the course. In 1845 the Highland Society insisted that all students must attend two years of instruction and that the six-month winter course (from November to April) should comprise a hundred lectures, increasing thereby the amount of instruction in anatomy, physiology, pathology and the medical treatment of cattle and sheep (Macdonald, Warwick and Johnston 2005). John Barlow (Figure 2.14a), who in 1844 had been the best student of his year (Figure 2.14b), worked hard to introduce into his teaching the modern methods of disease investigation being used in the medical schools, such as the use of the microscope and the study of pathology (Warwick and Macdonald 2006). In the early 1840s John Hughes Bennet (1812–75) had organised in Edinburgh the first British course in practical microscopy (Jacyna 2006). An indication of the scale of clinical teaching material to which the Edinburgh students were exposed is indicated by the monthly reports published in the *Veterinarian* through 1845 and 1846. These tabulate over 3,500 animals treated in the school in 1845, with the senior students having the opportunity to present details of individual cases (Table 2.2). Practical students also continued to have free access to classes given by the University's professors of anatomy and agriculture (Macdonald, Warwick and Johnston 2005).

Portraits of the Dick family

The 1850s was an important decade, artistically speaking, in the life of William Dick (Macdonald, St Leger and Warwick 2021). In 1850 William Shiels exhibited his painting *Portrait of Professor Dick* in the North Octagon at the 24th Royal Scottish Academy show. The following year, at the 25th RSA show, Tavenor Knott exhibited in the North Octagon his *Portrait of Professor Dick – Presentation to him by his Students of the Session 1850–51*.

Mary Dick was sixty years old in 1851, and two years later William Dick was also sixty years old. During the summer of 1853 a new lecture

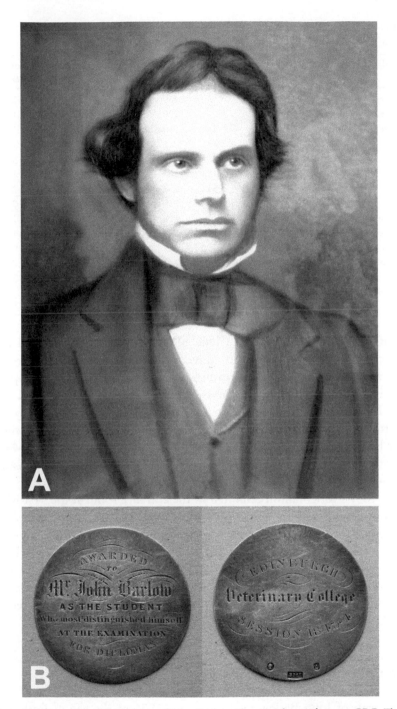

Figure 2.14   A. Retouched photo of John Barlow. Photographer: unknown. CRC, The University of Edinburgh. B. Silver medal (43 mm diameter) awarded to John Barlow in Session 1843–4. Photographer: Colin M. Warwick.

Table 2.2 Numbers of veterinary cases treated by senior students at the Edinburgh Veterinary College each month in 1845.

Month	Dogs	Cats	Pigs	Neat cattle	Horses	Total	Equine mortalities	Canine mortalities
January	20	2	2	18	269	311	10	2
February	13	5		7	229	254	7	1
March	29	4		24	270	327	9	1
April	41		1	48	246	336	8	1
May	31		1	22	272	326	8	3
June	35			13	268	316	5	1
July	23		18	34	257	332	9	2
August	18			11	235	264	6	0
September	17			12	229	258	9	1
October	13		19	27	228	287	10	1
November	9			46	242	297	5	0
December	7			24	237	268	5	0
Total	256	11	41	286	2982	3576	91	13
Monthly average	21			24	249	298	8	

room had been created at the Clyde Street Veterinary School and the old classroom was soon to be converted into an enlarged museum. A new dissecting room, better reading room and library were to be provided soon thereafter (Anonymous,1853). It was sometime in 1853 that Elizabeth Olden painted her portrait of William Dick, perhaps as a birthday gift from the Olden family. It could reasonably be presumed that her watercolour painting of a 'lady' might well have been of Mary Dick; both were exhibited in 1854 at the RSA (Macdonald, St Leger, and Warwick 2021).

In 1857 Clark Stanton exhibited in the entrance room at the 31st RSA exhibition his design for a *Bust of Professor Dick, Founder of the Edinburgh Veterinary College, To be executed in Marble, and presented to Mr. Dick, as a Testimonial from the Members of the Veterinary Profession*. The following year, in 'Sculpture', the completed *Bust in Marble of Professor Dick, Founder of the Edinburgh Veterinary College – a Testimonial to be presented to Mr. Dick from the Members of the Veterinary Profession* was exhibited at the 32nd RSA exhibition (Macdonald, St Leger and Warwick, 2021).

John Barlow and John Gamgee

The death of John Barlow on 22 January 1856 at the age of forty was widely felt in the veterinary profession (Warwick and Macdonald 2006). He had been an original thinker, a hard-working scientific investigator, seen by many as the man destined to advance and elevate veterinary medicine. He was also revered by his students for his almost paternal kindness and interest in them (Warwick and Macdonald 2006). It was a tragic personal and professional loss.

His death also set in train a series of unforeseen changes to veterinary education in Edinburgh. John Gamgee (1831–94) was a London graduate of 1852 who, after a year or two touring the Continent and visiting veterinary schools in France, Germany and Italy, had returned to London in 1855; he then gave extra-mural lectures on veterinary medicine and surgery at the Camden Hall, in Camden Town (Smith 1933). He was a brilliant young veterinary surgeon who, like Barlow, had a strong interest in science (Hall 1965). William Dick recognised Gamgee's writing talents and appointed him in 1856 to lecture on anatomy and physiology in Edinburgh. Dick also promoted his offer to edit veterinary contributions to the Highland Society, which resulted in the Society inviting Gamgee to write articles and review books. Gamgee also travelled around Scotland, taking up and extending one of Barlow's suggestions to study the sites of infections of cattle and sheep, and investigate the course of disease (Barlow 1856). The experience of contagious diseases in animals that he had already gained on the Continent served as the foundation of his research interests thereafter (Gamgee 1857; Smith 1933).

Gamgee strongly believed in the then minority view that germs were responsible for certain diseases (D'Arcy Thompson 1974). William Dick, however, now aged sixty three, although a highly experienced clinician, was somewhat set in his ways; he took the majority view that disease was produced by atmospheric causes (miasma) which appear at the same time each year. The opinions of the two men on such things as the causes of disease and their spread, and on veterinary education and whether the Royal College of Veterinary Surgeons should monopolise student examination, were irreconcilable (Smith 1933; Hall 1965). As a consequence, Gamgee's appointment was not extended beyond his first session in Edinburgh (Bradley 1923).

References

Anonymous, 1853. Edinburgh veterinary college. *The Scotsman*, 9 November 1853, p. 3, col. 4.

Anonymous, 1879. Historical account of the Veterinary Department of the Highland and Agricultural Society. *Transactions of the Highland and Agricultural Society of Scotland*, fourth series, 11, 121–89.

Ballingall, G. 1834. *Inventory of preparations in the veterinary museum. Report submitted to the Highland Society of Scotland.* Archives of the Royal Highland and Agricultural Society of Scotland.

Barlow, J. 1856. Note on the occurrence of paralysis and muscular atrophy in connection with arterial obstruction and obliteration/ by the late John Barlow. *Edinburgh Medical Journal*, 1 (12), 1087–9.

Bradley, O. C. 1923. *History of the Edinburgh Veterinary College*. Edinburgh: Oliver & Boyd.

Castley, J. 1830. Of the Edinburgh veterinary school, etc. *Veterinarian*, 3, 305–11.

Clarke, W. 1833. On the neglect of the medical treatment of cattle in the pages of *The Veterinarian*. *The Veterinarian*, 6, 179–84.

D'Arcy Thompson, R. 1974. *The Remarkable Gamgees: A story of achievement*. Edinburgh: Ramsay Head Press.

[Dick, W. 1817–18]. *Lecture notes on the anatomy, physiology and pathology of the horse delivered by E. Coleman at the London Veterinary College, Camden Town, taken down by W.D.* [1817–18]. 4 c.208 ff. Edinburgh University Library MS.2747.

Dick, W. 1839. In Youatt, W. (ed.). Professor Dick. *The Veterinarian*, 12, 127–9.

Dixon, H. H. 1870. *Saddle and Sirloin, or English Farm and Sporting Worthies*. London: Rogerson & Tuxford.

Dollar, T. A. 1894. *Inaugural address delivered by Thomas A. Dollar, M.R.C.V.S. at the opening of the 72nd session of Royal (Dick) Veterinary College Edinburgh, 3rd October 1894. Presentation to the trustees of Miss Dick's Portrait and report of the banquet given to the Lord Provost, Magistrates, and Town Council, and leading members of the medical and veterinary professions*. Edinburgh: Turnbull and Spears.

Gamgee, J. 1857. *Diseased meat sold in Edinburgh, and meat inspection, in connection with the public health and with the interests of agriculture: a letter to the Right Hon. the Lord Provost of Edinburgh*. Edinburgh, 3–13.

Gardner, A. 2007. Elephants and exclusivity: An episode from the 'pre-Dick' history of veterinary education in Edinburgh. *Veterinary History*, 13 (4), 299–309.

Hall, S. A. 1965. John Gamgee and the Edinburgh New Veterinary College. *Veterinary Record*, 77, 1237a–1241b.

HASS, 1840. Meeting of Directors, 24 April 1840, *Records of the Highland and Agricultural Society of Scotland*, 16, 514–17.

HASS, 1844. Minutes of the Veterinary Committee, 18 May 1844, *Records of the Highland and Agricultural Society of Scotland*, 19, 286–7.

Jacyna, L. S. 1994. *Philosophic Whigs: Medicine, Science and Citizenship in Edinburgh, 1789–1848*. London and New York: Routledge.

Jacyna, L. S. 2006. Medicine in transformation, 1800–1849. In Bynum, W. F., Hardy, A., Jacyna, S. and Lawrence, C. *The Western Medical Tradition. 1800–2000*. Cambridge: Cambridge University Press, 11–101.

Johnston, W. T. 2002. *Transcript of an inventory of preparations in the veterinary museum, 1834*. Edinburgh Research Archive (ERA), the University of Edinburgh, <era.ed.ac.uk /handle/1842/36672 > (accessed 9 September 2022).

Macdonald, A. A. 2013. The Royal (Dick) School of Veterinary Studies: what's in a name? *Veterinary History*, 17 (1), 33–65. <era.ed.ac.uk/handle/1842/7760> (accessed 9 September 2022).

Macdonald, A. A. 2020. Clyde Street 1833–1841: the veterinary teaching and learning environment. *Veterinary History*, 20 (3), 272–306. <era.ed.ac.uk/handle/1842/38679> (accessed 9 September 2022).

Macdonald, A. A., Johnston, W. T. and Warwick, C. M. 2022. The Edinburgh Veterinary Medical Society's library. *Veterinary History*, 21 (2), 168–93, also appendix 3, <era.ed .ac.uk/bitstream/handle/1842/38322/Appendix_3_1857_transcribed_catalogue.pdf ?sequence=4&isAllowed=y> (accessed 9 September 2022).

Macdonald, A. A., St Leger, A. and Warwick, C. 2020. The 1853 portrait of William Dick and the undelivered letters. *Veterinary History*, 21 (1), 60–3. <era.ed.ac.uk/handle/18 42/38664> (accessed 9 September 2022).

Macdonald, A. A. and Warwick, C. M. 2012. Early teaching of the 'veterinary art and science' in Edinburgh. *Veterinary History*, 16 (3), 227–73. <era.ed.ac.uk/handle/1842 /6277> (accessed 9 September 2022).

Macdonald, A. A. and Warwick, C. M. 2013. Preparations in Comparative Anatomy removed from Dr Knox's Premises (and written before 23 Sept. 1828 – an extract from Knox Old Catalogue, University of Edinburgh Anatomy Archives – CRC DA 50 Anat [905]. <era.ed.ac.uk/handle/1842/8306> (accessed 9 September 2022).

Macdonald, A. A and Warwick, C. M. 2014a. Dr John Barclay's teaching of comparative anatomy. *Veterinary History*, 17 (3), 202–37. <era.ed.ac.uk/handle/1842/9409> (accessed 9 September 2022).

Macdonald, A. A. and Warwick, C. M. 2014b. Barclean Museum Catalogue (Comparative Anatomy Specimens) extracted from: Knox, R. (1828). *Catalogue of the Barclean Museum*. In *The Deeds of Settlement and Catalogue of the Barclean Museum bequeathed to the Royal College of Surgeons of Edinburgh by John Barclay*. <era.ed.ac.uk/handle/18 42/8307> (accessed 9 September 2022).

Macdonald, A. A. and Warwick, C. M. 2019. A wee blether with Mary Dick. *Veterinary History*, 19, 341–69. <era.ed.ac.uk/handle/1842/38663> (accessed 9 September 2022).

Macdonald, A. A. and Warwick, C. M. 2023. The Highland Society's Veterinary School in Edinburgh 1823–1829. *Veterinary History* (in press).

Macdonald, A. A., Warwick, C. M. and Johnston, W. T. 2005. Locating veterinary education in Edinburgh in the nineteenth century. *Book of the Old Edinburgh Club*, New Series, 6, 41–71. <era.ed.ac.uk/handle/1842/2199> (accessed 9 September 2022).

Macdonald, A. A., Warwick, C. M. and Johnston, W. T. 2011. John Feron and his 'address' on a veterinary institution in Edinburgh. *Veterinary History*, 16 (1), 41–64. <era.ed.ac.uk/handle/1842/5264> (accessed 9 September 2022).

[Stewart, J.] 1834. *A concise account of veterinary surgery, its schools and practitioners, for the benefit of proprietors of domestic animals, by a veterinary surgeon*. Glasgow.

Warwick, C. M and Macdonald, A. A. 2006. Barlow: a mind of no common mould. *Veterinary History*, 13 (2), 100–10. <cra.ed.ac.uk/handle/1842/2197> (accessed 9 September 2022).

Chapter 3

John Gamgee's Edinburgh New Veterinary College (1857–65)

A new veterinary college is established

John Gamgee (Figure 3.1) remained in Edinburgh. He put into immediate effect the plans he had formulated during the previous year, to find financial backers and create a new veterinary school of his own (Syme 1858). He succeeded. On 4 November 1857 he opened his Edinburgh New Veterinary College in a stable courtyard at 6 Drummond Street, very close to the University (Figures 1.1g and 3.2). This was to be temporary accommodation that he had rented from Alex Stuart. Almost seventy years earlier, the ground in that area, then known as Dr Munro's Park, had been offered for sale, with the description: 'south part to be a large stable yard with coach houses and stables, to which there will be an entry by an arch in the middle of the houses fronting the north' on Drummond Street (Valuation, 1858–9).

For the first time in Edinburgh, veterinary students were offered a properly arranged course of study (Hunting 1894). Anatomy, Physiology, Medicine and Surgery, Materia Medica and Chemistry were taught in separate classes by different lecturers and demonstrators (Table 3.1). A dissecting room, museum and library were made available to the students. Although two winter sessions were compulsory, Gamgee recommended that they attend classes over three winters (Gamgee 1857a). He also indicated that an additional complete set of courses, with opportunities for the practical study of disease, would be made available from May until the end of July. The same year a horse infirmary was established in 206 West Rose Street under John Gamgee's father, Joseph Gamgee (1801–85), and clinical reports of a proportion of the cases seen by the students in 1857–8 were published (Gamgee 1858). These cases were mainly equine, but reference

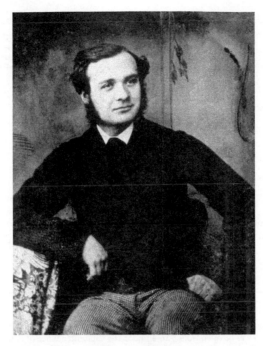

Figure 3.1 Photograph of John Gamgee. Photographer: unknown. Courtesy of the late Ruth D'Arcy Thompson and the Ramsay Head Press.

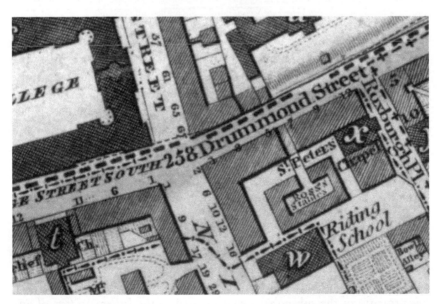

Figure 3.2 Detail from Kirkwood's new plan of the City of Edinburgh, 1821, showing the relationship of Ross's stable courtyard at 6 Drummond Street to the Riding School to the south (replaced by Playfair's Surgeons' Hall in 1829) and the University of Edinburgh to the north-west. Reproduced with the permission of the National Library of Scotland.

Table 3.1 Staff and courses of instruction offered during the 1857 winter and 1858 summer sessions at the Edinburgh New Veterinary College.

Staff name	Course of Instruction during the Winter Session
Dr A. Monastier	Descriptive Anatomy of the Domestic Animals
Mr John Gamgee	Physiological Anatomy and Physiology
Dr Stevenson MacAdam	Chemistry
Mr John Gamgee	Materia Medica and Practical Pharmacy applicable to Veterinary Purposes
Mr John Gamgee	Clinical Lectures
Mr James Law	Anatomical Demonstrations
	Course of Instruction during the Summer Session
Dr A. Monastier	Practical or Regional Anatomy
Dr Stevenson MacAdam	Practical Chemistry
Mr Carruthers	Geology and Botany Applicable to Veterinary Purposes
Mr John Gamgee	Principles of Veterinary Medicine and Surgery
Mr John Gamgee	Clinical Lectures
Mr James Law	Anatomical Demonstrations

The Winter Session commences on the 4th of November and ends on the 3rd week in April.
The Summer Session will open early on the 5th of May and terminate on the 31st of July.
The Dissecting Room will be open from 9 to 4 under the superintendence of Anatomy staff.
The Practical Department is conducted jointly by Mr Gamgee senior and Mr John Gamgee.

Reference: Gamgee, J. 1857. *On the study of veterinary medicine; being an inaugural address at the opening of the Edinburgh New Veterinary School.* Edinburgh: Sutherland & Knox.

was made to canine and on-farm bovine conditions (Gamgee 1858). The infirmary, although at first small, was increased to accommodate the admission of horses, cattle and dogs. The charges for the keeping of animals under treatment was: Horses, 3s. daily; Cattle, one shilling and six pence per day; Dogs, 3d. per night or eighteen pence per week, when small; and 4d. per night or two shillings per week, when large (Gamgee 1860a).

A list of subscribers to veterinary care, being 'any person or persons possessing either Horses, Cattle, Dogs or other domestic animals which he or they may at any time wish to consult the Professors of the [New Veterinary] College', attracted nearly a hundred horse proprietors in Edinburgh and Leith within a month of the issue of the Rules and Regulations relating to subscribers (Gamgee 1860a). The subscriptions charged are listed in Table 3.2. A Subscriber could have any number of horses or other animals examined for soundness. Sick animals, the *bona fide* property of the subscribers, were treated in the Infirmary free of any charge beyond their keep and medicines. All surgical operations on them were performed free. Medicines prepared in the Pharmacy of the College were supplied to subscribers and others at very moderate prices.

Table 3.2 Subscriptions for veterinary services at the Edinburgh New Veterinary College.

Subscribers at a distance from Edinburgh	
Life subscription	£21 0s. 0d.
Annual subscription	£2 2s. 0d.
Tenant farmers	£1 1s. 0d.
Subscribers in or within three miles of Edinburgh	
Noblemen, independent gentlemen, &c.	
Life subscription	£21 0s. 0d.
Annual subscription	£2 2s. 0d.
Proprietors of from one to three horses	
Life subscription	£10 10s. 0d.
Annual subscription	£1 1s. 0d.
Proprietors of from three to ten horses	
Life subscription	£21 0s. 0d.
Annual subscription	£2 2s. 0d.
Proprietors of from ten to twenty horses	
Life subscription	£31 10s. 0d.
Annual subscription	£3 3s. 0d.
Horse dealers	
Life subscription	£21 0s. 0d.
Annual subscription	£2 2s. 0d.
Cattle dealers	
Life subscription	£10 10s. 0d.
Annual subscription	£1 1s. 0d.

Proprietors of more than twenty horses are charged an additional ten guineas on a life subscription, or one additional guinea per annum for every ten horses.

Proprietors of smaller animals, such as dogs or cats, are admitted Subscribers for the annual payment of 10s. 6d.

Reference: Gamgee, J. 1860a. *Rules &c. of the New Veterinary College, Edinburgh*. Edinburgh: Black.

In 1858 John and his father established the vigorous monthly periodical, *Edinburgh Veterinary Review and Annals of Comparative Pathology*. It was used to publish lectures, statistics, information of veterinary interest and propaganda supportive of his new College and the modernising veterinary ethos that John Gamgee wished to project (Smith 1933).

Twenty students were reportedly (Syme 1858) enrolled for the first session of studies (1857–8), although it was suggested that less than half that number were paying fees for instruction (Dick 1858). Interestingly, some of those enrolled in 1857 had already had one session of veterinary training. This was indicated by the silver medals awarded to 'Senior Students' William Malcolm Reid and Thomas Sarginson for written examinations on descriptive anatomy and on veterinary medicine and surgery respectively. The first-year silver medal went to Joseph H. Welsby (Anonymous

1858). That the second-session students had begun to come from the Clyde Street College was subsequently made clear when legal questions were raised about the payment of course fees to Clyde Street; £8 8s. for one session and £16 16s. for 'perpetual' study (Anonymous 1860a). John Joss from Aberdeenshire was another of those who had spent his first session at the Clyde Street College and had moved to the New College for his second session.

The first two years of the New College stimulated a period of intense discussion and sometimes fierce argument inside and beyond the city, both in favour of and against the establishment in Edinburgh of this second Veterinary School north of the border. This was partly catalogued in the *Edinburgh Veterinary Review* and was also aired in the *Scotsman* newspaper. Considerable effort had to be expended by John Gamgee in first seeking influential sponsors and then courting recognition by Royal Sign-Manual in order that his students could eventually be examined by the Royal College of Veterinary Surgeons (Gamgee 1858–9; Hunting 1894). It was not until the end of March 1859 that this recognition was finally granted (Gamgee 1860b).

What impact this debate and associated uncertainty had on student recruitment to the Edinburgh New Veterinary College is hard to gauge accurately as there appear to be few extant records. Naturally, there is no evidence of any of the students from the New College taking the RCVS membership exams in the April of 1858. However, William Malcolm Reid, Joseph H. Welsby, Alexander C. Muir, William Appleton and James I. Lupton were all listed as having obtained MRCVS qualifications in 1859 (Anonymous 1859). Two of the men from the initial first session of New College intake, David Mackay and George Reilly, passed the MRCVS exam in 1860 (Anonymous 1860b). Thirty-nine students studied at the New Veterinary College in the 1859–60 session (Gamgee 1860b).

In his introductory lecture in 1859, John Gamgee recognised that the location of his New Veterinary College in Drummond Street was not ideal, and he indicated its obvious deficiencies to his students (Gamgee 1860b). His wishes for better facilities were outlined. He explained that efforts had been made to secure sufficient sponsorship for the construction of a new building elsewhere, but without success. In 1859 he and his wife Adeline moved from 4 Scotland Street to 2 St Cuthbert's Glebe, which lay on the east side of Lothian Road, south of the Castle Terrace intersection and St Cuthbert's Church. He rented an office nearby at 8 St Cuthbert's Glebe, and his postal address became 'New Veterinary College, Lothian Road, Edinburgh' (Macdonald, Warwick and Johnston 2005). This move brought him diagonally opposite the Scottish Naval and Military Academy (which was just south of St George's Free Church and

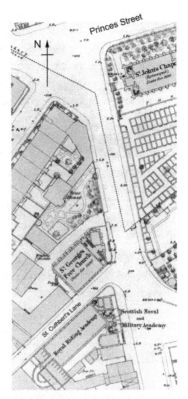

Figure 3.3 Detail from the 1852 Ordnance Survey map of Edinburgh showing the north end of Lothian Road, with the Royal Riding Academy and Scottish Naval and Military Academy buildings. Gamgee's Edinburgh New Veterinary College was sited here from 1862 to 1865. Reproduced with the permission of the National Library of Scotland.

St Cuthbert's Lane). Behind the Military Academy lay the former Royal Riding Academy. The neighbourhood was close to the more fashionable West End of Princes Street (Figure 3.3). An alternative to the physical construction of a veterinary college somewhere else in Edinburgh now lay before him.

The students were required to spend twenty-three weeks each winter session on veterinary study (Gamgee 1860b); thus, forty-six weeks to cover both winter sessions. Gamgee estimated that each weekday the students worked for ten hours, with lectures and examinations taking up 484 of the 1,242 hours available to them each session. He proposed that four hours should be worked on Saturdays. For physiology and dissection, he expected a minimum of two hours to be spent on each subject daily during the two sessions. He estimated that the study of chemistry would occupy almost four hundred hours, largely in one session. Materia Medica would occupy one hour per day for one session. Gamgee emphasised that veterinary therapeutics was being taught in his College by a veterinary surgeon rather than by a chemist. Courses being given on the principles and practice of horse shoeing, botany, the principles of veterinary medicine and surgery, and the clinical lectures were all seen as improvements to the way veterinary students had been taught up until then. Detailed synopses of these courses of lectures on veterinary medicine, surgery and obstetrics to be delivered in Session 1860–1 were published to indicate the breadth and depth of material covered at the Edinburgh New Veterinary College (Gamgee 1860c, d). However, Gamgee bemoaned the fact that veterinary medicine and surgery had to be presented as succinct digests in four hours per week, with occasional lectures in the evening (Gamgee 1860b). His analysis indicated that more learning time was required. He also strongly recommended that veterinary graduates should spend a year working in a large practice with a skilful veterinary surgeon immediately after obtaining their veterinary Diploma (Gamgee 1860b).

An unrecorded number of men put themselves forward for the MRCVS exams in 1861, of whom seven passed: John Joss, William Cope, Andrew Robbie, James Gordon, George Robertson, P. Galloway and David Clark Emmott (Anonymous 1861). An increased number, thirteen students, graduated MRCVS in 1862 (Anonymous 1862a).

The New Veterinary College moves west in Edinburgh

In 1862 the opportunity to access better accommodation presented itself. The continual growth in student numbers at Drummond Street had made it imperative to move. Gamgee rented from John Croall the large buildings on the west side of Lothian Road that had previously been used by the Scottish Naval and Military Academy (Gamgee 1862; Anonymous 1862b). He also rented from its trustees the former Royal Riding Academy that lay behind the Academy (Figures 1.1h, 3.3 and 3.4). These buildings offered much-improved teaching facilities, including large halls and excellent stables, as well as the increased status of being in the West End of Edinburgh. Gamgee transferred his Veterinary College there in 1862. The number of students who qualified MRCVS at the end of the 1862–3 Session increased again to twenty-two (Anonymous 1863). One of these was Robert Morris, from Wick (Figure 3.5). He was a very bright student, as indicated by two of the medals he was awarded (Figure 3.6).

The staff presenting the courses in the 1863–4 Session are listed in Table 3.3. It was during this Session that the first approaches were being made to John Gamgee by businessmen in London with a view to purchasing the College and transferring it to London (Anonymous 1865a). For

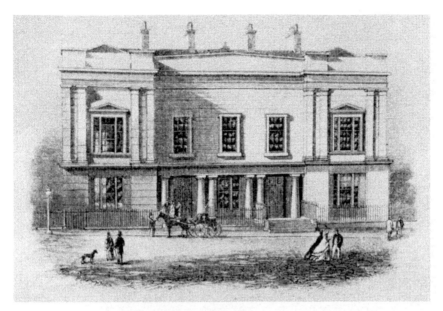

Figure 3.4 Façade of Gamgee's Edinburgh New Veterinary College at 8 Lothian Road. Illustration courtesy of the late Ruth D'Arcy Thompson and the Ramsay Head Press.

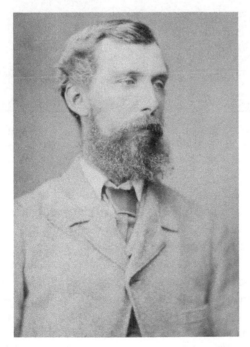

Figure 3.5 Robert Morris graduated from Gamgee's Edinburgh New Veterinary College in 1863. Photographer: Alexander Johnston. Permission granted by the Wick Society Johnston Collection.

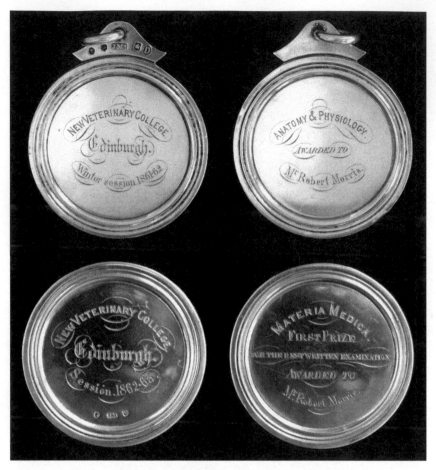

Figure 3.6 Medals (56 mm diameter) awarded by Gamgee's Edinburgh New Veterinary College to Robert Morris for Anatomy and Physiology in Session 1861–2 and Materia Medica the following Session. Photographer: Colin M. Warwick.

some time, the Caledonian Railway Company had been actively purchasing property in the area of Edinburgh neighbouring Gamgee's Veterinary College. Its intention was to extend the railway line and replace its temporary wooden Edinburgh terminus with something more substantial and closer to Princes Street. It is very likely that John Gamgee, as a resident in the area for some five years, and as a tenant of the former Riding Academy's buildings, was well aware of how temporary his occupancy of this college accommodation was likely to be. There were also indications that the income to the Edinburgh New Veterinary College was nowhere near matching the expenditures being incurred by Gamgee. It was rumoured that the annual loss since the establishment of the College had amounted to upwards of one thousand pounds (Anonymous 1865a).

Table 3.3 Staff and courses of instruction offered during the 1863 winter session at the Edinburgh New Veterinary College, Lothian Road.

Staff name	Course of Instruction during the Winter Session
Mr James Law	General and Descriptive Anatomy of the Domestic Animals
Mr James Law, and	Practical Anatomy
Mr W. Duguid, demonstrator	Anatomical Demonstrations
Mr Alfred Thomas Brett	Physiology of the Domestic Animals
Dr Stevenson MacAdam FRS	Chemistry
Dr Arthur Gamgee	Materia Medica and Practical Pharmacy applicable to Veterinary Purposes
Mr John Gamgee, and	Practical Chemistry
Mr Robert Morris, assistant	
Mr Alfred Thomas Brett	Veterinary Materia Medica
Mr Gamgee, Sen.	Principles and Practice of Shoeing
Mr John Gamgee	Veterinary Medicine and Surgery
Mr Gamgee, Sen., and	Clinical Instruction
Mr John Gamgee	

Introductory Lecture on Wednesday, the 4th of November 1863.

Reference: Gamgee, J. 1863. Advertisement.

No decision was made, but the increased cost of the more prestigious college premises would certainly have been a factor for consideration. Sixteen students passed the MRCVS examinations in 1864 (Anonymous 1864).

Teaching and research output

In addition to his teaching, John Gamgee researched productively and wrote education material prolifically: *The Veterinarian's Vade Mecum* was published by Sutherland and Knox in Edinburgh in 1858; *Our domestic animals in health and disease* was issued in four parts during 1861, 1862, 1863 and 1864 by Maclachlan & Stewart in Edinburgh; *Dairy stock, its selection, diseases and produce* in 1861 by T. C. Jack in Edinburgh; and together with James Law, his staff member and former student, Gamgee published *General and descriptive anatomy of the domestic animals* in two parts in 1861 and 1862, also issued by T. C. Jack. Via the columns of the national and international press he exposed to public view his research findings on the widespread traffic in diseased meat and the generally bad husbandry conditions in the city's cowsheds, and drew public and governmental attention to the then 'normality' of poor sanitary conditions (Gamgee 1857b, 1863a, b, c). He campaigned energetically on the methods by which animal disease spread, and employed the recent gathering of national statistics, national and international correspondence with veterinary colleagues and the columns of the press to bring attention to the need for government regulation of animal movement and veterinary inspection of animal markets and meat (Gamgee 1857, 1863d). Sadly, tragically, all to no avail; Gamgee was obstructed nationally and locally by culpable ignorance, neglect, greed and indifference (Hunting 1894; Smith 1933). Rinderpest, the cattle plague that he had long predicted would come from the Baltic, arrived in Hull in 1865 on the steamship *Tonning*. Its cargo of infected cattle had come from the ports of Revel and St Petersburg (Gamgee 1866). The disease travelled rapidly to London, where it was eventually identified (Gamgee 1866; Thompson 1974). The impact of the disease, between 1865 and 1867, was later recognised as the 'most dramatic episode in British agricultural history' (Orwin and Whetham 1964).

The College closes and moves to London

Perhaps it is not surprising, then, that when the company of influential men from London made Gamgee an offer to take over his Veterinary College, including 'his whole staff of professors, teachers, and students, museum, library, diagrams, apparatus etc.', and transfer it to London, he accepted (Anonymous 1865a, b, c). In May 1864 John Gamgee sold his house at 12 Castle Terrace but continued to occupy it as a tenant. The publication of the last part of Vol. 6 of the *Edinburgh Veterinary Review* came out in December 1864, after which its publication stopped. The last teaching session of the New Edinburgh Veterinary College terminated with the RCVS examinations in April 1865, at which fourteen students successfully obtained MRCVS (Anonymous 1865d). During the 1857–65 existence of the Edinburgh New Veterinary College a total of sixty-six students became qualified Members of the Royal College of Veterinary Surgeons.

The staff and students from the New Edinburgh College moved to London to re-establish the college under its new name, the Albert Veterinary College, Limited on Queen's Road, Bayswater (Gamgee 1865). Despite having many titled backers and friends, the 'whirlwind' created in the country's livestock population by the spreading devastation of rinderpest and the all-consuming diversion it represented to John Gamgee, the proper establishment of veterinary education in the Albert College was neglected; it ran into financial difficulties and closed in 1868 at great financial loss (Thompson 1974).

John Gamgee never received credit at the time for his foresight in grasping the principle of contagion as a cause of disease nor for his tenacious attention to explaining and spreading his warning of the consequences of failing to act to restrict the spread of the disease (Huntington 1894; Smith 1933). With John Barlow, John Gamgee may be said to have initiated the scientific era of veterinary teaching in Scotland (Hunting 1894). Before their time, veterinary teaching was rooted in personal experience. The lasting impact of the ripples of ideas that were promoted by the Edinburgh New Veterinary College can still be detected in the Royal (Dick) School of Veterinary Studies today, in the importance of research, the exploration of new ideas, and in an informed and informing awareness of the epidemiology of contagious animal diseases.

References

Anonymous, 1858. New Veterinary College – Session 1857–58. *Edinburgh Veterinary Review and Annals of Comparative Pathology*, 1, 243.

Anonymous, 1859. Examination of Students. *The Veterinarian*, 32, 357.

Anonymous, 1860a. Veterinary jurisprudence. *Edinburgh Veterinary Review and Annals of Comparative Pathology*, 1, 180–6.

Anonymous, 1860b. Examination of Students. *The Veterinarian*, 33, 368.

Anonymous, 1861. New members of the profession: Students of the New Veterinary College, Edinburgh. *The Veterinarian*, 34, 366–7.

Anonymous, 1862a. New members of the profession: Students of the New Veterinary College, Edinburgh. *The Veterinarian*, 35, 378–9.

Anonymous, 1862b. The New Veterinary College. *The Scotsman*, 28 March 1862, p. 2, col. 4.

Anonymous, 1863. New members of the profession: Students of the New Veterinary College, Edinburgh. *The Veterinarian*, 36, 388.

Anonymous, 1864. New members of the profession: Students of the New Veterinary College, Edinburgh. *The Veterinarian*, 37, 438.

Anonymous, 1865a. Removal to London of the New Veterinary College. *The Scotsman*, 19 June 1865, p. 2, col. 6.

Anonymous, 1865b. The New Veterinary College. *The Veterinarian*, 38, 373–5.

Anonymous, 1865c. Money market and city intelligence. *The Times*, 17 June 1865, p. 10, col. f.

Anonymous, 1865d. New members of the profession: Students of the New Veterinary College, Edinburgh. *The Veterinarian*, 38, 409.

Dick, W. 1858. Letter from Professor Dick to the Editor of the Scotsman, August 25. *Edinburgh Veterinary Review and Annals of Comparative Pathology*, 1, 249–52.

Gamgee, J. 1857a. *On the study of veterinary medicine being an inaugural address at the opening of the Edinburgh New Veterinary School*. Edinburgh: Sutherland & Knox.

Gamgee, J. 1857b. *Diseased meat sold in Edinburgh, and meat inspection, in connection with the public health and with the interests of agriculture: a letter to the Right Hon. the Lord Provost of Edinburgh*, Edinburgh: [s.n.].

Gamgee, 1858. Clinical report of the Edinburgh New Veterinary College, from 1st August, 1857, to 1st August, 1858. *Edinburgh Veterinary Review and Annals of Comparative Pathology*, 1, 139–56, 291–8.

Gamgee, J. 1858–9. [Editorials.] *Edinburgh Veterinary Review and Annals of Comparative Pathology*, 1, 190–2, 245–75, 354–60, 477–81.

Gamgee, J. 1860a. *Rules &c., of the New Veterinary College, Edinburgh*. Edinburgh: Black, 1–4.

Gamgee, J. 1860b. The Royal Sign-Manual. *Edinburgh Veterinary Review and Annals of Comparative Pathology*, 2, 63–4.

Gamgee, J. 1860c. Synopsis of lectures on veterinary medicine and surgery, delivered in the New Veterinary College. *Edinburgh Veterinary Review and Annals of Comparative Pathology*, 1, 237–45.

Gamgee, J. 1860d. Synopsis of course of lectures on operative veterinary surgery and veterinary obstetrics. *Edinburgh Veterinary Review and Annals of Comparative Pathology*, 1, 348–51.

Gamgee, J. 1862. The New Veterinary College. *Edinburgh Veterinary Review and Annals of Comparative Pathology*, 4, 250.

Gamgee, 1863a. The diseases of animals in relation to public health and prosperity: being a lecture delivered before the Metropolitan Association of Medical Officers of Health, on the 18th of April, 1863. *Edinburgh Veterinary Review and Annals of Comparative Pathology*, 5, 254–68.

Gamgee, 1863b. Health of stock. *Edinburgh Veterinary Review and Annals of Comparative Pathology*, 5, 269–97, 334–50.

Gamgee, 1863c. Health of stock in the United Kingdom during the year 1862. *Edinburgh Veterinary Review and Annals of Comparative Pathology*, 5, 401–18.

Gamgee, 1863d. The system of inspection in relation to the traffic in diseased animals or their produce. *Edinburgh Veterinary Review and Annals of Comparative Pathology*, 5, 663–70.

Gamgee, 1865. *Rules and regulations of the Albert Veterinary College Limited. Queen's Road, Bayswater*. London: A. H. Baily & Co.

Gamgee, J. 1866. *The cattle plague, with official reports of the International Veterinary Congresses, held in Hamburg, 1863, and in Vienna, 1865*. London: R. Hardwicke.

[Hunting, W.] 1894. Professor John Gamgee. *Veterinary Record*, 29 December 1894, 365–6.

Macdonald, A. A., Warwick, C. M. and Johnston, W. T. 2005. Locating veterinary education in Edinburgh in the nineteenth century. *Book of the Old Edinburgh Club*, New Series, 6, 41–71. <era.ed.ac.uk/handle/1842/2199> (accessed 9 September 2022).

Orwin, C. S. and Whetham, E. H. 1964. *History of British Agriculture, 1846–1914*. London: Longmans.

Smith, F. 1933. *The Early History of Veterinary Literature and its British Development*, 4 vols. London: Baillière, Tindall & Cox.

Syme, J. 1858. Letter to the Members of the Highland and Agricultural Society of Scotland. *Edinburgh Veterinary Review*, 1, 245–7.

Thompson, R. D. 1974. *The Remarkable Gamgees: A story of achievement*. Edinburgh: Ramsay Head Press.

Valuation, 1858–9. Valuation Rolls, Edinburgh Burgh, 1858–59. National Archives of Scotland, V.R. 100/23, Folio 284.

Chapter 4

Clyde Street College Developments (1857–74)

The presence of a second veterinary college in Edinburgh was not without impact on William Dick's veterinary college, or indeed on William Dick himself; he was outraged. The Edinburgh Veterinary Medical Association, which had been established in 1834 'for the advancement and diffusion of Veterinary Knowledge, particularly among veterinary students', had built up a large library (Macdonald, Johnston and Warwick 2022). A new list of those 361 book titles was published in 1857. However, the considerable ill feeling expressed by William Dick towards Gamgee's college during 1857 and 1858 prompted the passing of a by-law by the Edinburgh Veterinary Medical Association on 20 January 1858,

> providing that the Members shall consist of Veterinary Surgeons and Veterinary Students attending the London or Edinburgh Veterinary Colleges, and that if any member should attend any rival school or Society in Edinburgh, he should forfeit the membership and the whole privileges thereof . (Anonymous 1874a)

The right of students to become members of the Association was subsequently limited to those attending the Edinburgh Veterinary College based in Clyde Street.

Nevertheless, the heated controversy over the establishment of the Edinburgh New Veterinary College, its founder's choice of the RCVS for the examination of its students, and Gamgee's infusion of thoughts and ideas from veterinary colleagues on the Continent, all acted as stimuli to the way veterinary medicine was discussed and taught in Edinburgh. In addition, throughout this period, Dick and the graduates of his veterinary college were subjected to a continuous flow of barbed comment in the veterinary press to do better (Gamgee 1858, 1860).

The numbers of students attending the Clyde Street College did not seem to be much affected, however, fluctuating between about 60 and 100 as before (Figure 2.7). As indicated in chapter 3, some students attended the Clyde Street College in their first year and then moved to Gamgee's college for their second year. The numbers of Clyde Street students successfully obtaining their certificates from the Highland Society seemed to maintain an upward trend (Figure 2.6). In 1857 Thomas Strangeways (1824–69) graduated with a Highland Society medal and was immediately appointed Demonstrator of Anatomy for one year (Macdonald, Warwick and Johnston 2005). He was invited to return to Clyde Street in November 1859 to take the Anatomy Chair following James McCall's (1834–1915) departure from that post to go into veterinary practice in the West of Scotland. By 1862 McCall had established the Glasgow Veterinary College, the third veterinary college in Scotland and the fourth in Britain (Weipers 1976).

In April 1863 William Dick was seventy years old. At the end-of-session dinner he indicated that he would continue to teach for as long as he could (Figure 4.1). He noted, however, that it was no easy task to carry through a whole session with a class of some eighty or ninety young men, 'wild, sometimes, and riotous – careless, and sometimes stupid – sometimes

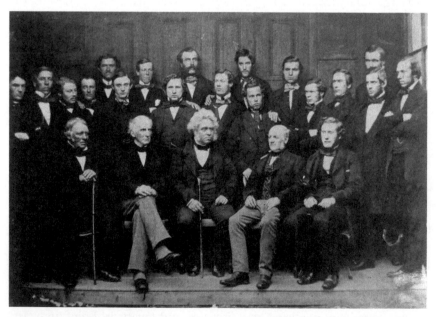

Figure 4.1 Photograph, probably taken inside the Clyde Street College, of staff and students, c. 1860. Seated left to right: Peter Young, Alan Dalzell, William Dick, William Worthington, Thomas Strangeways. Note the apparent range of ages of the students, whose identities were not recorded. Photographer: unknown.

high-spirited, and at other times taking up notions of their own'. He was clearly not feeling quite as supple as before (Anonymous 1879a). In the past he had 'prided himself on quelling offenders by the unaided power of his eye' (Dixon 1870). His students used to call him the 'old white lion'.

Nevertheless, during that session he had begun to publish in the *Transactions of the Highland and Agricultural Society of Scotland* a second series of accounts of the cases of disease and injuries seen by his students at Clyde Street; some 2,483 were seen in 1862 and 2,385 in 1863, the majority being horses, with the total for cattle, sheep, dogs and cats amounting to between three hundred and four hundred. Clinical notes were taken by the more advanced students, who were also given more or less personal management of the cases (Dick 1869). These accounts, Dick pointed out, proved that his range of teaching in Edinburgh was far more comprehensive than that of his London critics.

William Dick's teaching continued to be firmly based on his forty years of personal clinical experience and a good memory on the practice of the art of veterinary medicine. The application of science to veterinary medicine was still in its infancy. He had taken on practical farriers and farriers' apprentices, the so-called 'Professional' or 'Practical' pupils, people like himself, and trained large numbers of them to become experienced veterinary surgeons. He had kept his educational fees low to match the ability of these students to pay. He also attracted students of agriculture and had arranged classes for 'Amateur' pupils at more convenient times. The latter were gentlemen who had expressed interest in expanding their knowledge and understanding of the subject. They were not intent on taking up the practice of veterinary medicine. Dick was a proud man, and happy to point out to his students that the success which materially surrounded him was the result of his own hard labour (Dick 1863).

He had been appointed Veterinary Surgeon in Scotland to Queen Victoria in 1837, and the Royal Crest on the north wall of the college courtyard was put up perhaps as his sign of 'by appointment' (Plate 2.1). At the Highland Society meeting on 24 June 1863, it was reported that no fewer than 1,700 gentlemen had been educated at the Edinburgh College, and 740 had received Highland Society diplomas (McLagan 1863). Nevertheless, an atmosphere of unease at the way students were being taught and examined was beginning to gain currency in the country (Gamgee 1864).

On 16 February 1864, just as William Dick was about to commence his 4 pm lecture, a fire broke out under the classroom seating. It caused the destruction of the lecture theatre and the roof above it. It also somewhat damaged the contents of the adjacent museum. Fortunately, the students' book collection was not harmed. Repairs were speedily made, but home

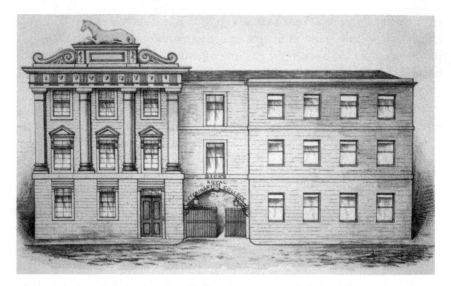

Figure 4.2 New housing accommodation, three storeys in height, built in 1865 at 10 Clyde Street and attached to the east side of the 1833 College building. Detail from a Diploma awarded by the Edinburgh Veterinary Medical Society. Photographer: Colin M. Warwick.

life in the College was disrupted by the accident (Anonymous 1864a, b). True to character, Dick took the rebuilding as an opportunity to knock down the old tenement next door at number 10 and replace it with new housing accommodation, three storeys in height (Figure 4.2). Designed by John Chalmers, this tenement was constructed in the summer of 1865 (Macdonald, Warwick and Johnston 2005).

The death of William Dick

As indicated in chapter 3, that summer the epidemic of cattle plague, rinderpest, which had been introduced via Hull into the South of England, soon swept north, consuming the time and efforts of the staff at the Clyde Street College. The 1865–6 Session was the last one taught by William Dick (Macdonald, Warwick and Johnston 2005). He was sent to London by the Highland Society to investigate the course of the disease, and subsequently was appointed by the Government as the Inspector of Foreign Cattle for Midlothian. However, despite his extensive clinical experience, it was his lack of understanding of the nature of infectious disease which no longer fitted him for this task. He had also been putting on weight and was having occasional breathless episodes (Macdonald and Warwick 2019). For much of March 1866 he was confined to the house with pains in his chest and difficulty with his breathing. The stress to him caused by the cattle epidemic and a heart problem were together too much. He died on 4 April 1866 (Anonymous 1866a, b). The doctor said that his dropsical symptoms and ascites (oedema) were due to heart failure. He was buried in the family plot in New Calton Cemetery, about a hundred metres from his birthplace (Bradley 1923; Macdonald and Warwick 2019).

As well as establishing, largely with his own funds, the first veterinary college in Scotland, lecturing and running an extensive practice, William Dick had been editor of *The Veterinarian* for twelve years and frequently wrote papers on clinical subjects (Pringle 1869). He was also public-spirited and well-connected to the Edinburgh political establishment (Jacyna 1994). For fifteen years he was Honorary Treasurer of the Royal Physical Society. He was also Justice of the Peace, Moderator of the High Constables, Dean of Guild, Deacon of the Hammermen Guild and Deacon-convenor of Trades, which entitled him to sit on the Town Council (Bradley 1923). In his will he left his estate in trust, the interest to be used to maintain his college; the Lord Provost, Magistrates and Council of the City of Edinburgh were appointed as Trustees (Bradley 1923).

William was survived by his elder sister, Mary Dick (1791–1883), who never ceased to take a lively interest in the welfare of the College (Figure 4.3). She had never married, but looked after her parents and her short-lived brother, John (Macdonald and Warwick 2019). Thomas Dollar, a former student and old family friend, wrote that she concerned herself with everything that went on within the college walls, took the greatest interest in the welfare of every student. Her anxiety for the real good of her protégées made her kindly and helpful when they were in sickness or trouble (Dollar 1894). Following the death of William, Mary moved immediately from 8 Clyde Street to her house on Craigkennockie Terrace, Burntisland, Fife and thereafter resided there. William Worthington, William Dick's long-time clinical assistant, retired in 1867. He moved from his small house in the north-east corner of the Clyde Street courtyard to his newly built house, also on Craigkennockie Terrace, to continue as a neighbour of his old friend (Macdonald et al 2022).

James Herbert Brockencote Hallen appointed Principal

Following the transfer of the College to its Trustees, James Herbert Brockencote Hallen (1829–1901) (Figure 4.4), formerly Principal Veterinary Surgeon to Her Majesty's Bombay Army, was appointed by the Lord Provost and Magistrates of Edinburgh to be Principal of the

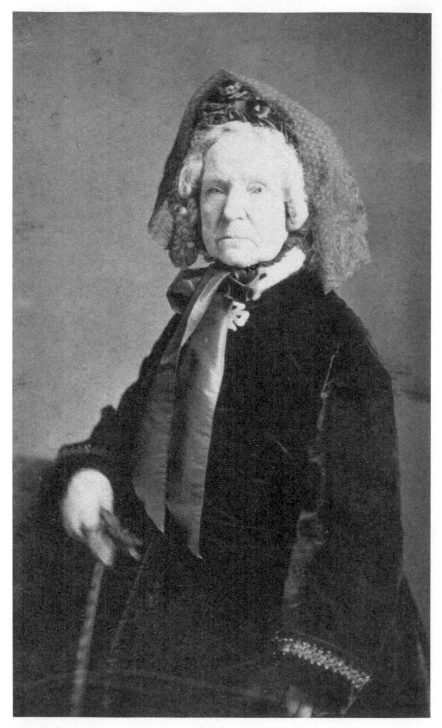

Figure 4.3 Carte de visite of Mary Dick. Photographer: Alexander Asher.

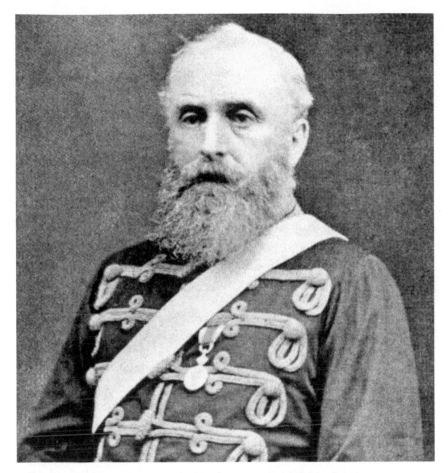

Figure 4.4 Photograph of James Herbert Brockencote Hallen in uniform. Photographer: unknown. Public domain <https://commons.wikimedia.org/wiki/File:JHB_Hallen.jpg>

Edinburgh Veterinary College for the 1866–7 Session (Bradley 1923). Hallen brought a fine military and administrative mind to the College. He introduced innovation at the Diploma examinations; students were required to examine four horses not previously seen, write a diagnostic report on them and identify their ailments. This was the first example of practical skills in clinical examination being tested in a British veterinary college (Anonymous 1879a) and it acted as a stimulus for practical tuition. Hallen taught Histopathology, and together with William Worthington gave Clinical Instruction. His staff included Thomas Strangeways teaching both Anatomy and Cattle Pathology, Peter Young teaching Physiology and Allan Dalzell teaching both Chemistry and Veterinary Materia Medica (Anonymous 1866c).

It was with regret that Hallen had to be urgently recalled to his military duties in India to investigate an outbreak of Indian cattle plague, subsequently also identified as rinderpest (Bradley 1923; Scott 2000). However, his short time in Clyde Street did enable him to list a number of recommendations for the Trustees and the Highland Society (Hallen 1867). These included:

1. Examine students prior to matriculation.
2. Students should attend an additional three months of lectures on chemistry.
3. Veterinary students should have knowledge of the sciences of botany and agriculture, lectures on which to be timed during a summer session.
4. Lectures on pathological anatomy, not hitherto considered in the curriculum of study in any British veterinary college, should be introduced.
5. A chair of Cattle Pathology should be endowed.
6. Students should attend at least three winter sessions and one or two summer sessions.
7. The hospital accommodation for sick and lame animals is currently very insufficient in the college. The available stabling is not well adapted for sick horses – and as a consequence they are seldom seen in them. There is currently no hospital accommodation for sick cattle and dogs. These are required so that students can see disease in its various phases.
8. The absence of an operating theatre means that operations are carried out in the open yard and only those students close to the patients operated on can learn or see how an operation is performed.
9. The dissection room is now too small for the number of students. It should be at least twice as large as at present and be better lighted.

In 1867 the Lord Provost, William Chambers, published a detailed description of the veterinary college property which had been entrusted to the City (Chambers 1867):

> The buildings are disposed in the form of a quadrangle, with an open court in the centre, and having a dwelling house in front which formed the residence of Mr Dick . . . The buildings around the courtyard appear to have been erected or acquired at different times, and pieced together with interior connections in the best way possible, . . . The buildings are on a slope, and accordingly at various levels. Some parts are reached from the court-yard by outside stairs. The northern or lower range of building contains the old and well-known Clyde Street Hall, which is now employed for the annual examinations, the interior being decorated with a good portrait of Mr Dick . . . (Plate 4.1)
> The museum is so small as to be insufficient for the proper exhibition of anatomical and pathological specimens, a matter greatly to be regretted; for

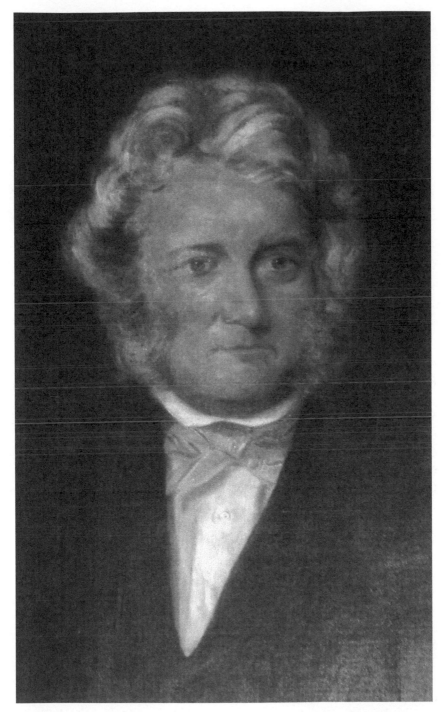

Plate 4.1 Painting of William Dick by Tavernor Knott dated 1851. Photographer: Colin M. Warwick.

a number of the specimens, illustrative of the diseases of horses and other animals, are in excellent condition, and full of interest. The Class or Lecture Room is also, I should imagine, inconveniently small. The infirmary for horses, which ought to be a leading feature in the establishment, consists of some dingy and ill-ventilated loose-boxes, entered by different doorways; whereas the loose-boxes should be well-lighted, airy, and cheerful, with all suitable accommodation as regards water etc. I believe there is no Infirmary for Dogs, or other small animals, needing temporary treatment. The premises do not allow of the proper arrangements for a thorough examination of horses. Ordinary investigation and operations seem to go on in the open court-yard, within view of the street, which is generally complained of. The dissecting Room is over the Forge, so that the heat of the fires, and the effluvia from singeing, aggravate the unpleasant odour from the dissecting operations; this Dissecting Room should be improved in ventilation as soon as possible. A larger and more comfortable Reading and Lounging Room is required for the Students. The central quadrangle [which is approached by an arched gateway in front] is on a slope, and open; whereas it should be level, and covered with a spacious glass roof, to allow of horses being walked about and exercised in all weathers.

. . . One small portion of the quadrangular block, consisting of a workshop, at the north-west exterior angle, and facing a lane from St Andrew's Street, does not belong to Mr Dick's property . . .

Chambers felt that there was the possibility of transferring the College from Clyde Street to new buildings. These could be erected on a quadrangular piece of ground, 250 by 150 feet (76.2 m x 45.7 m), between College Wynd and Horse Wynd, which fronted onto North College Street, soon to be renamed Chambers Street, opposite the University. However, the college staff at that time did not have the necessary leadership driving force to act rapidly enough, and Edinburgh University bought the land instead (Macdonald, Lad, Hunzinger and Warwick 2023).

William Williams appointed Principal

In June 1867 William Williams (1832–1900), who had been one of William Dick's star students, was appointed as Principal. He had enrolled at the Clyde Street College in 1855 and after two years' study obtained both a Diploma and the first Highland and Agricultural Society's Gold Medal for proficiency in Veterinary Science (Warwick and Macdonald 2003). Williams concurred with the Lord Provost's views that improvements needed to be made, not only to the college buildings, but also in the pre-college education of the veterinary students. An increase in the time students spent studying veterinary medicine was also required. These opinions were further discussed at the National Veterinary Congress held in London in May 1867. George Armitage, from the Glasgow Veterinary College, had proposed there should be preliminary examinations, a longer course to permit both practical and theoretical instruction and an examination that included both written as well as verbal components. This stimulated considerable debate on the topic within the profession (Armitage 1867). It also coincided with discussions within the Senatus of the University of Edinburgh. Consideration was being given to a scheme for granting degrees in veterinary science which could have brought the Veterinary College into 'direct educational communion with the University'. However, the failure in 1868 of a second attempt to obtain a veterinary charter for Scotland, co-promoted by the Town Council of Edinburgh and the Highland Society, contributed to the demise of this initiative (Anonymous 1879b).

Williams held the post of Principal at the Clyde Street College until July 1873. However, during that period there were a number of problems, the factors underlying which can now only be surmised. Two of these may be identifiable: the death in 1867 of Williams's first wife, Charlotte Owens; and the culture changes resulting from the new staff and management at the Veterinary College, from a brother and sister 'family-run' private business to one managed by a group of Trustees in the form of the Lord Provost, Magistrates and Council of the City of Edinburgh (Warwick and Macdonald 2003). In 1868, 1870 and 1873 a series of comprehensively reported disagreements took place, among the staff members of the College, between the clerk to the Trustees and Mary Dick (William Dick's redoubtable sister retained, under the terms of his will, a large say in the finances of the College), and between Principal Williams and some of the Trustees (Smith 1981; Warwick and Macdonald 2003). As a consequence of this apparently never-ending train of events, which also involved student unrest and significant legal and other costs, the majority of Trustees perceived that the underlying reason for these troubles was Williams's inability to adequately control his staff. There were also indications that Williams was unhappy with the job he had because of his inability to run the Veterinary College exactly as he wanted (Bradley 1923). On 16 July 1873 it was finally agreed that he would be asked to resign for 'want of harmony between the Principal and professors' (Warwick and Macdonald 2003). The way that the decision was reached and delivered to him had a large and negative impact on Williams. This substantial hurt was reflected in public speeches he made throughout the remaining twenty-seven years of his life (Warwick and Macdonald 2003). However, William Williams did not give up. Instead, he followed the example set during his student days, when his former anatomy teacher in Clyde Street, John Gamgee, departed in 1857 to establish the first Edinburgh New Veterinary College

(Bradley 1923; Hall 1965). In 1873 Williams took with him from the Clyde Street College most of the clinical material and more than forty of the students he had been teaching (Warwick and Macdonald 2003).

William Fearnley appointed Principal

William Fearnley (1843–1927) from Leeds was appointed Principal in Williams's place in 1873 (Bradley 1923). However, the lack of students, teaching material and farriery equipment that Fearnley found when he took up the job at Clyde Street made his task very difficult. In addition, his handling of the students who comprised the membership of the Edinburgh Veterinary Medical Society was incorrect (Macdonald, Johnston and Warwick 2022). The students' Society owned the books in the library. As the majority of the students had moved to Williams's New Veterinary College in Gayfield House, they requested that the books go there too. Fearnley and the Trustees refused to comply. After a legal battle, the students succeeded and took with them the whole library of 374 published items, eighteen titles listed as 'Text Books' and six others listed as 'various books' (Macdonald, Johnston and Warwick 2022).

The state of disorganised college affairs, coupled with the ongoing interference and lack of support from the Trustees during the 1873–4 Session, resulted in Fearnley's abrupt resignation, less than a year after taking up office (Anonymous 1874b). He had been unable to cope with the material, financial, political and administrative chaos left by Williams's departure. Fearnley remained in Edinburgh for a short time. He enrolled to study medicine at the Royal College of Surgeons of Edinburgh and, after graduating in 1875 as a licentiate of that college, went south to become a general medical practitioner in London. Ironically, in October 1873 a significant number of structural improvements had been recommended to be made to the Clyde Street College. However, these were not carried out until the 1874–5 Session (Macdonald et al. 2022).

References

Anonymous, 1864a. Alarming fire at Edinburgh Veterinary College. *North British Agriculturist*, 16, 104.

Anonymous, 1864b. Fire at the Edinburgh Veterinary College. *The Veterinarian*, 37, 195–6.

Anonymous, 1866a. Death of Professor Dick. *North British Agriculturist*, 18, 228.

Anonymous, 1866b. Obituary. *The Veterinarian*, 39, 439–40.

Anonymous, 1866c. Edinburgh Veterinary College [advert]. *The Scotsman*, 15 September 1866, p. 4, col. 3.

Anonymous, 1874a. [*Veterinary Medical Association history.*] Sederunt Books, Professor Dick's Trust Petition, 2, 713–15.

Anonymous, 1874b. Edinburgh Veterinary College – Resignation of Principal Fearnley. *The Veterinarian*, 47, 557.

Anonymous, 1879a. Historical account of the Veterinary Department of the Highland and Agricultural Society. *Transactions of the Highland and Agricultural Society of Scotland*, Fourth Series 4, 11, 160–8.

Anonymous, 1879b. Appendix No. 3. – Proceedings relative to a Veterinary Charter for Scotland. In Historical account of the Veterinary Department of the Highland and Agricultural Society, *Transactions of the Highland and Agricultural Society of Scotland*, Series 4, 11, 182–9.

Armitage, G. 1867. The education of the veterinary surgeon; The importance of the apprenticeship clause; the preliminary examination, and a lengthened period of matriculation at college. *The Veterinarian*, 40, 505–14.

Bradley, O. C. 1923. *History of the Edinburgh Veterinary College*. Edinburgh: Oliver and Boyd, 68–70.

[Chambers, W.] 1867. *Some observations on the Edinburgh Veterinary College by the Lord Provost*. Edinburgh: Neill and Company, 1–16.

Dick, W. 1863. Inaugural address, 1863. The appendix in [William Chambers's] *Some observations on the Edinburgh Veterinary College by the Lord Provost* (Edinburgh, 1867).

Dick, W. 1869. Proceedings in the Edinburgh Veterinary College. In *Occasional papers on veterinary subjects; with a memoir by R. O. Pringle*. Edinburgh: William Blackwood and Sons, 442–501.

Dixon, H. H. 1870. *Saddle and Sirloin, or English Farm and Sporting Worthies*. London: Rogerson & Tuxford.

Dollar, T. A. 1894. *Inaugural address delivered by Thomas A. Dollar, M.R.C.V.S. at the opening of the 72nd session of Royal (Dick) Veterinary College Edinburgh, 3rd October 1894. Presentation to the trustees of Miss Dick's Portrait and report of the banquet given to the Lord Provost, Magistrates, and Town Council, and leading members of the medical and veterinary professions*. Edinburgh: Turnbull and Spears.

Gamgee, J. 1858. Monopoly incompatible with progress. *Edinburgh Veterinary Review and Annals of Comparative Pathology*, 1, 188–90.

Gamgee, J. 1860. Rival examining boards. *Edinburgh Veterinary Review and Annals of Comparative Pathology*, 2, 164–6.

Gamgee, J. 1864. Preliminary examinations. *Edinburgh Veterinary Review and Annals of Comparative Pathology*, 6, 731–2.

Hall, S. A. 1965. John Gamgee and the Edinburgh New Veterinary College. *Veterinary Record*, 77, 1237–41.

Hallen, J. H. B. 1867. [*Letter and suggestions from J. H. B. Hallen*], Minutes of [the] meeting of the sub-committee of the Lord Provost's committee in charge of the management of Professor Dick's Trust, . . . 13th November 1867. Sederunt Books, Professor Dick's Trust, 3 vols (1866–77) 1, 248–52, Edinburgh City Archives, Handlist of Historical Records.

Jacyna, L. S. 1994. *Philosophic Whigs. Medicine, Science and Citizenship in Edinburgh, 1789–1848*. London and New York: Routledge.

Macdonald, A. A., Johnston, W. T. and Warwick, C. 2022. The Edinburgh Veterinary Medical Society's library. *Veterinary History*, 21 (2), 168–93.

Macdonald, A. A., Lad, K., Hunzinger, V. and Warwick, C. 2023. The Edinburgh Veterinary College 1866–1886. *Veterinary History* (in press).

Macdonald, A. A. and Warwick, C. 2019. A wee blether with Mary Dick. *Veterinary History*, 19 (4), 341–69. <era.ed.ac.uk/handle/1842/38663> (accessed 9 September 2022).

Macdonald, A. A., Warwick, C. and Johnston, W. T. 2005. Locating veterinary education in Edinburgh in the nineteenth century. *The Book of the Old Edinburgh Club*, New Series, 6, 41–71. <era.ed.ac.uk/handle/1842/2199> (accessed 11 September 2022).

McLagan, P. 1863. Report to the General Meeting 24th June 1863. *Highland and Agricultural Society of Scotland*, 24, 53.

Pringle, R. O. 1869. Memoir. In W. Dick, *Occasional papers on veterinary subjects; with a Memoir by R.O. Pringle*. Edinburgh: William Blackwood and Sons, i–xci.

Scott, G. R. 2000. The Murrain now known as 'Rinderpest'. *Newsletter of the Tropical Agriculture Association, UK*, 20 (4), 14–16.

Smith, R. N. 1981. Dr J. A. McBride, MRCVS 1843? – 1889 itinerant professor extraordinary. *Veterinary History*, NS 2 (1), 3–25.

Warwick, C. and Macdonald, A. A. 2003. The New Veterinary College, Edinburgh, 1873–1904. *The Veterinary Record*, 153, 380–6. <era.ed.ac.uk/handle/1842/2198> (accessed 9 September 2022).

Weipers, W. L. 1976. The development of veterinary education in the west of Scotland. *Veterinary History*, 7, 9–19.

Note: Despite detailed and exhaustive searches by O. Charnock Bradley in 1922–3 and T. James, C. M. Warwick and A. A. Macdonald in 2006–7 and 2014–15, no photographs of William Fearnley have been found.

Chapter 5

William Williams's New Veterinary College (1873–1904)

Gayfield House (1873–83)

William Williams (Figure 5.1) established his New Veterinary College in 1873, 'at the request of numerous students of veterinary science, veterinary surgeons and agriculturists' (Anonymous 1873), in Gayfield House, a large villa on East London Street, at the east end of Edinburgh's New Town (Figure 5.2). The house had been built by Charles and William Butter between 1761 and 1765, before the New Town of Edinburgh was planned (Warwick and Macdonald 2005). The property comprised a five-roomed basement, two storeys of four rooms each (Figure 5.3) and a two-roomed attic. There was a separate, single-storey office block in the garden comprising six rooms. In addition, across the road, there was a coach house and stables with a hayloft. No evidence was found that Williams purchased the property (Warwick and Macdonald 2005).

On 1 and 3 October 1873, the following announcement, dated Edinburgh, 29 September 1873, was inserted in *The Scotsman* newspaper:

> NEW VETERINARY COLLEGE EDINBURGH,
> Professor Williams begs to intimate that he has
> REMOVED his PRACTICE to the NEW VETERINARY
> COLLEGE, Gayfield House, East London Street, where he
> may be consulted.
> The SHOEING DEPARTMENT is at present carried on at the
> West End of Rose Street, adjoining the Tontine Stables

Originally designed for family life, the adaptation of Gayfield House for use as a college, particularly for animal dissection and the reception

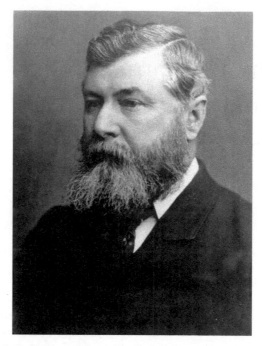

Figure 5.1 Professor William Williams. From O. Charnock Bradley, *Edinburgh Veterinary College*, 1923.

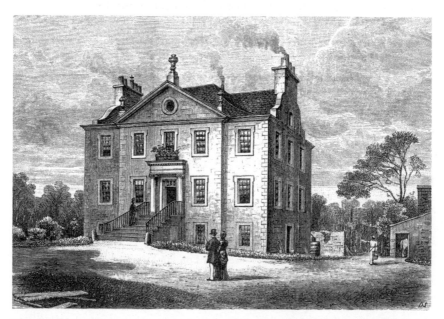

Figure 5.2 Gayfield House viewed from the south. The single-storey outside office block can be seen in the garden to the right of the house. Illustration from Grant, J. 1880–3. *Cassell's Old and New Edinburgh*. London: Cassell & Co.

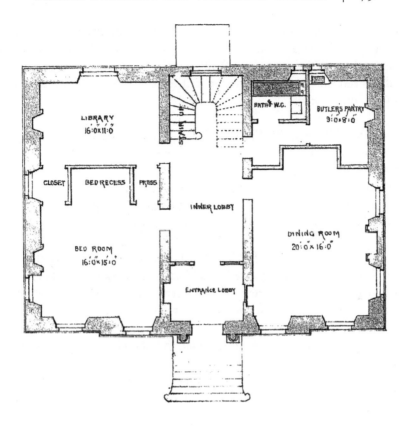

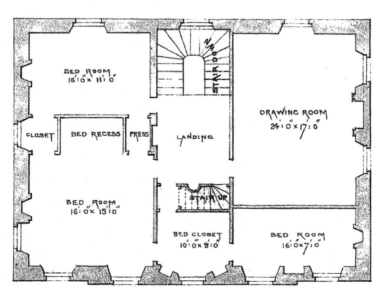

Figure 5.3 Plans of the ground floor and first floor of Gayfield House. Illustration from Blanc, 1870.

of clinical material, must have been difficult. Nevertheless, the New Veterinary College was formally opened on Wednesday, 22 October 1873 (Anonymous 1873). It remained Williams's home of veterinary education in Edinburgh for the next ten years. In the same advert the members of staff were announced:

Prof. W. Williams, FRSE, MRCVS	Veterinary Medicine & Surgery
Prof. Melville, FRPhSE	Physiology
Prof. I. Vaughan, MRCVS	Anatomy
Dr Stevenson Macadam, FRSE	Chemistry
Mr A. Balfour, MRCVS	Practical Pharmacy
Mr T. J. Simpson	Secretary

Following the death of Melville, Peter Young transferred from Clyde Street to Gayfield House in 1875 to teach Physiology there. This signalled the start of a pattern of long-term stability among the teaching staff. At the opening of the 1875 Session, Williams listed the men trained by William Dick or himself in Edinburgh who were now professors in the veterinary colleges of Canada and the United States, such as James Law, Andrew Smith and Duncan McNab McEachran, or who held high positions in India and Australia. He also noted that all but one of the veterinary textbooks published in the last twenty years had been written by Edinburgh graduates (Williams 1875). The two veterinary colleges, situated less than two hundred metres from one another, settled down to attract and train veterinary students in an atmosphere of constructive and friendly rivalry. Both Principals were aware of the changes they needed to introduce to improve the educational levels of the students they enrolled and the training they subsequently received. It was commented upon by Williams in 1876 that 'there has never been one word of discord between any professors nor has there been any unpleasantness among the students themselves or between them and their teachers' (Williams 1876).

In 1881 Anatomy teaching was transferred from I. Vaughan to T. H. Lewis, who remained until 1891, to be followed by D. C. Longden and then from 1894 to 1900 by O. Charnock Bradley. In 1882 the Physiology post passed to James Hunter, who remained with the College until it closed in 1904. Chemistry was taught by Stevenson Macadam from 1873 to 1884, and his son, W. Ivison Macadam, from 1885 until his early death in 1902. Daniel McAlpine taught Natural History and Botany from 1879 until his departure for Australia in 1884, when he was succeeded for the following six years by Archibald N. McAlpine. Williams's eldest son, William Owen Williams (1860–1911), completed the veterinary course in

April 1881, and after a study period in Alfort, returned to work first as his father's assistant and then to teach in his own right in 1886 (Warwick and Macdonald 2005).

The news in 1873 of the requested resignation of Principal Williams from the Clyde Street College was received 'with great surprise' by the students, and twenty-seven of them unanimously passed a vote of confidence in him (Faulkner 1873). Many of these students subsequently followed Williams to Gayfield House. However, a number of students took fright at the prospect of losing a session of study and transferred from Edinburgh to study elsewhere. It was not clear to them that Williams would obtain the necessary authority for them to sit the examinations set by the Royal College of Veterinary Surgeons (Williams 1874). Nevertheless, sixty-one students attended during the year 1873–4 (Lewis 1882). Moreover, at the opening of the new Session in 1874, Captain Tod reported that forty-six students from Gayfield House had taken the examinations before the Highland and Agricultural Society of Scotland in April that year (Williams 1874). The numbers of students attending grew each year. In order to maintain this increase in student numbers, Williams chose not to alter student fees in 1876, when the length of the course was increased from two to three years (Williams 1876). At the prize-giving ceremony in 1882, Williams declared that his classes had grown to such a degree (145 students on the roll) that larger and more suitable premises were required (Williams 1882). Student numbers had reached 154 by the 1882–3 Session (Williams 1883a).

During the ten years at Gayfield House, student esteem for Williams the teacher was manifest in a number of ways, of which the following is a good example. At the prize-giving in April 1878 the students presented a large photograph of those attending the 1877–8 Session to the Principal (Anonymous 1878). At the same meeting, and on behalf of members of the veterinary profession, General Fizwygram, President of the RCVS, presented to Principal Williams a full-sized head portrait of himself by J. M. Barclay, RSA. Although the current whereabouts of these gifts is unknown, a photograph taken by Patrick of staff and students about 1883 has been found (Figure 5.4). The one student in the group that can be identified is William Gilholm Berry, at the bottom of the stairs in a bowler hat (Hawryluk 2003).

Until 1987 Gayfield House retained four signatures scratched onto several glass windowpanes. These were: 'Professor W. Williams'; 'W.O Williams, Esq., M.R.C.V.S., The New Veterinary College, Edinburgh'; 'John Young, Cockermouth, Cumberland, 1883' and 'J.W. Bennett, Leigh, Lancashire'. These panes were removed for safekeeping, and sadly have not yet been traced.

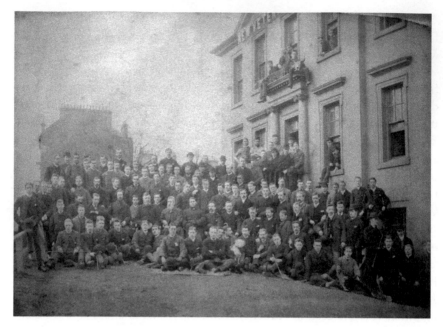

Figure 5.4 Photograph taken c. 1883 of Gayfield House with Williams, his staff and students. Photographer: J. Patrick. Courtesy of Mrs Daisy Hawryluk.

41 Elm Row (1883–1904)

On 24 October 1883, 300 metres to the east of Gayfield House, a custom-built Veterinary College (Figure 5.5), designed by Hamilton Beattie, was officially opened on Elm Row, Leith Walk (Anonymous 1883). Williams indicated that the chief aim of the design of the building was:

> to secure accommodation not only for the students, but to enable us to demonstrate clinically our treatment of disease, and to show the higher value we attach to physiological principles and sanitary measures than to mere medical remedies, and also to give facilities for the scientific investigation both of healthy and diseased structures and processes; in fact, we aspire not only to encourage a desire for research in our students, but also, as is the case in continental laboratories, to give facilities to those members of the profession who have already been engaged in its arduous toils and duties, and who may wish to improve their knowledge, and perhaps to unravel, with the assistance of scientific applications, some mysterious problems which may have repeatedly arisen in the course of their ordinary practice. (Williams 1883b)

The new buildings were described in the local press (*Edinburgh Courant* 1883; *The Scotsman* 1883):

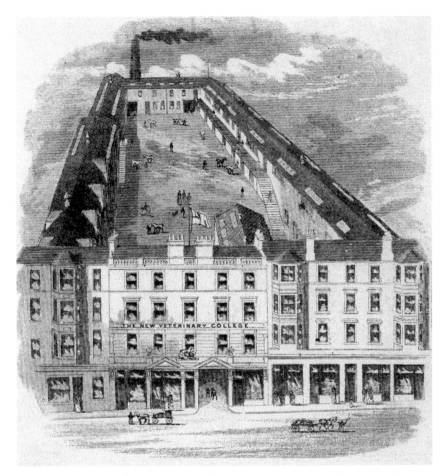

Figure 5.5 Bird's-eye view of the New Veterinary College, built in 1882–3 at 41 Elm Row, Leith Walk, Edinburgh, seen from the north-west. Illustration from the *New Veterinary College Prospectus 1903–04*.

extend about 80 yards backwards from Leith Walk, and, speaking roughly, cover four sides of a square, to the height of two storeys, leaving a large open space in the centre [Figure 5.6]. This open space or yard is covered with [lithite] concrete cement, with the exception of the central portion of its entire length, which has been causewayed, so as to give a length of fifty yards of 'trotting stone' as it is called – a stone course upon which horses are trotted to test their soundness. The elevation of the building towards Leith Walk presents a bold and massive yet ornamental appearance – a frontage [of polished ashlar] in which boldly-pedimented windows are a feature, being surmounted by a handsome stone balustrade [Figure 5.5].

On the street floor, the pier heads are decorated with carved representations of various animals. The upper flats of this block are to be occupied partly by resident professors, and partly as students' boarding-houses.

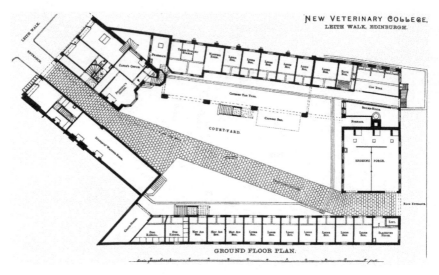

Figure 5.6 Ground-floor plan of the New Veterinary College, Edinburgh. Illustration from the *New Veterinary College Prospectus 1903–04*.

In connection with the College, a restaurant, with a saloon at back, and having an entrance from Leith Walk, has been provided for the students.

Entering by [the] principal doorway – (there is another doorway at the opposite end of the yard, opening on Windsor Street) we have immediately to the left on the ground floor the Principal's office [with a bow window, commanding a view of the courtyard] and consulting room, with the College offices adjoining, and the pharmacy next, farther on [Figure 5.6]. Making up the remainder of the northern line of the buildings are a six-stalled stable with saddle-room, six horse-boxes (including an extra large one for any particularly violent animal), and a six-stalled cow house; while a covered shed, laid with bark, and intended for the exercise of horses, extends along the greater part of the front of these boxes and stalls.

A concrete bath for animals, with shower and spray apparatus, and an inclined entrance were constructed in the courtyard on the north side. Horses could have a hot or a cold bath there according to the nature of their ailments.

A large boiler house occupied most of the floor level of the eastern block. This heated the whole building by means of hot-water pipes, with the radiators extending to some of the horseboxes, where the temperature could be raised as high as 21 degrees Centigrade. Beside and to the south of the boiler house was the shoeing forge, fitted with three forges 'of the most modern construction'. The boiler house was large enough to accommodate ten horses for shoeing at any one time.

The post-mortem room was situated at the east end of the southern line of buildings. Animals could be elevated from there by a hoist to the dis-

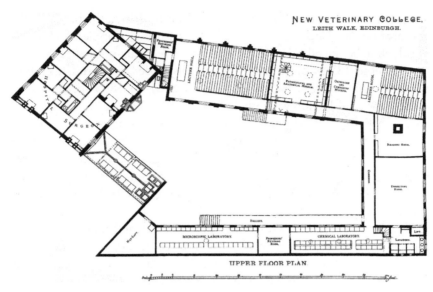

Figure 5.7 Upper-floor plan of the New Veterinary College, Edinburgh. Illustration from the *New Veterinary College Prospectus 1903–04*.

secting room above, and by means of small overhead carriages with chains, running on rails attached to the roof, could be moved from one part of the room to another as required. Beside the post-mortem room were ten horse-boxes, boxes to accommodate about a score of dogs, and a coach house.

The upper storey was reached by two flights of steps, one on each side of the yard. These led to an open balcony which ran round three sides of the square (Figure 5.7). On the northern side there was a large lecture hall, with tiers of seats for 192 students. Beside this was the College museum, around which ran an interior gallery. There was also a public museum or 'bone room' for the students, and a smaller lecture hall which seated 125 (Anonymous 1893). Fitted to the walls of the museum were glass cases containing

> numerous and rare specimens of animals both in the diseased and healthy conditions, there being a large and varied collection preserved in spirits. There are specimens of dissected parts of animals, wax and papier maché models, monstrosities, anatomical collections and specimens illustrating various diseases of the bones, a collection of teeth, etc. On the ground floor in the centre, are numerous complete skeletons of animals, and in one of the glass cases are skeletons of a man and of a monkey. Other cases contain grasses and feeding stuffs, drugs, English and foreign horse-shoes, etc. (Anonymous 1893)

The students' reading room and library were located on the upper level at the eastern end of the courtyard (Figure 5.7). Disastrously, not very long after the move from Gayfield House to Elm Row, a fire broke out in this area during a fierce storm on 26 January 1884, completely destroying the fine book collection of the Edinburgh Veterinary Medical Society (Anonymous 1884a, b, c). Following appeals made by the students to the profession for replacement books (Purdy 1884), in 1885 the library of John Greaves of Flixton was donated to the New College and formed the core of a new library (Robinson 1885). The dissecting room completed the east wing. The chemical laboratory was situated in the western block adjacent to a professors' 'retiring-room'. The pathological and histological laboratories were then further to the west. An open-air laboratory was sited on the roof, 'where chemical experiments giving forth bad odours may be conducted'.

On the wall to the left of the wide main entrance on Elm Row was sited a pedestal upon which was placed a sculptured group, two metres high, consisting of a horse, bull and dog carvings, attributed to John Rhind (Figures 5.5 and 5.8). The logo on the front of the prospectuses for sessions 1895–6 and 1903–4 (Prospectus 1895, 1903) show the group more clearly (Figure 5.9). The logo was printed on the certificates issued by the Edinburgh Veterinary Medical Society to William G. Burndred in 1900. The currently available evidence suggests that these animal sculptures

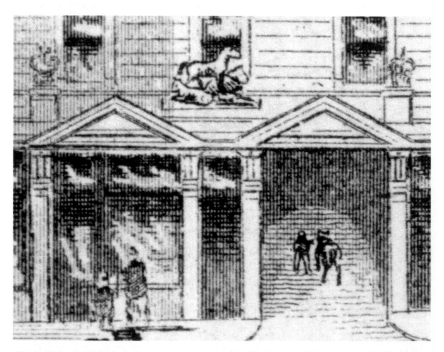

Figure 5.8 Detail from Figure 5.5 showing the appearance of the horse, bull and dog in the etching. From the *New Veterinary College Prospectus 1903–04*.

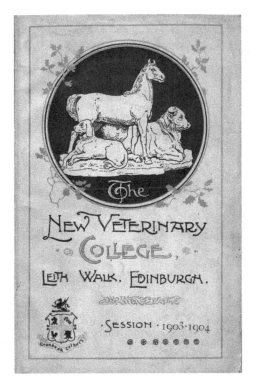

Figure 5.9 The front cover of the prospectus of the New Veterinary College, Edinburgh, for its final year, 1903–4.

disappeared from sight after the building ceased to be used as a Veterinary College. However, the statue of the dog from the Elm Row façade was rediscovered in the garden of a private house in the Scottish Borders countryside (Figure 5.10). It is of a recumbent hound, attractively carved from sandstone, and measures approximately 100 cm long and 75 cm high. In its present location it sits on a red-sandstone plinth. The back of the sculpture has an unfinished appearance, which helped confirm its authenticity. Other recent research has suggested a rather different, and perhaps more convoluted, path had been taken by the sculpted horse (Macdonald, Forrest and Warwick 2021). Most recently, in 1914 and 1919, a very similarly posed equine statue was photographed above the frontage of the Royal Riding Academy at 8 Home Street, Tollcross, Edinburgh. Since then, the trail of that sculpture has gone cold. However, the provenance and present whereabouts of the sculpted bull are the topics of ongoing investigations.

The number of students that attended the Elm Row College during the 1883–4 Session was 164. As had been the custom at Gayfield House, they showed their appreciation to the Principal by presenting, in 1884, a

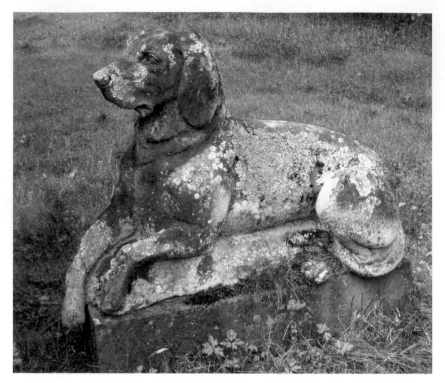

Figure 5.10 Carving of the dog by John Rhind, which formerly formed part of the sculpted group including a horse and a bull on the front of the New Veterinary College, Edinburgh. Photographer: Colin M. Warwick.

clock and illuminated address (Warwick and Macdonald 2005). The clock donated by the students of the 1883–4 Session was installed in the college yard on the east wall opposite the main entry. It was shown in a photograph of students and staff (Figure 5.11) taken at 2.51 pm on 20 April 1893. The number of students increased to 196 by 1887 and to nearly two hundred the following year (Williams 1887, 1888). In 1890–1 there appeared to be about 180 students, and two years later, the figure of 190 on the roll included agriculture as well as veterinary students (Williams 1891, 1893). Two reasons were repeatedly blamed for the drop in recruits; the more demanding 'prelim' (entrance) exams in 1892 and the simultaneous start of the more costly four-year course (Williams 1898, 1899, 1900). The opening of the Veterinary College in Dublin was also alleged to have further reduced the student intake to the two veterinary colleges in Edinburgh (Anonymous 1900a; Shennan 1900).

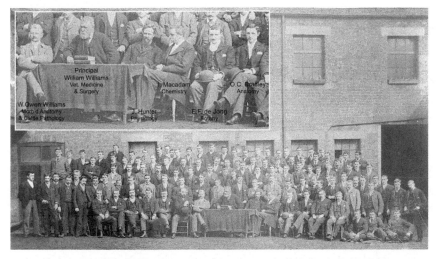

Figure 5.11 Photograph taken in 1893 of students and staff at the New Veterinary College, Edinburgh. Insert: enlargement to show the members of staff present. Photographer: unknown. Photo S2957/1 by courtesy of the University of Liverpool library.

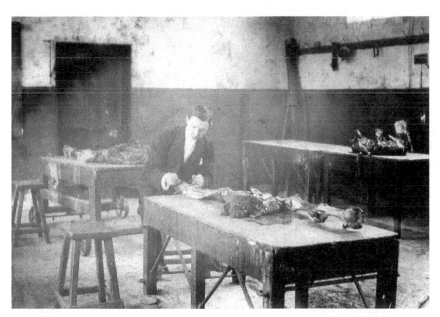

Figure 5.12 O. Charnock Bradley in the Anatomy Dissection Room, New Veterinary College, Edinburgh, c. 1892. Photographer: unknown. Photo courtesy of Frances and Jon Harrison, Rhydymwyn, Wales.

Two significant students: O. C. Bradley and A. I. Cust

Within this time period, two students merit particular attention. Orlando Charnock Bradley matriculated in 1889. He had been such an exceptional and ambitious student that Williams, in the spring of 1892, had enlisted him onto his teaching staff (Figures 5.11 and 5.12) while he was still a student (Warwick and Macdonald 2010). As well as being appointed Lecturer in Comparative Anatomy in 1894, Bradley taught Meat Inspection and supervised the Clinical Hospital. His days as a young anatomy demonstrator in 1892–3 were recalled by one of his students, R. Craig Robinson: 'From the first, Mr Bradley as he then was, gained the confidence and respect of the new students of that session' (Robinson 1937). On 22 October 1895, Bradley registered as a medical student and matriculated at the University of Edinburgh. This may have been because he was young (twenty-four), very bright and keen to learn more from the academic environment of Edinburgh which surrounded him. The medical degree would certainly have given him access to more rapid advancement, better access to the prominent research staff in Edinburgh University, and very likely a better status within the Edinburgh academic community. On 30 June 1900 he passed his medical 'finals' with distinction ('much to my surprise') and graduated MBChB on 28 July 1900 (Warwick and Macdonald 2010).

The list of staff and the subjects that were taught in the college during the 1895–6 Session are shown in Table 5.1 (Prospectus 1895). The four years' scheme of veterinary professional education came into force after 7 April 1895. The fee for the first Session, including a 1 guinea Matriculation Fee, was £18 18s. The fee for the second Session was £15 15s. The fee for the third Session was £13 13s. And for the fourth Session £10 10s. Amateur students could purchase single tickets for the Winter Session: Veterinary Medicine and Surgery, with Clinical Instruction £7 7s.; Anatomy £4 4s.; Physiology £4 4s.; Chemistry £4 4s.; Analytical Chemistry £2 per month, or £5 for three months; Natural History £3 3s. Senior veterinary students were appointed in rotation as 'Dressers', 'Dispensers' and 'Visitors', and (under the supervision of the Principal and staff) were required to medically attend all patients in the Infirmary. Horses, cows, sheep and pigs were kept at the College for the practical instruction of the students. Senior students also had the privilege of visiting, with the Principal and other members of staff, the cases in the city and neighbourhood occurring in the College veterinary practice and in branch veterinary practices.

Among the veterinary student intake that Charnock Bradley tutored was the first woman student, Aleen Isobel Cust (1868–1937) (Figure 5.13).

Table 5.1 Staff and courses taught at the New Edinburgh Veterinary College, Leith Walk, Edinburgh, during Session 1895–6.

Staff of Professors	Subjects Taught
Professor W. Williams	Veterinary Medicine and Surgery
Professor James Hunter	Physiology and Practical Histology
Professor O. Charnock Bradley	Anatomy of the Domesticated Animals
Professor W. Owen Williams	Diseases of the Ox, Sheep, Pig and Dog
Professor Ivison MacAdam	Chemistry, Practical Chemistry
Professor W. R. Davis	Materia Medica, Therapeutics, and Toxicology
Professor R. S. MacDougall	Botany
Professor W. Owen Williams	Morbid Anatomy
Professor O. Charnock Bradley	Bacteriology
Professor R. S. MacDougall	Parasites of the Domestic Animals
	Junior Anatomy
Members of the Veterinary Staff	Stable Management
Professor W. R. Davis	Practical Pharmacy
Professor R. S. MacDougall	Natural History, Zoology, Ornithology, & Mammalogy
Professor W. Owen Williams	Gynaecology
Members of the Veterinary Staff	Clinical Instruction
Professor O. Charnock Bradley	Meat Inspection
Professor W. R. Davis	Principles of Shoeing
Professor James Hunter	Elementary Physics
Professor W. R. Davis	Hygiene

She had been born in Cordangan Manor, County Tipperary into an aristocratic family, the great-granddaughter of Lord Brownlow (Ford 1990; Warwick and Macdonald 2005). Her father was Sir Leopold Cust, and following his death in March 1878, Major Widdrington of Newton Hall was appointed her guardian. Whether Charnock Bradley persuaded Aleen to enrol in Williams's New Veterinary College rather than at the Dick Vet in the autumn of 1894 is not indicated. Aleen had enrolled in the College under the name A. I. Custance, although her name thereafter appeared in a number of forms: for example, Miss Corstorphine and Arno Constance (Anonymous 1895, 1898). She was a good student. In 1895 she won the New Veterinary College medal for Junior Anatomy (Anonymous 1895), as had Charnock Bradley, and in 1897 was presented with the silver medal for Zoology from the Highland and Agricultural Society (Anonymous 1897, 1898). However, that same year she was unfairly denied access to the RCVS examinations by legal sleight of hand (Editorial 1897).

Charnock Bradley came to know Aleen ('AC') well. They met almost daily from 20 to 30 August 1895 (the first days of his diary), and on 28 September 1895 he wrote that he had seen her off to Germany. She was the only female veterinary student in Britain at that time. The closeness of their relationship over the following five years was indicated in part by the

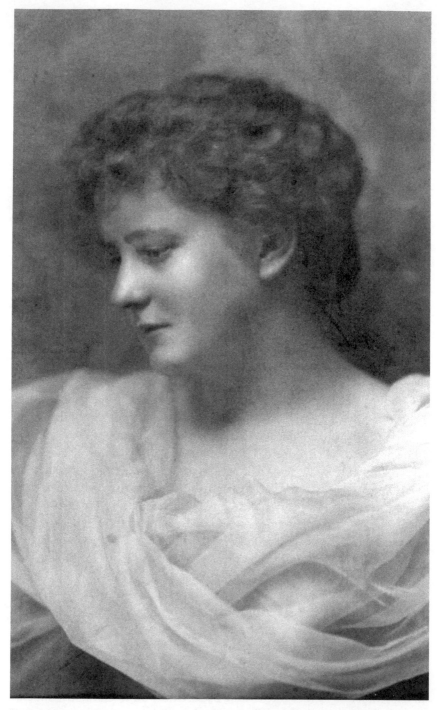

Figure 5.13 Aleen Cust, probably as a student at the New Veterinary College, Edinburgh. Photographer: W. Crooke.

frequency during the 1896 and 1897 sessions with which Bradley visited her home at Northfield (a farmhouse near Duddingston) for the purpose of 'coaching A.C.', by their walks together, and by their lunch and tea appointments in the newly rebuilt Jenner's department store on Princes Street (Bradley 1896–7).

Although Aleen Cust went on to complete her studies in 1900 and, with the help of a testimonial to that effect from William Williams, went into practice in Ireland, she was not admitted to membership of the RCVS for a further twenty-two years (Ford 1990). It is also of interest that a letter, dated 25 May 1900, which Williams received about one week after the RCVS final exams in Scotland, was published in the veterinary press and elsewhere (An old student 1900; Prospectus 1903):

> Remembering the many kindnesses which I have received from you, and also the fact that to you I owe the present position which I now occupy, I would like in some way to express my gratitude. Therefore, if you will kindly allow me, I will give a Prize of £25 annually for the next four years, to be competed for by students of the New Veterinary College, Edinburgh. I would suggest that the Prize should be given to the student who obtains the highest aggregate number of marks in his A B C and D examinations of the Royal College of Veterinary Surgeons; also that the student must have been regular in his attendance, and of good behaviour during the time he has attended the New Veterinary College . . . signed an old student.

Death of William Williams and the transfer to Liverpool University

William Williams died suddenly and quite unexpectedly of heart failure on 12 November 1900, aged eighty-six. Tributes flowed in and were republished in December by the *Veterinary Journal*. It was repeatedly noted that Williams had been the author of two standard textbooks in use in veterinary colleges throughout the world: *The Principles and Practice of Veterinary Surgery* had run to nine editions, and *The Principles and Practice of Veterinary Medicine* had reached its eighth edition. As a mark of respect, Aleen Cust sent a floral wreath to Williams's funeral on 15 November at Warriston Cemetery (Anonymous 1900b). A portrait of Williams by John D. Bowie was presented to the Royal College of Veterinary Surgeons on 3 April 1903 (Williams 1903a).

Later that year, the thirtieth session of the New Veterinary College began. The available evidence indicates that, within a year or two of his father's death, partly due to inadequate college finances, Owen Williams had begun to engage in discussions with Liverpool University about its invitation to transfer the New Veterinary College to Liverpool (Anonymous

1904; Williams 1904; Kraft 2004). At a meeting of the North of Scotland Veterinary Medical Society in Aberdeen, he indicated that within twelve months various universities would open their doors to veterinary students, and in addition to a licence to practise as a veterinary surgeon, these students would thereby have university degrees (Williams 1903b, c). In fact, the New Veterinary College held its final prize-giving ceremony on Monday 16 May 1904 (Williams 1904). Comments were made in the veterinary press that it was not the College that was moving from Edinburgh to Liverpool, but only Professor Owen Williams; the rest of the staff would stay in Edinburgh (Fiat Justitia 1904). This was not so. At least eleven of the Edinburgh New Veterinary College students also went to Liverpool; for example, James R. Rigby, whose lecture notes from the New Veterinary College, Edinburgh and the Faculty of Veterinary Medicine, Liverpool, remain extant, together with the diplomas and medals awarded to him (University Archives Liverpool 1992). The other New Veterinary College students transferred to the remaining Edinburgh, Glasgow and London colleges to complete their four-year coursework (Rutherford 1903, 1904; Veterinary Register 1910). Owen Williams was installed in Liverpool as the first Professor of the Principles and Practice of Veterinary Medicine and Surgery. The New Veterinary College was incorporated with Liverpool University and formally opened on 13 December 1904 (Kraft 2004).

Searches within the city of Edinburgh and the University of Liverpool for accumulated records of the New Veterinary College have failed to reveal any large body of archive material. These may have been destroyed prior to the move to Liverpool (Warwick and Macdonald 2005).

References

An old student, 1900. Gratitude. *Veterinary Journal*, 1, 342.

Anonymous, 1873. The New Veterinary College, Edinburgh. *The Scotsman*, Thursday, 25 September 1873, p. 2, col. 2.

Anonymous, 1878. Edinburgh New Veterinary College – Presentation to Prof. Williams, and award of class prizes. *The Veterinarian*, 51, 408–11.

Anonymous, 1883. New Veterinary College, Edinburgh. *The Veterinarian*, 56, 822–32.

Anonymous, 1884a. Fire at the New Veterinary College. *The Scotsman*, Monday, 28 January 1884, p. 4, col. 5.

Anonymous, 1884b. Disastrous storm. *Edinburgh Evening News*, 28 January 1884, p. 2, col. 5.

Anonymous, 1884c. Fire at the new veterinary college, Edinburgh. *The Veterinarian*, 57, 141.

Anonymous, [1893]. The New Veterinary College, Leith Walk, affiliated by Her Majesty's Royal Sign-Manual with the Royal College of Veterinary Surgeons. Founded by W. Williams, F.R.S.E., F.R.C.V.S, etc. in 1873, at Gayfield. In *A Descriptive Account of Edinburgh – Illustrated*. Brighton and London: Robinson, Son & Pike, 111.

Anonymous, 1895. Extracts and notes: New Veterinary College, Edinburgh. *The Veterinary Record*, 7, 650.

Anonymous, 1897. The New Veterinary College. *Edinburgh Evening News*, 12 May 1897, p. 3, col. 4.

Anonymous, 1898. Veterinary Department: Class examinations – 1897. *Transactions of the Highland and Agricultural Society of Scotland*, Series 5, 10, 487.

Anonymous, 1900a. Veterinary colleges. *The Veterinary Journal*, ns. 1, 348–9.

Anonymous, 1900b. Funeral of Principal Williams. *North British Agriculturist*, 21 November 1900, p. 752, cols 3–4.

Anonymous, 1904. Veterinary education in Liverpool. *The Times*, 24 May 1904, p. 13, col. e.

Blanc, H. J. 1870. *Gayfield House: Plans of dwelling house and offices, also stables and coach house*. Edinburgh: Hippolyte J. Blanc. National Archives of Scotland, West Register House, RHP 11114.

Bradley, O. C. 1896–7. Manuscript diary entries. [Nineteen visits at the end of 1896, twenty-eight in February/March/April 1897]. Royal (Dick) School of Veterinary Studies Archive.

Edinburgh Courant, 1883. New Veterinary College, Leith Walk. *Edinburgh Courant*, Thursday, 27 September 1883, p. 2, col. 1.

Editorial, 1897. Lady students. *The Veterinary Record*, 10, 407.

Faulkner, E. 1873. Letter to the Editor. *Edinburgh Courant*, Thursday, 17 July 1873, p. 5, col. 1.

Fiat Justitia, 1904. The New Veterinary College. *The Veterinary Record*, 16, 696.

Ford, C. 1990. *M. Aleen Cust, Veterinary Surgeon*. Bristol: Biopress.

Grant, J. 1880–3. *Cassell's Old and New Edinburgh*. London: Cassell & Co., Vol. 3, 165.

Hawryluk, D. 2003. Personal communication.

Kraft, A. 2004. Liverpool veterinary school: The first 100 years. *The Veterinary Record*, 155, 620–4.

Lewis, T. H. 1882. Edinburgh New Veterinary College: Opening of session. *The Veterinarian*, 55, 844–6.

Liverpool University Archive. Photograph of staff and students, New Veterinary College, Edinburgh. Special Collections and Archives, University of Liverpool Library, reference S.2957/1.

Macdonald, A. A., Forrest, J. and Warwick, C. 2021. Whispers in Edinburgh: Horse sculptures with veterinary connections. *Veterinary History*, 20 (4), 457–75. <era.ed.ac.uk/handle/1842/37747> (accessed 9 September 2022).

Prospectus, 1895. *The New Veterinary College, Leith Walk, Edinburgh. Session 1895–96*. Edinburgh, 42 pages.

Prospectus, 1903. *The New Veterinary College, Leith Walk, Edinburgh, founded in 1873 by the late W. Williams, F.R.C.V.S., F.R.S.E., J.P., and affiliated by Royal Sign-Manual to the Royal College of Veterinary Surgeons; 1903–14*. Edinburgh, 32 pages.

Purdy, 1884. The late fire at the new veterinary college, Edinburgh. *The Veterinarian*, 57, 151.

Robinson, 1885. Edinburgh Veterinary Medical Society. *The Veterinarian*, 58, 376.

Robinson, R. C. 1937. Personal tributes. *The Veterinary Record*, 49, 1550.

Rutherford, R. 1903. Examinations in Scotland. *The Veterinary Record*, 15, 427–8.

Rutherford, R. 1904. The May examinations in Scotland. *The Veterinary Record*, 16, 780.

Shennan, T. 1900. The New Veterinary College, Edinburgh. *The Veterinary Journal*, ns. 2, 272–8.

The Scotsman, 1883. Building operations in Leith Walk. *The Scotsman*, Monday, 22 October 1883, p. 5, col. 1.

University Archives Liverpool, 1992. Summary list of papers, certificates, medals, and publications of the late Mr J.R. Rigby, M.R.C.V.S., of Lytham St. Annes [a student at the New Veterinary College, Edinburgh, later at the University of Liverpool's Veterinary

School until 1907] deposited by his daughter, Miss B. Rigby, Lytham, Lytham St. Annes, Lancashire, FY8 5LL, 5 September, 21 November 1989 and 22 June 1992. D.492.

Veterinary register, 1910. *The Register of Veterinary Surgeons*. London: Royal College of Veterinary Surgeons.

Warwick, C. M. and Macdonald, A. A. 2005. The New Veterinary College, Edinburgh, 1873 to 1904. *The Veterinary Record*, 153, 380–6. <era.ed.ac.uk/handle/1842/2198> (accessed 9 September 2022).

Warwick, C. M. and Macdonald, A. A. 2010. The Life of Professor Orlando Charnock Bradley, (1871–1937): Diary entries 1895–1923. *Veterinary History*, 15, 205–20. <era .ed.ac.uk/handle/1842/3643> (accessed 9 September 2022).

Williams, W. 1874. New Veterinary College. *Edinburgh Courant*, Thursday, 29 October 1874, p. 3, cols 3–4.

Williams, W. 1875. The veterinary profession – the Scotch Colleges. *North British Agriculturist*, 26, p. 701, cols a–c.

Williams, W. 1876. New Veterinary College. *Edinburgh Courant*, Thursday, 26 October 1876, p. 2, cols 5–6.

Williams, W. 1882. New Veterinary College, Edinburgh: Prize list. *The Veterinary Journal*, 14, 455–6.

Williams, W. 1883a. New Veterinary College, Edinburgh. *The Veterinarian*, 56, 370–1.

Williams, W. 1883b. [Opening address] *The Veterinarian*, 56, 823–9.

Williams, W. 1887. New Veterinary College, Edinburgh: Principal Williams on the situation. *The Veterinarian*, 60, 372–6.

Williams, W. 1888. New Veterinary College, Edinburgh. *The Veterinarian*, 61, 421–3.

Williams, W. 1891. New Veterinary College, Edinburgh. *Veterinary Journal*, 33, 35–6.

Williams, W. 1893. New Veterinary College, Edinburgh. *The Veterinarian*, 66, 503.

Williams, W. 1898. Medal day at the New Veterinary College. *North British Agriculturist*, 50, 312 (col. 4)–313 (col. 1).

Williams, W. 1899. The New Veterinary College. *North British Agriculturist*, 51, p. 656, cols 3–5.

Williams, W. 1900. New Veterinary College, Edinburgh. *Veterinary Journal*, ns. 1, 340–1.

Williams, W. O. 1903a. The late Principal Williams. *Veterinary Journal*, ns. 7, 243–4.

Williams, W. O. 1903b. Address by Principal Williams – The proposed veterinary degree. *Veterinary Journal*, ns. 8, 123–8.

Williams, W. O. 1903c. [Vote of thanks] New Veterinary College, Edinburgh. *Veterinary Journal*, ns. 8, 238–9.

Williams, W. O. 1904. Close of Edinburgh New Veterinary College. *Veterinary Journal*, ns. 9, 290–2.

Chapter 6

Clyde Street College Developments (1874–1916)

Thomas Walley becomes Principal

The next phase in the history of the Dick Vet can be characterised largely as a period of structural and constitutional reconstruction. Thomas Walley (1842–94), who had been appointed Professor of Cattle Pathology at Clyde Street in Session 1871–2, was now offered the job of Principal and accepted (Figure 6.1). He began by re-establishing a teaching team of staff who worked well together. To the students he gave detailed instruction on animal diseases and meat inspection, and reintroduced practical work on the microscope. Bradley (1923) commented that the Principalship of Thomas Walley,

> compared with that of his predecessors, was one of peace and tranquillity. The reputation of the College as a teaching institution of high standard was maintained – thanks to an enthusiastic and efficient staff – and the wise and calm administration that was essential was forthcoming.

The two veterinary colleges, situated about three hundred metres from one another, settled down to attract and train veterinary students in an atmosphere of constructive and friendly rivalry (Macdonald, Warwick and Johnston 2005). Both Principals were aware of the changes they needed to introduce to improve the educational levels of the students they enrolled and the training that they subsequently received. A summer term of two months had been instituted in Session 1873–4, and in 1876 the period of study was further increased nationally to three years, comprising two winter terms of not less than eleven weeks each and a summer term of not less than eight weeks. Students were examined by the RCVS at the end of each year. Both Walley and Williams knew in 1873 that the college

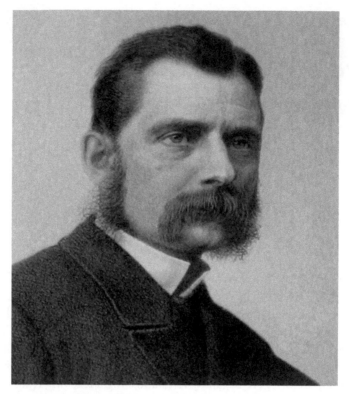

Figure 6.1 Thomas Walley (1842–94). Photographer: unknown.

facilities they had at their disposal were not fit for purpose. In addition, it was also clear that their personalities offered opportunities to resolve the problems of bitter antagonism and distrust which had been generated and nurtured between the London and Edinburgh colleges over the previous thirty to forty years. The discord within the young veterinary profession would only be resolved when it became generally accepted that accreditation by the Royal College of Veterinary Surgeons was the only way to become a veterinary surgeon in Britain (Macdonald, Warwick and Johnston 2005).

The timing was propitious. Major General Sir Frederick W. J. Fitzwygram, 4th Bart. (1823–1904), a graduate in 1854 of William Dick's College who subsequently passed the RCVS examinations in 1871, was elected President of the RCVS in 1875. He was well qualified, by military training, veterinary qualifications (both Highland certificate and MRCVS Diploma), common sense and nobility, to draw the profession together. After careful and considerate discussion and assisted by George Fleming (1833–1901) on the RCVS Council, agreement was reached with the Highland Society that no new applicants for the Society's veterinary examinations would be accepted after 1 January 1879. The last of the Highland Society's veterinary examinations were held in April 1881. A few months later, on 27 August, the Veterinary Surgeons Bill received Royal Assent. It established the rules governing the registration of veterinary surgeons in Britain and had as its main purpose the ready and public differentiation between qualified and unqualified practitioners. Up to the end of December 1883, anyone could style themselves a veterinary surgeon. There would now only be one portal through which well-educated students could enter the veterinary profession (Macdonald, Warwick and Johnston 2005).

Building works at the Clyde Street College

By the autumn of 1873 the Trustees allocated £150 to put the Clyde Street College and museum in a proper state of repair. A students' room was created on the ground floor of the small house on the north-east side of the courtyard. It provided a new space for the thirty-six students attending the 1874–5 Session (Macdonald et al. 2023). Above this room, a new connecting doorway was built through the wall into the dissecting room.

On the west side of the courtyard, the museum was lengthened to about 8.5 metres and redesigned. In 1853 it had already been extended from its original length of 3 metres, into part of what had been the old classroom (Macdonald 2020). In 1853 a new semicircular lecture theatre had been constructed above the stables to the north of the museum (Anonymous 1864). The two rows of new six-shelved storage cases that were installed there greatly increased the availability of dry- and wet-specimen storage space. The room was also well lit. Adequate floor space remained for mounted skeletal specimens beneath the six windows and against the north wall. Through this wall to the south of the museum, the remaining space of the original 1833 classroom was converted into a bone room. A new access stairway was constructed from what in 1833 had been a stable below (Macdonald et al. 2023).

On the east side of the courtyard, increased sun-lighting of the dissecting room was achieved by removing two of the small original glazed panels and fitting seven enlarged glazed panels into its roof. In addition, two eighteen-section compartmentalised storage cupboards were built near the fireplace on the south wall of the dissecting room. These may have been to provide the equivalent of personal locker space for the students. A small ground-floor room on the east side of the courtyard was identified for the reception of pet dogs, as requested by Professor Walley (Anonymous 1874a). The opportunity was also taken to build a small assay laboratory, increase the number of toilet facilities and build an indoor 'dung heap' in that general location with access from the east side of Clyde Street Lane. At the same meeting of the Trustees, Professor Walley asked for some of the seating in the lecture theatre to be removed to allow skeletons to be moved between the museum and the theatre. He also requested that the exterior walls around the courtyard be whitewashed prior to the start of the 1874 Session (Anonymous 1874a). In December 1873 the name of the College had been changed to the Dick Veterinary College, following a request to the Trustees from Mary Dick. Four years later, the College became known as the Royal (Dick's) Veterinary College (Macdonald 2013). Gradually, in local parlance, the college came to be known as 'the Dick Vet'.

The course content

On 3 September 1874 the Committee of Management approved the Prospectus for Session 1874–5 and ordered it be printed and distributed (Anonymous 1874b). The Prospectus (1874) said that the lectures were:

> so arranged as to allow of the hours from 10 to 12 for Junior, and from 10 to 1 for Senior Students being left open for practical work under the direction of the Veterinary Staff, such as Dissection, Patient Visiting, Clinical instruction, Examination of horses as to Soundness, Experimental and Operative Surgery, post-mortem Examinations, Microscopical and Anatomical demonstrations, Dispensing, Practical Examination of Feet for Lameness, &c.

The Winter Session commenced on 21 October and closed at the end of April. The Summer Session began on the first Monday in May and closed early in July. The courses included Veterinary Medicine, Surgical Pathology, Practical and Military Veterinary Surgery, Comparative Pathology, Anatomy, Functional and Pathological Physiology, Histology, Organic and Inorganic Chemistry, Materia Medica and Therapeutical and Toxicological lectures. Weekly Saturday visits were made to the Edinburgh slaughterhouses for practical demonstrations on healthy and diseased internal organs and flesh of cattle, sheep and pigs. Botany was a summer course conducted in the Botanical Gardens. Two winter sessions and one summer session were required before examination, but it was recommended, when practicable, that students should take three winter sessions and one summer session. In the intervals between College sessions the students were encouraged to engage in practice. During the first fortnight of the Winter Session, examination of the Senior Students was held to select those most qualified to fill the respective offices of Hospital Surgeon, Dispenser and Prosector. Those coming second in these competitions received the titles of Assistant Hospital Surgeon, Dispenser or Prosector. All second-year students were eligible as Clinical Clerks, Dressers and Visitors.

The Matriculation Fee was 10s 6d. To students possessing recognised educational certificates, this fee was not charged. Tickets for attendance at the classes necessary to qualify for the Diploma were on two scales: 1) by annual payment of £13 5s. for the two years (winter and summer included) and £5 5s. for each subsequent sessional year; 2) by payment of one sum of £25 for two sessional years, a further fee of £5 5s. being charged for each year beyond the second. Practical Chemistry cost an additional £1 1s. and the Garden Fee for Botany was 2s. 6d. Amateur students paid for single tickets: Pathological Classes, with Clinical Instruction £5 5s. each or £7 7s. for both; Anatomy, Physiology and Chemistry, £3 3s. each.

The number of students attracted to study at the Clyde Street College increased to about forty in 1876–7, to more than fifty the following year, and to seventy-three in 1878–9. By 1882–3 there were more than 130 and in 1883–4 there were 136 students (Macdonald et al. 2023). These numbers corresponded to a period of stability within the College. In his introductory lecture in 1875, the new Professor of Physiology, J. G. McKendrick, had stated that

> within two years from the time of entering the college, the student is expected to have acquired an elementary knowledge of chemistry, botany, the anatomy of the domestic animals, physiology, pathology, materia medica, and veterinary medicine and surgery. In addition to this, he endeavours to acquire a practical knowledge of disease and its treatment, by the examination of sick animals, and also he must be familiar with all the operations practised in veterinary surgery. Much the same course of study occupies the student of medicine for at least four years.

Two sessions and two examinations remained until 1876. However, from 1876 this was increased to three sessions and three examinations. From 1 January 1884 the Royal College of Veterinary Surgeons demanded that all students should pass an entrance examination in general knowledge. Nine years later, the regulations and standard of the examination were revised. They were brought into line with those framed by the General Medical Council for intending medical students.

Further accommodation adjustments

Despite the adjustments to the college property made in the 1870s, the new spaces were still too small and not sufficient. Principal William Williams had built a brand-new veterinary college in Elm Row near the top of

Leith Walk in Edinburgh (Chapter 5). Its facilities completely eclipsed the Clyde Street Veterinary College. As a consequence, in October 1883 the Edinburgh Dean of Guild Court granted warrant to the Trustees to make further 'minor alterations in the interior of the College buildings in Clyde Street'. In fact, significant modifications were made to the houses at 10 Clyde Street (Macdonald et al. 2023). At the north-east end of the courtyard, the ground-floor former students' room was reconverted into a saddle room and smoking room. The ground-floor rooms in the south-east corner were converted into a pharmacy, Materia Medica room, an extension of the dissecting room and a preparation room (Figure 6.2). The pressure on available lecture classroom space was dealt with by creating an additional lecture room out of the dining room and a small bedroom on the first floor. The first floor also contained Professor McFadyean's room, a Botany preparation room and a senior students' room. On the two floors above the entrance to the college courtyard was the College Janitor's dwelling house. There was a mezzanine storey on the east side of the courtyard, and it was occupied by an animal room and a macerating room. In 1881 the domestic part of the original 1833 Veterinary School building was partially occupied as a dwelling house by the clinical Professor Colin C. Baird and his wife Helen, as well as by Margaret H. Campbell, the cook, and Jessie MacKinlay, the housemaid (Macdonald et al. 2023). However, the top-floor bedrooms of the former domestic building had already been converted into Botany and Chemistry teaching rooms.

By 1883 the ground floor on the west side of the courtyard housed a dry store, stables, dog kennels and a coach house (Macdonald et al. 2023). On the first floor were located the bone room, museum, library, semicircular lecture room, a hayloft, a chemical laboratory and an apparatus room. At the north-west end of the courtyard, on the second floor were a library, gymnasium, smoking rooms and lavatories. The building along the north end of the courtyard, which had been the Clyde Street Hall, now contained a chemical laboratory and lumber room on the ground floor and a chemical laboratory and professors' room on the first floor (Macdonald et al. 2023). The appearance of the north end of the courtyard was captured in a photo of staff and students by James Howie Jr (Figure 6.3). Taken about 1880, the chemical laboratories formed the backdrop wall. The stairs led up to the back entrance into the semicircular lecture theatre built in 1853.

By 1885, space for an aviary had been found within the rooms on the south-east side of the courtyard (Macdonald et al. 2023). By that time too, on the ground floor in the south-east corner of the courtyard, the clinical Professor had a surgery. The top floor of the south-east side of the courtyard was converted into a chemistry classroom and a pathology laboratory.

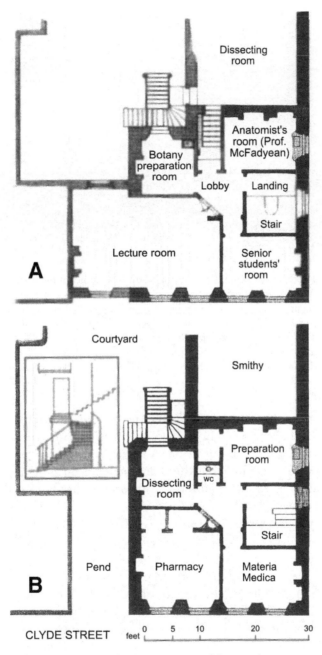

Figure 6.2 Plans made in 1883 for the conversion of the rented tenement accommodation at 10 Clyde Street into teaching space. A. The second-floor (south-east) lecture room, the botany preparation room, Professor McFadyean's room and the senior students' room; B. The ground-floor pharmacy, the Materia Medica room, a preparation room and an extension of the dissecting room. Images modified from Edinburgh City Archives.

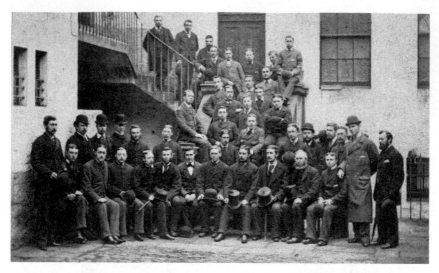

Figure 6.3 Photograph, taken c. 1880, of the north-west corner of the Royal (Dick) Veterinary College courtyard, with forty-three staff and students on and around the stairway leading up to the semicircular lecture theatre. Thomas Walley, the Head of College and Professor of Anatomy, is sitting in the front row, legs apart, with a top hat on his knees. On his left is possibly Prof. Daniel John Cunningham (Physiology), also with a top hat, resting on a walking stick. On his left is the bearded Prof. Colin C. Baird (Clinical), with his top hat resting on his right leg. Photographer: James Howie Jr.

The discussion of how best to commemorate the memory of William Dick had begun shortly after his death (Anonymous 1866a, b). Professor Walley raised the issue again in 1878 (Walley 1878). However, it was not until 1883 that a decision was made. A statue of the late Professor Dick was cut from freestone by John Rhind and unveiled on 24 October 1883 (Macdonald et al. 2023) (Figure 6.4). Its location has been deduced to have been at the north end of the courtyard, sheltered from the wind and bathed in sunlight. Through the entrance to the courtyard (Plate 6.1A) the sculpted seated figure of William Dick can be glimpsed. Regretfully, Mary Dick had died three months earlier, on 14 July 1883.

It was possible to extract from the architect's building plans for the new 1886–7 building the structural element of the 1885 building (Morham 1886a, b). Based on this information, a three-dimensional virtual copy of the old Clyde Street College was constructed. Its structural 'skeleton' was clad with wall and roof surfaces, including details such as the roof lights above the dissecting room (Plate 6.1B). It also enabled the old Clyde Street College buildings to be viewed from different perspectives. The result is currently the best available image of the most likely appearance of the Royal (Dick) Veterinary College in 1885 (Macdonald et al. 2023).

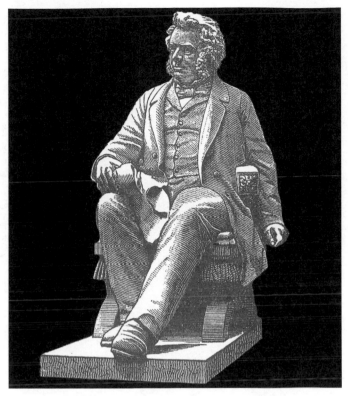

Figure 6.4 Etching of the statue of William Dick, cut in freestone in 1883 by John Rhind, and published in 1883 by the *Veterinary Journal*, 17, 443. The image was probably made from a photograph taken before the statue was erected onto its six-foot-high pedestal in the Clyde Street courtyard.

The 1886–7 Clyde Street College rebuild

Virtual reconstruction of the 1886–7 Clyde Street building then followed. The following architect drawings were assembled and copied: the 1833 construction of the original Edinburgh Veterinary School (RCAHMS 1832); the 1865 reconstruction of the tenement on Clyde Street adjoining and to the east of the Veterinary College (Edinburgh City Archives 1865); and the 1883 drawings for the remodelling of the interior of the tenement and other buildings in the courtyard (Anonymous 1883a). The published floor plans of the new building and the architectural drawings for the 1886 reconstruction of the Royal Dick Veterinary College provided vital and detailed support for its virtual reconstruction (Prospectus 1888; RCAHMS 1883). The data for the computer-based rebuild were extracted from the architectural drawings prepared by Mr Morham, the City

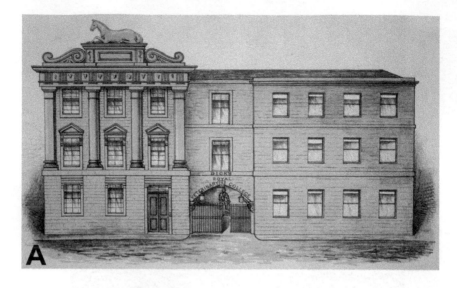

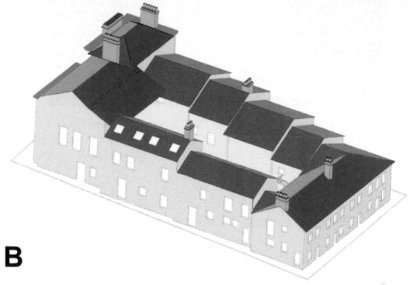

Plate 6.1 A. Façade of the Royal (Dick) Veterinary College, published in the prospectus for 1886–7, illustrating, through the entrance gateway, the sculpture of William Dick. This image suggests that the sculpture was on its pedestal at the north end of the courtyard and situated to the east of the stairway leading up to the semicircular lecture theatre. Photographer: Colin M. Warwick; B. Aerial view from the north-east illustrating the outer surfaces of the virtually reconstructed 1885 Royal (Dick) Veterinary College buildings. The colour palette used was chosen to aid clarity of structure. Image: Ketan Lad, Valentin J. Hunzinger and Alastair A. Macdonald.

Superintendent of Works (Morham 1886a, b). The computer-aided design (CAD) tool used in 2004 by the then students Ketan Lad and Valentin Hunzinger in this project was 'form-z v4.2' developed by AutoDesSys.

The initial phase of the digital reconstruction was to create a base model from the historic sectional and plan drawings. The base reconstruction of the interior of the building relied on both the architectural drawings prepared by Mr Morham and the photographs of the classrooms taken by Professor O. Charnock Bradley (Anonymous 1905). From Bradley's diary, the entry for 11 July 1905 says: 'Otherwise the whole of the day at the College. In the afternoon was photographing the class-rooms.' Study of these photographs allowed the accurate capturing of internal partition wall positions as well as door and window composition. Balconies and their intricate railings and balusters, light fittings and other ironwork typical of that era were also reconstructed with the use of detailed drawings and photographs. Seating, tables and other furniture were then constructed and placed as per the photographic information to capture the use and atmosphere of the spaces (Anonymous 1905). Intricate details were added where appropriate to show extra fittings, teaching tools and miscellaneous items visible in the photographs.

Following completion of the details of these reconstructions, a series of video fly-through presentations of the building were made (Videos). The main entrance was as before in the form of an archway, opening off Clyde Street. It was high and wide enough to admit a horse and open carriage. To the left of the entrance was the College office and waiting rooms, and to the right of the entrance was a house provided for the janitor and a small additional office (Macdonald et al. 2005). No internal details of these rooms and accommodation were available for study.

With respect to the actual building, by the start of the 1886 Session (28 October) much of the east side of the construction had been completed. At ground level, the east side was occupied mainly by stables, but it also comprised a pharmacy, an operating theatre and the post-mortem room (Figures 6.5 and 6.6; Macdonald et al. 2005). On the north side it comprised a horse-shoeing forge as well as hospital accommodation in the form of dog kennels. The lower part of the staircase at the north end of the courtyard was in the form of an arcade (Videos – The Courtyard), in the central niche of which was placed the recently unveiled memorial statue of Professor Dick (Anonymous 1886d). A harness room, storeroom, loose boxes, kennels and stables were built along the west side of the courtyard (Macdonald et al. 2005). No photographic details of the interiors of these rooms were available for study.

The virtual reconstruction illustrated for the first time the view towards the Clyde Street entrance from the north end of the central courtyard

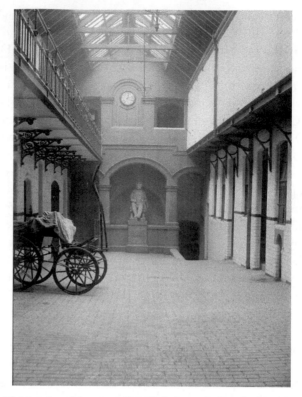

Figure 6.5 The interior of the post-1887 Clyde Street College building looking north towards the statue of William Dick. Photographer: O. C. Bradley.

(Plate 6.2A). The courtyard itself was entirely roofed over with glass. An open stairway led up from the first-floor level to the teaching laboratories on the Top Level. A balcony corridor ran along the west side of the first floor (Plates 6.2A and B). Additional architectural aspects of the court-yard, extracted from the architectural drawings, were illustrated in (Videos – The Courtyard).

One stairway from the ground floor to the first floor was situated to the left of the entrance from Clyde Street (Videos – The Courtyard; Macdonald et al. 2005). The appearance of these stairs is further illus-trated at the start of the video fly-through, which also shows the few steps leading to the anatomical museum, pathological museum and bone room (Videos – The Balcony; Macdonald et al. 2005). Photographs of these three rooms were very likely taken by Professor Bradley but sadly have not been located. However, photographs of the practical chemistry classroom (Plate 6.3A), the adjacent practical physiology and pathology classroom (Plate 6.3B) and the pathology laboratory which were above them on the Top Level, do exist (Macdonald et al. 2005); the first two

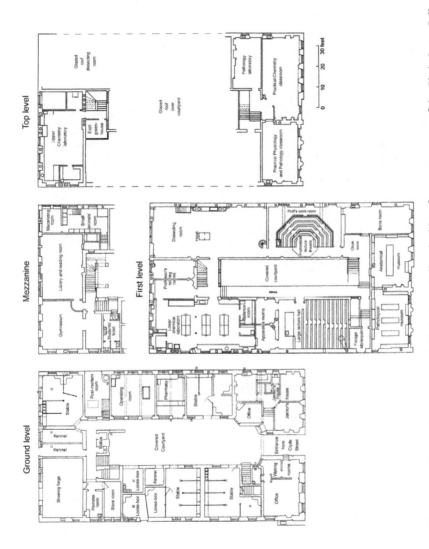

Figure 6.6 Annotated floor plans of the newly reconstructed Clyde Street College building from a prospectus of the Clyde Street College.

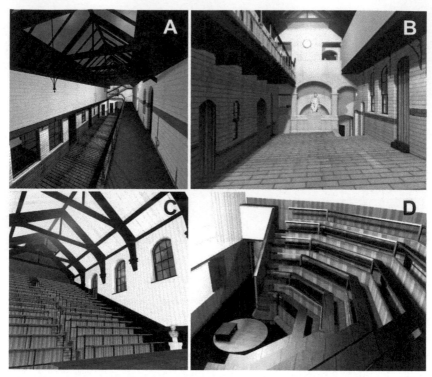

Plate 6.2 Virtual reconstruction of the interior of the new Clyde Street College building: A. View of the glass ceiling and courtyard looking south from the first-floor balcony; B. View of the courtyard from the entrance looking north (compare Figure 6.7); C. View of the large West Lecture Hall from the doorway; D. View of the Anatomical Lecture Theatre. Images: Ketan Lad and Valentin J. Hunzinger.

were published over a hundred years ago (Anonymous 1905). The second one of these (Plate 6.3b) shows that routine practical microscope work was undertaken in connection with the classes in Physiology, Pathology and Parasitology.

Halfway along the balcony, overlooking the covered central courtyard, was the door to the large west lecture theatre (Videos – West Lecture Hall). This classroom could seat two hundred students (Plate 6.2C; Macdonald et al. 2005). The walk-through gives a clear impression of the climb up through the 'chicane' in the steps leading to the back of the classroom. It gives views of the room from the perspective of the lecturer as well as from those at the top of the class. The question has arisen: Why was the chicane designed into the theatre staircase? Although one suggested answer was connected to the disturbance of lectures that golf balls descending the steps might have caused, it is more likely to have been a safety feature when two hundred students were leaving.

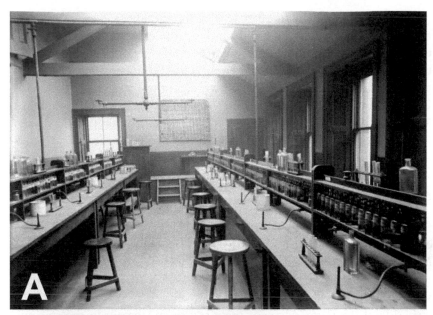

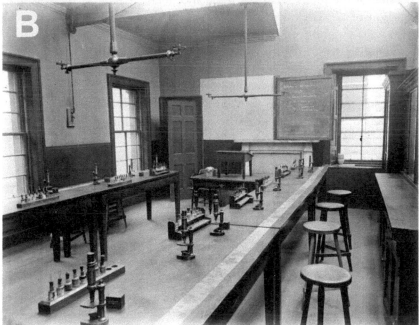

Plate 6.3 A. View, looking east, of the Practical Chemistry classroom on the Top Level of the new Clyde Street College building; B. View, looking west, of the Practical Physiology and Pathology classroom on the Top Level of the new Clyde Street College building. Photographs: O. C. Bradley, colorised by Alastair A. Macdonald.

At the north end of the first level were the lower chemical laboratory, the professors' retiring rooms and, on the mezzanine, the students' toilet, gymnasium, library and reading room, the small animals room and the macerating room (Macdonald et al. 2005). Unfortunately, no photographs of any of these were found. However, at the Top Level of the building on the north side was the Upper Chemistry laboratory (Figure 6.6) and its photograph was very helpful to the reconstruction of that room (Macdonald et al. 2005). A walk-through was created of the stairway leading up to the laboratory and around the bench at its centre (Videos – The Upper Chemistry Laboratory). Adjacent to it was a small experimental greenhouse.

The anatomy department occupied the rooms on the east side of the first level (Macdonald et al. 2005). The dissecting room was modelled on the design of the then new dissecting room in Edinburgh University Medical School (Anonymous 1886c). It was lit entirely from the north through a glazed roof (Videos – The Dissecting Room). A spiral stairway led up to a gallery for the display of preserved specimens along the west side of the room. Many of these specimens remain in the teaching collection of the Dick Vet today. A hoist brought the dissection specimens from ground level up through a trapdoor in the floor. A drawing of the students at work dissecting a horse carcass in this room (see Figure 14.5) was created by William Gordon Burn Murdoch and published by Dollar (1894). The computerised walk-through of the dissecting room takes the observer up this spiral stairway onto the balcony gallery of glazed cupboards containing the preserved specimens (Videos – The Dissecting Room). It then brings the observer back down the stairway to the adjacent connecting doorway into the anatomical lecture theatre.

The design of the anatomical lecture theatre retained the semicircular layout of the pre-1886 theatre (Anonymous 1864) and had seating for 150 students (Plate 6.2D). Dissected subjects could be wheeled in from the dissecting room and transferred onto a circular revolving table, so that the parts being lectured upon could be turned in succession to be viewed by different parts of the room. The lecture theatre also connected to the anatomical museum on the south side of the building (Macdonald et al. 2005). The fly-through (Videos – Anatomy Lecture Theatre) illustrates the overall form of the room. The video ends in the seat occupied by Professor Bradley when he took the photograph that we have.

The completed building was a huge improvement (Figure 6.7a–d). It was finished in time for the 1887 intake of students, and a detailed description of the new facilities was given in the prospectus for 1888–9 (R(D)VC 1888). Edinburgh Town Council, although by its very nature poorly equipped to struggle with the management of the Clyde Street

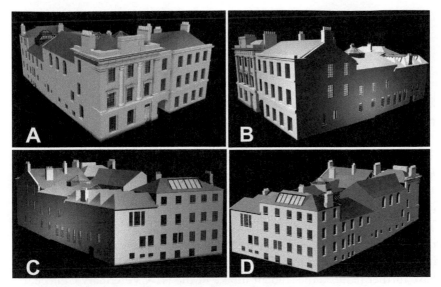

Figure 6.7 Virtual reconstruction of the outside of the new Clyde Street College building viewed from the four corners: A. South-west; B. South-east; C. North-east; D. North-west. Images: Ketan Lad and Valentin J. Hunzinger.

College, had managed to harness the available resources to pay for the construction of the new buildings in 1886–7.

Both veterinary colleges in Edinburgh now had new facilities specifically designed for their active staff and increasing numbers of students. The 1880s could be largely characterised by a sense of 'normality' and improvement. A more detailed understanding of the sciences of medicine and veterinary medicine was being encouraged to develop rapidly. However, as a consequence, increasing pressure was being put, firstly, on the educational background of the students being enrolled and, secondly, on the proposed number of years designated by the RCVS for their veterinary studies. Only a very small proportion of the students (15 per cent or less) succeeded in going through the curriculum in the currently specified time of three sessions (Walley 1892).

In July 1892 a conference of veterinary teachers, examiners and members of the RCVS Council met to discuss and agree the teaching content of the new course. How was the subject material to be distributed throughout a lengthened, four-year course of instruction? The first group of students to take the new course enrolled in 1893. In addition, however, it had also been agreed that from September 1893 those students who wished to study veterinary medicine should also pass the tougher preliminary general educational examination required by the General Medical Council for its students. There was evidence to suggest that pre-warning of this increase in the severity of the entrance examinations led to a rush for veterinary college places in the years before 1893, and to fewer applicants thereafter (Dewar 1902).

Expansion of course length and creation of new management structure

There was certainly a drop in the numbers of students presenting for RCVS examinations in Edinburgh and elsewhere in the country from 1894. Williams repeatedly blamed the 1893 innovations for the reduced numbers of veterinary students attracted to the New Veterinary College. The numbers graduating from his College progressively dropped, from thirty-two in 1894 to eighteen in 1896 and eleven in 1898. The opening of the Royal Veterinary College in Dublin in 1900 was perceived to have further reduced the student intake to the New Veterinary College in Edinburgh (Macdonald, Warwick and Johnston 2005).

The impact on the veterinary profession of this decreased output of college graduates was dramatic. Whereas during the six years prior to the 1893 changes the number of veterinary surgeons on the register had increased by 385, in the four years thereafter the net increase was only seven (McFadyean 1901).

On 10 December 1894 Walley died from tuberculosis, probably self-inoculated during his experimental studies with the disease. His death coincided with a marked decline in student intake and the resulting increase in financial difficulties. A small and vociferous group of people in Edinburgh began to campaign publicly for the amalgamation of the two Edinburgh veterinary colleges, favouring the New Veterinary College site on Leith Walk, and consequently the appointment of a new Principal was delayed. The subject was discussed in committee, and by the Town Council; both rejected the idea. John R. U. Dewar (1850–1919) was appointed Principal (Figure 6.8) on 7 May 1895 and held the post for sixteen years (Bradley 1923). The same year the course length was increased to four sessions, with four examinations.

As both veterinary colleges in Edinburgh struggled to minimise the drop in student numbers, individuals continued to air the case for amalgamation. The income from student fees was clearly insufficient to cover the running costs. There was a Matriculation Fee of 1 guinea for all students entering the Clyde Street College for the first time. The Curriculum Fee for Class A (first year) was 17 guineas, for class B 15 guineas, for class C 13 guineas and for class D (final year) 10 guineas (Prospectus 1895). Income from the private or public veterinary practices of the college professors,

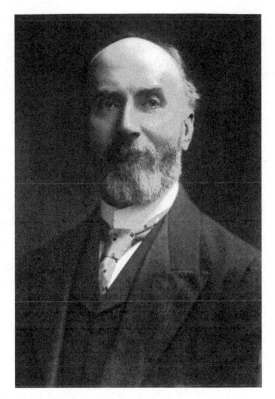

Figure 6.8 John R. U. Dewar. Photographer: unknown.

which had until then sustained the Scottish veterinary colleges financially and provided the material for clinical tuition, was no longer sufficient (Macdonald, Warwick and Johnston 2005). Although the financial status of the Clyde Street College was not as bad as published figures implied, the controversy stimulated a search for alternative means of support. Exploring government funding during the Anglo-Boer war (1899–1902) was not successful. The question of finding benefactors who might financially assist the College was raised. Under the will of Mary Dick, the residue of her estate was to be retained until it amounted to £20,000, when it was to be divided into two equal portions; one was for the furtherance of veterinary science in the Clyde Street College, and the other to found a professorship, either of comparative anatomy or of surgical anatomy, in the University of Edinburgh, in memory of the late Dr John Barclay and the late Professor John Goodsir (Anonymous 1883b). Publicity was given to the fact that the Principals of all five veterinary colleges in the United Kingdom had been educated at the Clyde Street College.

Earlier questions were recalled, asking whether it might not be possible for universities to confer degrees in veterinary medicine in the way that the four Scottish universities already did for medicine. On 21 November the following letter (Macdonald, Warwick and Johnston 2005) from Principal Dewar at the Clyde Street College was put before the Senatus of the University of Edinburgh:

> We look on Universities as the seats of learning, the sources of education and enlightenment to the communities around them, and in this progressive age, the centres of scientific investigation, and as the University of Edinburgh now grants degrees in Science and Engineering, in Agriculture etc. it has occurred to me that it might also grant a degree in Veterinary Science.
>
> As those studying for our profession have now, for several years, been required to pass a preliminary examination equal to that required from students studying for Medical and Science degrees, and as our students have to study for four years before they can graduate as members of the profession, – during that time studying Botany, Natural History, Chemistry, Anatomy, Physiology, Pathology, Materia Medica, Meat Inspection, and subjects more purely veterinary, it seems to me that the University of Edinburgh might well consider the propriety of recognising our profession by granting a degree to those fully qualified to receive it.
>
> Whatever time this may take place I feel confident that the day is not far distant when our profession will obtain university recognition, and taking the deep interest in it [as] I do I would naturally prefer that Edinburgh should take the lead rather than have to follow in the wake of others.

A joint committee of the faculties of Science and Medicine made the following recommendation, which was accepted on 22 February 1902 (Macdonald, Warwick and Johnston 2005):

> The Senatus to request the Court to take into favourable consideration the propriety of applying for an ordinance, under Section XXI of the Universities (Scotland) Act 1889, to enable the University of Edinburgh to grant Degrees in Veterinary Science . . .
>
> [The committee] took for granted that every candidate would be required (1) to pass the Preliminary Examination prescribed for degrees in Pure Science: (2) to attend at least half of the required courses of instruction during a period of not less than three academical years in the University: and (3) that every candidate, before appearing for the Final B.Sc. Examination in Veterinary Science, would be required to have obtained a qualification to practice from the Royal College of Veterinary Surgeons. In other words, it was assumed the Degree in Veterinary Science, if instituted would be of the nature of an Honours Degree.

A proposed 'reconstruction' of the Royal (Dick) Veterinary College was made on 16 June 1903. A new Administrative Board would take over the College from the trusteeship of Edinburgh Town Council and the College would become an extramural school of Edinburgh University. Veterinary students would take classes either in the University of Edinburgh, or at

Clyde Street, or both, towards a degree in veterinary science. The General Council meeting of the University in October that year approved the draft ordinance of the University Court for the institution of the degrees of Bachelor and Doctor of Veterinary Medicine and Surgery (Macdonald, Warwick and Johnston 2005).

On 24 July 1905 the first meeting of the Representative Board for the Royal (Dick) Veterinary College met in preparation for taking over the administration of the College from the Town Council. The 83rd Session of the Clyde Street College was opened on 3 October 1905, with Sir William Turner (1832–1916), Principal of Edinburgh University (and one of the original Trustees appointed by Mary Dick), in the chair, and the new management of the College was inaugurated. The new independent board contained two representatives of the City Corporation, two from the University of Edinburgh, three members of the veterinary profession practising in Scotland, one representative from the (Royal) Highland and Agricultural Society of Scotland, one representative each from the three colleges of agriculture, one trustee of Miss Mary Dick and Alex I. MacCallum (1846–1921) and was incorporated by Act of Parliament in 1906. Student numbers had by then been increasing for some years. Veterinary education in Edinburgh had entered a new phase of growth and development (Macdonald, Warwick and Johnston 2005).

Within weeks of the Board's first meeting, the senior staff at Clyde Street had been asked what they thought of the facilities in the College. They had replied that they were unsatisfactory. The Chairman, Sir William Turner, concurred and reported that the lighting of the College was defective partly on account of the small size of the windows and the narrowness of the streets which surrounded the College. The heating arrangements required revision. The condition of the drainage was much complained of, and an adequate water supply was essential for cleanliness (Warwick and Macdonald 2011).

The search for new premises

Initially the idea was to alter the existing building on Clyde Street and to reconstruct the adjoining buildings belonging to the College; outline plans were drawn up to that effect. However, an alternative proposal, to find another site and construct larger premises, began to gain ground. This was not the first time that thoughts of finding new premises for the College had been discussed. In the nineteenth century several suggestions had been made to move away from Clyde Street to alternative locations within Edinburgh; nothing, however, had come of these ideas. It was not surprising, therefore, that in 1907 one of the first practical steps taken by the new Board was to

> enquire privately whether the subjects in Leith Walk formerly occupied as a Veterinary College [the Williams' New Veterinary College buildings, which were vacated in 1904] were in the market and as to the terms on which they could be acquired.

The investigation was unfruitful (Warwick and Macdonald 2011). Within a few weeks, various alternative sites in Edinburgh had been investigated. Charnock Bradley recorded, 'In the afternoon went out to see what Gorgie House Farm was like – it is there it is proposed to remove the College' (Bradley 1907a). Alternative areas on the Gorgie site (in the west of Edinburgh) were discussed and their relative sizes and costs assessed. Selection progressed to an advanced stage and sketch plans were prepared. Again, Charnock Bradley noted: 'Had an hour with McCarthy [sic], the architect, going over the plans of the anatomy department of the proposed new College at Gorgie.' David McArthy (c. 1854–1926) was the architect subsequently chosen to design the Summerhall building. 'In the afternoon, went with Linton to Gorgie to see the most recently contemplated site for a new College. There we unexpectedly came across Gofton, bent on the same errand' (Bradley 1907b). Arthur Gofton was first Professor of Surgery (1905–12) and then Professor of Medicine (1912–14) at Clyde Street.

Once again, the proposed alternative sites were deemed unsuitable. It took more than a year for the Board to reach a decision, in November 1908, about a better alternative. Charnock Bradley observed:

> Meeting unanimously decided that, provided money could be raised the site for the new College Buildings should be in proximity to the university in preference to Slateford or any other site on the outskirts of the city and that the Summerhall site should be acquired if possible. (Warwick and Macdonald 2011)

Thus, it was during the Principalship of John R. U. Dewar (known affectionately as 'Tam' by his students) that the decision was made for the Dick Vet to be transferred from its original Edinburgh New Town site in Clyde Street to the Summerhall Brewery site of about one and a half acres, due south of the University, at the east end of the Meadows (Figure 6.9).

Another year was to pass as various discussions, negotiations and draft plans for the new buildings were made. Each department was asked to list the staff retiring rooms, laboratories, storerooms, museums, dissecting room, histology room, consulting and waiting rooms as well as lavatories, smoking rooms, library and reading rooms and the sundry administrative

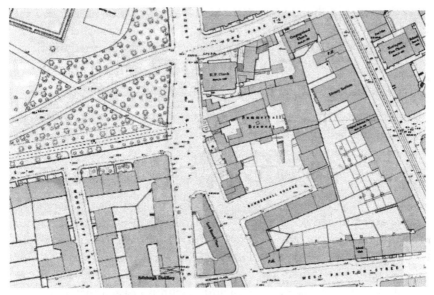

Figure 6.9 Summerhall Brewery site at the east end of the Meadows. Ordnance Survey, 1895. Reproduced with the permission of the National Library of Scotland.

rooms required. On 21 October 1909 *The Scotsman* announced to the public that plans had been made to move the College to Summerhall, and a description of that stage in the design of the building was given. Yet another year passed before the Secretary to the Board was 'instructed to intimate to Messrs Davidson & Syme, W.S., agents for the United Breweries Company Ltd. (the proprietors of the Summerhall site) that the Board was prepared to purchase the site on the terms already arranged' (Warwick and Macdonald 2010). Charnock Bradley reported in his diary of 7 December 1910: 'Today, the Board of Management finally decided to build a new College at the East end of the Meadows' (Bradley 1910). As it happened, Charnock Bradley lived nearby, at Argyle Park Terrace, about two hundred metres to the west of Summerhall.

Charnock Bradley had transferred from Williams' New College to the Clyde Street College in 1900, following graduation with a medical degree. On 18 September he received a telegram from Dewar saying that 'the Town Council had confirmed my appointment to the Dick Chair' (Warwick and Macdonald 2010). He was keen to develop his interest in research at once. Early in December 1902 he 'Received official notice of permission granted by the Senatus of the University to prosecute research as a Research Student; the subject of the research to be, "The Development & Morphology of the Mammalian Cerebellum".' Success followed success. On 2 March 1903 Charnock Bradley was elected a Fellow of the

Royal Society of Edinburgh and on 23 July that year he was awarded the Goodsir Memorial Fellowship. On 7 April 1905: 'Today is a red-letter day; having received the D.Sc.' On 9 February 1907 he mused in his diary, 'Am more or less seriously thinking of trying for the M.D.', and by 26 July that year, after researching the development of the mammalian liver and passing Clinical Medical exams, 'Got the M.D. degree in the morning' (Warwick and Macdonald 2010). Between 1893 and 1908 Charnock Bradley published forty-seven original scientific communications, principally on anatomical, genetical and historical subjects (Greig 1939). In 1908 he was awarded the John Henry Steel memorial medal by the Royal College of Veterinary Surgeons.

During the last years of Dewar's service as Principal, the detailed investigative work undertaken in the College on the meat industry reached a fitting conclusion (Anonymous 1910). In 1910 Professor Gerald R. Leighton and Mr Loudon M. Douglas published a comprehensive five-volume textbook entitled *The Meat Industry and Meat Inspection*. Farm animal meat was discussed in detail and Leighton insisted that a uniform system and standard of meat inspection for the whole country must be provided in the future. The defects of the various British systems when compared to the better-organised continental methods were plainly stated. Fish and poultry meats were also dealt with, together with the conditions that rendered these unfit for human food or dangerous for consumption. This encyclopaedic work echoed the calls for improvement made in Edinburgh some sixty years earlier by Gamgee. The Professorial Chair of Pathology, Bacteriology and Meat Inspection, which Leighton had occupied since 1908, had been founded in the Dick Vet in 1905 by a £15,000 donation from Alexander Inglis McCallum. John Dewar retired at the end of the 1910–11 Session.

References

Anonymous, 1864. Alarming fire in Clyde Street. *The Scotsman*, 17 February 1864, p. 2, col. 5.

Anonymous, 1866a. Memorial to Professor Dick. *The Scotsman*, 14 June 1866, p. 3, col. 2.

Anonymous, 1866b. The Dick Memorial. *The Scotsman*, 4 October 1866, p. 6, col. 6.

Anonymous, 1874a. Sederunt Books, Professor Dick's Trust Minutes of a meeting of the Committee of Management of the Trustees of the late Professor Dick, 3rd September 1874. Vol. 2, p. 35. CRC, The University of Edinburgh.

Anonymous, 1874b. Sederunt Books, Professor Dick's Trust Minutes of a meeting of the Committee of Management of the Trustees of the late Professor Dick, 3rd September 1874. Vol. 2, p. 32. CRC, The University of Edinburgh.

Anonymous, 1883a. Edinburgh Dean of Guild Court. *The Scotsman*, 5 October, p. 4, col. 6; The Royal Commission on the Ancient & Historical Monuments of

Scotland. Edinburgh, Clyde Street, Royal Dick Veterinary College, [Architect's plans] E/2113 (DC/7760), E/21114/CN (DC/7760), E/21115 (DC/7759), E/231116/CN (DC/7759), E/21118/CN (DC/7758), E/21119 (DC/7761), E/21120/CN (DC/7761).

Anonymous, 1883b. Bequest to the Dick Veterinary College and the University of Edinburgh by the late Miss Dick. *The Veterinarian*, 56, 663–4.

Anonymous, 1886c. The (Royal) Dick Veterinary College. *The Veterinary Journal*, 23, 264–5.

Anonymous, 1886d. Unveiling of a statue of the late Professor Dick. *Edinburgh Evening Courant*, 25 October. [Reprinted] The Royal (Dick's) Veterinary College: Unveiling of Professor Dick's statue. *The Veterinary Journal*, 17, 440–4.

Anonymous, 1905. Royal (Dick) Veterinary College, Edinburgh. *The Veterinary Journal*, 61 (8), 91–100.

Anonymous, 1910. The meat industry and meat inspection. An important new work. *The Scotsman*, 2 September 1910, p. 8, col. 4.

Bradley, O. C. 1907a. Diary account, Vol. 3, 1907 Oct 27th. RDSVS Archive, CRC, The University of Edinburgh.

Bradley, O. C. 1907b. Diary account, Vol. 3, 1907 Dec 15th. RDSVS Archive, CRC, The University of Edinburgh.

Bradley, O. C. 1910. Diary account, Vol. 3, 1910 Dec 7th. RDSVS Archive, CRC, The University of Edinburgh.

Bradley, O. C. 1923. *History of the Edinburgh Veterinary College*. Edinburgh: Oliver and Boyd.

Dewar, J. R. U. 1902. Royal (Dick) Veterinary College; opening address. *Veterinary Record*, 15, 215a.

Dollar, T. A. 1894. *Inaugural address delivered by Thomas A. Dollar, M.R.C.V.S. at the opening of the 72nd session of Royal (Dick) Veterinary College Edinburgh, 3rd October 1894. Presentation to the trustees of Miss Dick's Portrait and report of the banquet given to the Lord Provost, Magistrates, and Town Council, and leading members of the medical and veterinary professions.* Edinburgh: Turnbull and Spears.

Edinburgh City Archives, 1865. *The petition of William Dick Esquire.* Plan Room, Location C47, Clyde Street, William Dick, 3 June 1865. Edinburgh City Archives.

Greig, J. R. 1939. Obituary Notice: Orlando Charnock Bradley, M.D., D.Sc., F.R.C.V.S. *Proceedings of the Royal Society of Edinburgh*, 58, 254–7.

Macdonald, A. A. 2013. The Royal (Dick) School of Veterinary Studies – what's in a name? *Veterinary History*, 17, 33–65. <era.ed.ac.uk/handle/1842/7760> (accessed 9 September 2022).

Macdonald, A. A. 2020. Clyde Street 1833–1841: The veterinary teaching and learning environment. *Veterinary History*, 20 (3), 272–306. <era.ed.ac.uk/handle/1842/38679> (accessed 9 September 2022).

Macdonald A. A., Lad, K., Hunzinger, V. J. and Warwick, C. M. 2023. The Edinburgh Veterinary College 1866–1886. *Veterinary History* (in press).

Macdonald, A. A., Warwick, C. M. and Johnston, W. T. 2005. Locating veterinary education in Edinburgh in the nineteenth century. *Book of the Old Edinburgh Club*, New Series, 6, 41–71. <era.ed.ac.uk/handle/1842/2199> (accessed 9 September 2022).

McFadyean, J. 1901. The general education of the veterinary student. *Veterinary Journal*, NS 3, 13–20.

McKendrick, J. G. 1875. *Introductory lecture at the opening of the session 1875–76 of the Edinburgh Royal Veterinary College, 27th October 1875.* Edinburgh: R. & R. Clark.

Morham, R. 1886a. *Edinburgh, Clyde Street, Royal Dick Veterinary College [west elevation].* The Royal Commission on the Ancient & Historical Monuments of Scotland: National Monuments Record of Scotland E/21088 (DC/7773).

Morham, R. 1886b. *Dick Veterinary College. Clyde Street. Proposed Reconstruction.* City Chambers Edinburgh. 10 June 1886.

Prospectus, 1874. *Prospectus 1874–75. Edinburgh Royal Veterinary College. Edinburgh.* CRC, The University of Edinburgh.

Prospectus, 1888. *Prospectus 1888–89, Royal (Dick's) Veterinary College, Clyde Street, Edinburgh.* CRC, The University of Edinburgh.

Prospectus, 1895. *Prospectus 1895–96. Royal (Dick's) Veterinary College. Edinburgh.* CRC, The University of Edinburgh.

RCAHMS, 1832. *Richard and Robert Dickson, Plans of buildings proposed to be erected in Clyde Street by Mr Dick, 1832, E1868-69, E21871, E21873, E21876-77.* Royal Commission of Ancient and Historic Monuments of Scotland.

RCAHMS, 1883. *Edinburgh, Clyde Street, Royal Dick Veterinary College, proposed alterations,* 1883, DC/7758-DC/7761. Royal Commission of Ancient and Historic Monuments of Scotland.

Walley, T. 1878. Opening of the veterinary colleges: Royal Dick College. *The Scotsman,* 24 October 1878, p. 3, col. 5.

[Walley, T.] 1878. Edinburgh Veterinary College: An address. *The Veterinarian,* 51, 829–34.

Walley, T. 1892. *Inaugural address delivered on the occasion of the opening of the 70th session of the Royal (Dick) Veterinary College Edinburgh.* [Edinburgh, 1892], p. 16.

Warwick, C. M. and Macdonald A. A. 2010. The life of Professor Orlando Charnock Bradley, (1871–1937): Diary entries 1895–1923. Part 1. *Veterinary History,* 15 (3), 205–20. <era.ed.ac.uk/handle/1842/3643> (accessed 9 September 2022).

Warwick, C. M. and Macdonald, A. A. 2011. The life of Professor Orlando Charnock Bradley, (1871–1937): Building the Summerhall site. Part 2. *Veterinary History,* 15 (4), 309–34. <era.ed.ac.uk/handle/1842/4837> (accessed 9 September 2022).

Videos – Clyde Street virtual tour. <www.ed.ac.uk/vet/about/history/clyde-street/clyde-tour> (accessed 9 September 2022).

Anatomy Lecture Theatre
The Courtyard
The Balcony
The Dissecting Room
Upper Chemistry Laboratory
West Lecture Theatre

Chapter 7

The Dick Vet at Summerhall (1911–47)

Orlando Charnock Bradley installed as Principal

On 12 June 1911 Orlando Charnock Bradley took up the duties of Principal as well as those of Professor of Anatomy and Histology at the Royal (Dick) Veterinary College (Figure 7.1). That same year, he was offered the Mary Dick-endowed Barclay and Goodsir Lectureship in Comparative Anatomy in the University of Edinburgh, thereby sustaining and increasing the link between the Royal (Dick) Veterinary College and the University. He was also elected to the Council of the Royal College of Veterinary Surgeons, where he subsequently served twice as Vice-President (1912 and 1919) before being elected as President on 1 July 1920 (Warwick and Macdonald 2010). The story of the development of the Dick Vet was entering a new phase. It was under strong academic leadership with modern teaching facilities, research encouragement, expanding international links and testing social environmental circumstances. These were the core 'threads' running through the next three decades. Much of this can be learned from the diary entries made by Charnock Bradley (Warwick and Macdonald 2011). Charnock Bradley's staff in 1911 comprised Arthur Gofton, Professor of Medicine and Materia Medica; Ainsworth Wilson, Professor of Surgery and Obstetrics; Gerald Leighton, Professor of Pathology, Bacteriology, and Meat Inspection; David A. Farquharson, Professor of Physiology; George H. Gemmell, Professor of Chemistry and Physic; R. Stewart MacDougall, Professor of Biology (Zoology and Botany); and J. Basil Buxton, Hospital Surgeon and Lecturer on Hygiene and Dietetics, and Stable Management (Calendar 1911). The assistant to the Professor of Anatomy was William M. Mitchell. All third- and fourth-year students were required to act as Dressers, Dispensers and Visitors, and would receive, on obtaining their

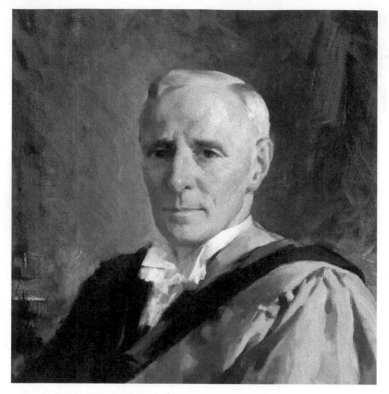

Figure 7.1 Detail of the portrait of Orlando Charnock Bradley in academic gown painted by Stanley Cursiter (1887–1976) in 1936. Photographer: Colin M. Warwick.

diplomas, Certificates of Merit, if their duties had been performed to the satisfaction of the Clinical Instructors (Calendar 1911).

Almost immediately it became clear to Charnock Bradley that the plans of the College, as drafted so far, were not sufficiently modern in outlook. From his diary we learn: 'The Board of the College are sending the architect – McArthy – and myself to see the schools at Brussels & Hanover' (Warwick and Macdonald 2011). On 5 September 1911 Charnock Bradley and McArthy got their bearings in Brussels, and 'after lunch we went to the veterinary school & went over part of it', and on the following day, 'the veterinary school was again visited in the morning'. On 9 September 'an inspection of the Hanover veterinary school occupied the whole of the morning' and on 13 September 'nearly the whole day was occupied by a visit to Aldershot to look at the Army Veterinary School there' (Warwick and Macdonald 2011). This search for new ideas in veterinary college design was much the same as William Dick had undertaken almost a century earlier (Macdonald, Warwick and Johnston 2005). That autumn, in his inaugural address, Charnock Bradley drew on all the strands of his College and University training to establish the foundations of his time as Principal, research promoter and link between Veterinary Medicine and Medicine:

> It is clear that the health of the community is constantly menaced by danger of a double origin. Not only may disease and death have a human source: there is an animal source as well . . . From his knowledge of all the phases of diseases in animals, no one is better fitted than the veterinary surgeon to assist in the safeguarding of man from disease of animal origin.(Bradley 1911)

College links to the University were further strengthened by the institution of the degrees of Bachelor and Doctor of Science in Veterinary Science within the University in 1911 (Warwick and Macdonald 2011).

On 3 April 1912 Charnock Bradley attended the Board meeting at which plans for the new building were passed (Figures 7.2, 7.3). The building was designed for the four-year course of training and an average yearly total number of 150 students, an approximate doubling of the then current student numbers (Mitchell 1951). A Building Fund was initiated to raise the money required to build the Veterinary College at Summerhall; an estimated total of £65,000 was required. Half of this sum was to be funded by the national government and the rest raised by public subscription (Warwick and Macdonald 2011). Examples of the 'public' donors included: Alex I. MacCallum (grad. Dick Vet 1867), who gave £10,000; Edinburgh Town Council, £3,000; the Carnegie Trustees, £3,000; the Guarantors of the Exhibition of 1908, £2,000; both the Midlothian County Council and the Highland and Agricultural Society of Scotland gave £600; the County Council of Aberdeen donated £250; the staff of the College gave £212 12s. Additional money was raised by an appeal to the alumni: 'Home all evening, trying to draft an appeal to old students for subscriptions to the building-fund.' A 'For Sale' sign was placed on the College buildings in Clyde Street in February 1913 (Warwick and Macdonald 2011). Total student numbers in the Clyde Street College remained fairly steady during Charnock Bradley's first three years as Principal: 74 in 1911–12, 78 in 1912–13 and 77 in 1913–14.

Construction of the Summerhall buildings

Charnock Bradley's diaries show that he was personally involved in the detailed planning of Summerhall, initially consulting with the architect: 'Down at McArthy's from 6 onwards going over sketch plans of the new College buildings. Had the staff of the College to meet the architect in

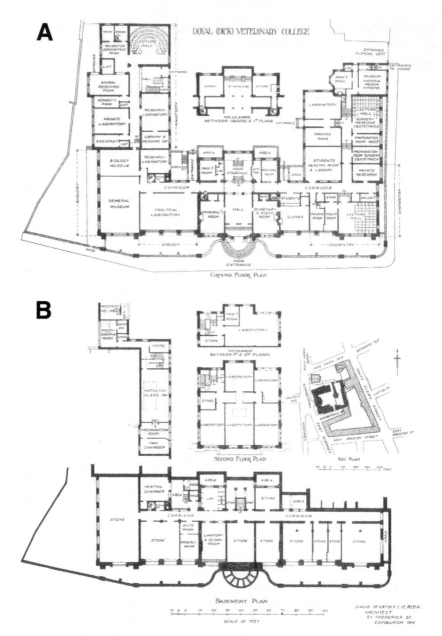

Figure 7.2 Plans of Summerhall Veterinary College by architect David McArthy in 1914. A. The ground floor and first mezzanine; B. The basement, second floor and second mezzanine.

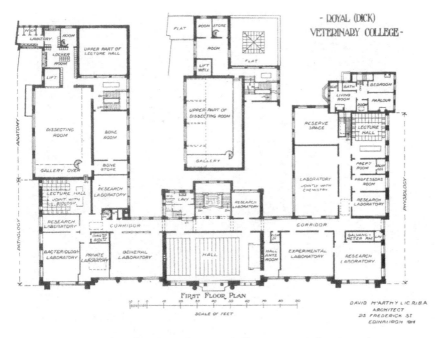

Figure 7.3 Plans of the first floor of Summerhall Veterinary College by architect David McArthy in 1914.

order to consider the plans of the new buildings.' By 1913 tenders for the new building had been submitted, Mr J. H. Lightbody, the Surveyor, appointed, and the old buildings on the site were demolished. Charnock Bradley paid 'a visit to Summerhall at 12.30 [on 23 October] to see the big chimney felled'. Less than four weeks later, on 11 November 1913, he 'found the actual building has begun' (his underlining). Later in November, Charnock Bradley was 'taking steps regarding the foundation-stone of the new buildings' (Warwick and Macdonald 2011).

He wrote that 21 July 1914 was 'A red-letter day. The Marquis [sic] of Linlithgow laid the Memorial Stone of the new buildings at Summerhall. The weather was perfect, the sun hot; & the ceremony is said to have gone off well' (Figure 7.4). Charnock Bradley had a particular aptitude for organising such ceremonial occasions, as indicated in the minutes of the Property, Law and Finance Committee: 'Stand accommodation decorations etc. to cost £130 ... the Secretary to arrange for the attendance of a good brass band [from Kirkcaldy] at a cost not exceeding £15:15/-, and to accept Messers McVittie Guest & Co's estimate for tea, coffee and ices at 1/3d per head', as was later recounted by the College secretary (Doull 1937). The ceremony was presided over by the Lord Provost of Edinburgh, Sir Robert Kirk Inches, wearing his official robes and regalia. Others on

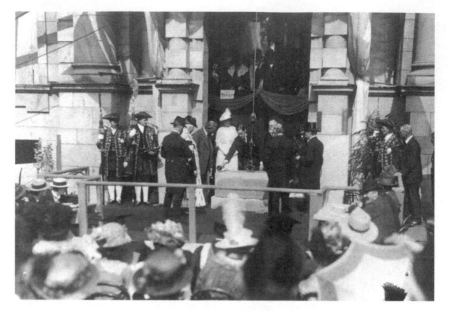

Figure 7.4 The ceremonial laying of the Memorial Stone at the main entrance of the Summerhall Veterinary College, 21 July 1914. Photographer: unknown.

the platform included the Marquess and Marchioness of Linlithgow, the Chairman of the Board of Management, Professor Sir John Rankine, and other Board members. Many attended the ceremony in addition to representatives of the Board of Agriculture, the Highland and Agriculture Society, the Scottish Universities and other Scottish educational and public bodies. Under the Memorial Stone was 'deposited a sealed lead casket containing a copy of the Scotsman, a portrait of the Founder, a copy of the current College Calendar, and coins of the realm' (Bradley 1923). Despite the fact that seven days later, on 28 July 1914, war was declared between Great Britain and Germany, building continued throughout 1914 and 1915 (Figure 7.5). On 12 December 1914, 'at 9 o'clock the last stone was set at the top of the front block of the new buildings' (Warwick and Macdonald 2011).

On 21 July 1914 *The Scotsman* described the building under construction in the following terms:

> The front, in the Renaissance style, is divided into a central and slightly projecting block, 60 feet in length; two sections, one on each side, each 40 feet in length; and two wings, 33 feet each. In the main portion is placed the principal entrance, approached by a semicircular flight of stairs. The entrance door is flanked by two Ionic columns, which rise two storeys; over the doorway is a large triple-light window surmounted by a cornice and semicircular pediment with carving, and at the height of another storey the wall head is

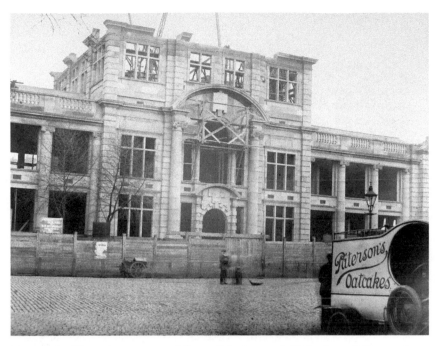

Figure 7.5 The main entrance and front of the Summerhall Veterinary College under construction. Photographer: O. C. Bradley.

finished by a plain-moulded cornice, open balustrade, and vases [Figure 7.6]. The two sections of the building on each side of the entrance are divided into three bays by Ionic columns, the two ranges of windows being of a large size, so as to give the maximum of light to the rooms. The wings are marked off from the main building by rusticated pilasters and columns, and are surmounted by moulded pediments with carvings. (Anonymous 1914)

Sadly, wartime financial constraints prevented the creation of the large 'carving' mentioned.

The main buildings are three storeys in height, the central part rising to a height of four storeys ... The south wing is two storeys high and the north wing three ... there are provided seventeen laboratories, five lecture theatres ... large dissection room to accommodate sixty-two students, a hall for special functions seated for three hundred persons ... There is a large general museum and several departmental museums ... In the clinical department [Figure 7.7] ... the accommodation includes post-mortem room, stocks and 'X'-Ray apartment, and rooms for teaching pharmacy and giving surgical demonstrations ... and there are waiting and consulting rooms. (Anonymous 1914)

Much remained to be done. Charnock Bradley's diary records that he personally oversaw the progress of construction with regular, almost daily

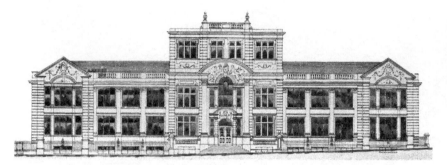

Figure 7.6 Architect's drawing of the proposed façade of the Summerhall Veterinary College. From the 1915–16 Calendar.

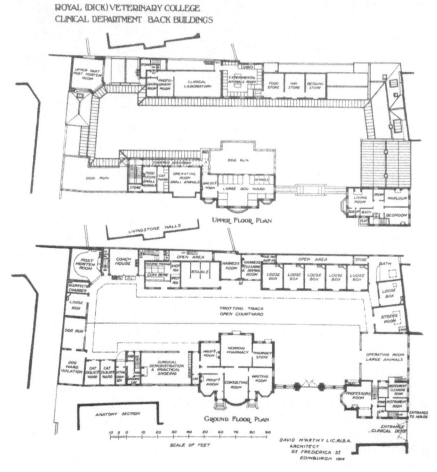

Figure 7.7 Plan of the Clinical Buildings of the Summerhall Veterinary College by architect David McArthy in 1914.

Number of students

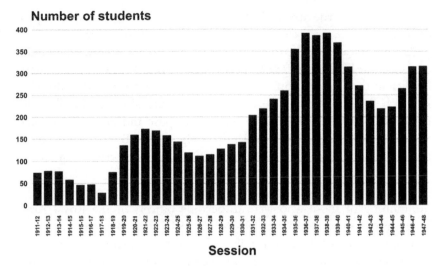

Figure 7.8 Annual account of the total number of undergraduate students attending the Royal (Dick) Veterinary College, 1911–49.

visits to the new buildings, accompanied by his pet dog, Tinker. Despite the hostilities in France, the building of Summerhall continued relatively unimpeded, as did general life in Edinburgh. However, there were problems with reduced student intake (Figure 7.8). In 1915, 'As a result of the [war] recruiting effort, Class B is now reduced to <u>one</u> student!' (Warwick and Macdonald 2010).

Summerhall occupied but not completed

Throughout 1915, Charnock Bradley and the Board were beset with financial worries resulting from the construction (Warwick and Macdonald 2011). In September the Board considered it was 'very advisable that as many classes as practicable should be transferred to the new buildings at the soonest date possible'. By January 1916 the buildings were sufficiently ready for occupation. On the 17th, 'Classes A, B & C were transferred today to the new buildings at Summerhall Square.' On 15 April, Charnock Bradley records: 'Today the clinical department was transferred from Clyde St to the new buildings at Summerhall. This means that the removal of the College is now complete.' Only two weeks before, on 3 April, during a Zeppelin raid, a bomb fell on nearby Causewayside. Charnock Bradley recorded this event but did not register any concern he may have had about the possible destruction of his new College buildings (Warwick and Macdonald 2011). At about that time the statue of William Dick was removed from Clyde Street, cleaned and re-erected onto a renovated pedestal near the Anatomy entrance in the Summerhall courtyard.

During these difficult years, J. Russell Greig (1889–1963), who graduated from the Dick Vet in 1911, became Professor of Medicine and Materia Medica in the College from 1919 to 1930 and Director of the Moredun Research Institute from 1930 to 1954. He wrote of O. C. Bradley: 'his dominant qualities, quiet steadfastness to purpose and unswerving determination were most clearly evident' (Greig 1939). By 1917 the building debt had shrunk to £1,700 and the balance was written off by the Agriculture (Scotland) Fund (Anonymous 1917).

Since the outbreak of war the College had been solely concerned with the training of those who were to become officers in the Royal Army Veterinary Corps (Rankine 1917). In 1915 the Board's Education Committee recorded: 'the possibility of holding an extra Summer Term was under consideration (owing to the demand for Veterinary Officers)'. After the war, on 17 March 1919, Charnock Bradley noted: 'Though the normal Term has ended, we are carrying on for the benefit of demobilised students.' The War Department had taken possession of the Clyde Street buildings on 16 June 1916 for sixty men of the Army Veterinary Corps, but it was understood that the occupation would be of a very short duration. In fact, the army remained there for over three years. At about the same time, the new Summerhall buildings were inspected with a view to them being requisitioned for use as a military hospital. Correspondence during the following twelve months stressed that 'interruption of or interfering with the training of Veterinary Students at this critical time would be most serious from a National point of view and would cripple the work of the college for many years to come'. However, it was not until May 1917 that this possibility was finally removed (Warwick and Macdonald 2011). Nevertheless, on 28 February 1918 Charnock Bradley wrote: 'Returned to Edinburgh. Found that the National Service people have taken the empty rooms at the College for temporary offices.' The National Service staff formally occupied the rooms from 13 March 1918 at a rent of £300 per year. When they moved out, staff from the Board of Agriculture took their place, on the College Board's understanding that this occupation would not extend beyond Whitsunday (8 June 1919). However, the Agriculture staff remained, and did not leave until 11 February 1921, at which time the temporary partitions segregating them from the teaching accommodation were removed (Warwick and Macdonald 2011).

The possibilities for future College development were not ignored during the war. On 29 January 1917 Charnock Bradley noted: 'Went with a deputation to the Board of Agriculture from the College Board to try to get a Research Station'; and on 5 February: 'Then out to Colinton with

Sir Robert Wright to look at a place for research animals.' On 15 August 1917 Charnock Bradley wrote: 'We are starting a Sheep Diseases Research laboratory at the College. Rich & Petrie are to do the work.' A year later, on 16 September 1918, he recorded: 'revising some notes relating to desirable post-bellum development at the College'; and five weeks later, on 21 October: 'The evening was passed preparing a skeleton memorandum of how the College should be developed, post-bellum.' One element of this, his interest in promoting animal disease research, took another step forward when on 28 February 1919, 'At 1.30 there was a meeting at the H.&A. Soc [Highland and Agricultural Society] rooms, previous to going as a deputation to the Board of Agriculture to press for a scheme of research in animal diseases.' This scheme was detailed in the Board's minutes, with the following as part of the introduction: 'The Royal (Dick) Veterinary College in Edinburgh is the most suitable Institution to form the nucleus of the movement. The new College Buildings are devised with this end in view and are provided with laboratories in which a start can be made' (Warwick and Macdonald 2011).

Post-war College developments

At the end of the war Charnock Bradley reported to the Board of Management that the increase in student numbers (Figure 7.8) and the large numbers of students in the junior classes had placed a severe tax on the resources of the College (Bradley 1920). In certain practical courses it had been necessary to divide the classes into sections. In this way the efficiency of the teaching had been maintained. He indicated that it was very probable that this method of dealing with large classes would have to be adopted to an even larger extent during the next Session. The Matriculation Fee had remained at 1 guinea, but the Class Fees had been raised: for the first period of thirty weeks, £19 19s. 0d.; for the second period of thirty weeks, £18 18s. 0d.; for the third period of thirty weeks, £16 16s 0d.; and for the fourth period of thirty weeks, £15 15s. 0d. (Prospectus 1918–19). There was an urgent need for additional equipment, especially microscopes. A new course of lectures on Veterinary Jurisprudence had been given during the Session by Mr J. R. Gibb, Advocate, and the first course for the Diploma in Veterinary State Medicine, recently instituted by the RCVS, was held during the Session. The reorganisation of the Clinical Department had enabled an increase in the number of operations performed. During Session 1920–1 the usual short courses in Pathology, Bacteriology and Protozoology were held and a six-month course of instruction leading to the Diploma in Veterinary State Medicine was given for the second time.

During the last week of the Summer Vacation in 1921, a one-week course for Practitioners was given for the first time. Though only six Practitioners attended, the course was so well received as to justify repetition.

Within a week of the staff from the Board of Agriculture moving out of the College's Summerhall buildings, on 11 February 1921:

> A letter was read from the Interim Secretary of the Animal Diseases Research Association [ADRA] asking if the College would be willing to grant the use of laboratories for Research and to absorb the Research Workers as Members of the College Staff.

The Board agreed. On 24 April 1922 Charnock Bradley 'visited three places with Milne, Gaiger & Dalling – looking for land for research animals', and on 1 May recorded: 'journey in the course of the morning to see Moredun Dairy with the Secretary of the A.D.R.A'. By January 1925, Professor Sydney H. Gaiger, Principal of Glasgow Veterinary College and the first Director of ADRA, Moredun, had accepted the invitation to become an Honorary Research Professor in Animal Pathology in the College. Three years later the top floor of the central block of the main College building at Summerhall had been prepared as research laboratories for ADRA, at a nominal rent of £5 per year (plus heating, lighting, water, etc.) (Warwick and Macdonald 2011).

The blight cast on the physical development of the College by the war was not lifted immediately thereafter. The Summerhall buildings were still far from complete. The laboratories were not fully furnished or fitted out. Money was raised in 1922 to establish a War Memorial Library (Anonymous 1922), and the Clyde Street alumni paid for stained-glass windows (Plate 7.1A) to go on the stairway leading up from the entrance hallway to the first floor (Figure 7.9) (Warwick and Macdonald 2011). The centenary celebrations on 27 and 28 November 1923, when Sir John McFadyean delivered the William Dick Oration, were considered a great success and it was agreed that an Annual Oration, or Founder's Day, would be an institution from which nothing but good would arise (Bradley 1924). The Oration brought people to the College who otherwise would have remained in ignorance of its functions and activities.

In 1924–5, by arrangement with ADRA and with the consent of the Board of Agriculture for Scotland, Prof. Sidney H. Gaiger, FRCVS, was appointed Honorary Research Professor in Animal Pathology in the College. This enabled an additional Assistant, Mr H. Preston, to be appointed in that department, with his primary duty being connected with the diagnosis of diseases of poultry.

Twelve years after its inception, the Veterinary College at Summerhall was completed on 17 October 1925. Charnock Bradley excitedly recorded:

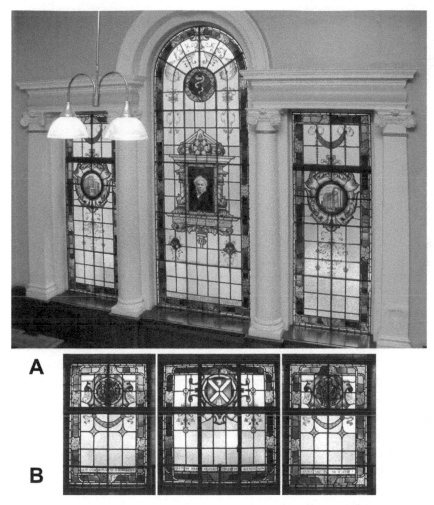

Plate 7.1 A. Photograph of the three large commemorative windows lighting the stairway from the Entrance Hall to the first floor, installed in 1923; B. Photograph of the three commemorative windows 'below the stairs' unveiled on 27 June 1928. Photographer: Colin M. Warwick.

the morning was mainly occupied making arrangements for the formal 'Opening' of the College new buildings on Monday next. [And on that Monday] The formal 'Opening' of the College new buildings at 2.30 by the Secretary for Scotland [Sir John Gilmour] – a great day. Hall full to overflowing.

As a result of work undertaken during the summer of 1925, all the classrooms and laboratories were now provided with permanent fittings, and additions had been made to the equipment (Bradley 1926). However, Charnock Bradley, in his vote of thanks, indicated gently that he had plans

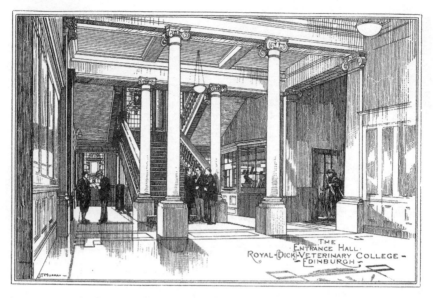

Figure 7.9 The Summerhall Entrance Hall drawing by J. T. Murray. From the 1936–7 Calendar.

for expansion in the future. True to his word, on 22 December 1926 he 'called at the College to meet Nasmyth & McCallum to talk over the possible purchase of land for an extension of the college'. More than a decade earlier, in 1913, the Board had noted 'Mr Alston's proposal to sell buildings and ground in Hope Park Terrace' but had decided not to do anything in the meantime (Warwick and Macdonald 2011). This ground lay immediately to the north of the College, between the United Free Church and the Congregational Church in Hope Park Terrace, and was then occupied by a miscellaneous collection of one-storey shops, stables and sheds (Figure 6.9).

In Session 1926–7 the number of students attending classes leading to the Diploma of MRCVS was only seven fewer than during the previous Session (Figure 7.8). The number of new entrants about equalled the average for the preceding five years. The intake for the following year was thirty-seven, among whom was a graduate in Veterinary Science from an Italian University. The Matriculation Fee was now half a guinea, and the class fee was 25 guineas for each session of three terms.

In the spring of 1927 'the question of a suitable Coat of Arms for the College was remitted to the Principal, to consult with the Principal of the Edinburgh College of Art [Gerald Moira, 1867–1959] as to a suitable design' (Board 1927). Eight months later a design was submitted to the Board of Management and approved, subject to an alteration being made to the design for the horse's head (Plate 7.2A). At the same meeting

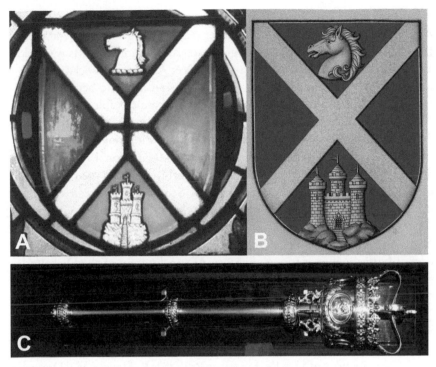

Plate 7.2   A. Image in stained glass of the design for the Coat of Arms approved in 1928; B. The Coat of Arms of the Royal (Dick) Veterinary College awarded on 12 January 1931 by the Lord Lyon King of Arms; C. The College mace presented by Emeritus Professor R. Stewart MacDougall in 1930. Photographer: Colin M. Warwick.

Charnock Bradley submitted drawings for three additional stained-glass windows, the central one of which carried the approved design for the Coat of Arms. He proposed that these should be installed over the windows at the rear of the main entrance to the College, behind the main staircase. These designs were also approved (Plate 7.1B). The total cost would be borne by the gentlemen who had graduated since the new Summerhall buildings had been erected. The windows were unveiled on 27 June 1928 by Viscount Novar (Bradley 1928). The Coat of Arms for the Veterinary College that had been petitioned by Orlando Charnock Bradley (Principal) and Alexander Campbell Doull (Secretary) was awarded by the Lord Lyon King of Arms on 12 January 1931, and recorded (Lord Lyon 1931). It was described as 'Azure, a saltire between a horse's head couped in chief and in base a triple towered castle all Argent, masoned Sable, windows, flags and portcullis gules, situate on a rock proper' (Plate 7.2B).

During Session 1927–8 additional staff resources were obtained; Dr T. H. Cameron lectured on Helminthology, Mr W. C. Miller lectured on Genetics, Mr W. P. Blount was appointed as Demonstrator of Anatomy and Mr W. L. Weipers was appointed as a Senior Clinical Assistant. Sadly, two years later the latter resigned to go into general practice. On 9 May 1930 a meeting of graduates and senior students was held at which it was agreed to establish a Dick Vet Alumnus Association. The number of enrolled members of the Association and the occurrence of the recent International Veterinary Congress 'made possible a highly successful reunion of graduates from all parts of the Empire' (Bradley 1930). The First Annual Meeting, on 7 August 1930, in the Zoological Gardens, London, was attended by over eighty members (Cameron 1930). During Session 1927–8 Bradley reported that the various classes were attended by students from twenty-two counties in Scotland; seventeen counties in England and Wales; nine counties in Ireland; and from Guernsey, Australia, India, Palestine, China, Italy, South Africa, the Gold Coast, Nyasaland and Southern Rhodesia (Bradley 1928). This was a clear indication of both the intra-national and international nature of the Dick Vet's veterinary education.

The College mace

In 1930, in memory of his wife, Emeritus Professor R. Stewart MacDougall presented a mace to the College (Figure 7.2c). Designed and constructed by Messrs. Brook & Son, Goldsmiths to His Majesty the King, 87 George Street, Edinburgh, the following is their description of the mace:

> The Mace is made of Silver, gilded all over, and measures three feet in length.
> The head is hemi-spherical in form and is richly embossed with thistle ornament in its lower portion, which also serves to separate four circular medallions. These are filled respectively with (1) The arms of the Royal (Dick) Veterinary College, Edinburgh, (2) St. Andrew, the patron saint of Scotland, (3) The Lion Rampant, Scotland's national emblem, and (4) the inscription which reads as follows:-
> 'Presented to the Royal (Dick) Veterinary College by Robert Stewart MacDougall in dear memory of his wife Eliza H. Stewart MacDougall 1930'
> The upper portion of the head [of the mace] forms the fillet of the crown and consists of a broad raised band of ornament, and above a row of fleur de lys and crosses alternately. From these spring four arches which are surmounted at their junction by the orb and cross, the whole being an adaptation of the ancient Royal Crown of Scotland which reposes with other pieces of the regalia in Edinburgh Castle. The Staff of the Mace consists of a plain cylindrical tube divided into two portions and a neckband by two beaded bands and a terminal and chased above and below with panels of Celtic ornament.
> Further evidence of the Scottish character of the design is seen in the four scroll-shaped brackets with unicorns' heads that enrich the neckband.
> (Brook & Son 1930; Bradley 1931)

This mace was treasured by the College and for many decades was paraded at graduation and other important College ceremonies.

An unusually large number (seventy-seven) of students entered the College for the first time during Session 1931–2 (Figure 7.8). This was due, partly at least, to the fact that the Royal College of Veterinary Surgeons had decreed that those students entering the Veterinary Colleges after the beginning of the Summer Term in 1932 must undergo training extending over five years, with five examinations, instead of four as formerly. However, although the intention may have been to give both student and teacher more leisure, the addition and extension of subjects to study did not make the class timetables any less congested. The acquisition of a Country Clinical Station at Dalkeith, donated in December 1930 by John Aitken of Dalkeith, greatly assisted the provision of additional larger farm animal teaching material. The new Department of Diseases of Poultry had developed considerably; during the 1931–2 season over 80,000 agglutination tests for bacillary white diarrhoea had been carried out, as against 13,500 in the previous season. The number of poultry post-mortem examinations had also materially increased, and, at the request of the Department of Agriculture for Scotland, the preparation of fowlpox vaccine had been undertaken. Although the preparation of the vaccine only began in October 1931, 15,500 doses were distributed between that date and 30 June 1932.

The number of matriculated students (219) attending classes during Session 1932–3 was the largest for any year for which the Dick Vet had definite records (Figure 7.8). The large and abnormal influx during the previous Session – the last Session permitting entry under the regulations for the four-year curriculum – contributed materially to this result. The unexpectedly large entry at the beginning of the Autumn Term helped considerably. The number (forty-nine) of new entrants was in excess of that for any previous year except the one immediately following the end of the war. It is noteworthy that twelve of the new entrants were admitted to the Second Year Classes by virtue of their possession of University Degrees or of having passed in the subjects of Chemistry, Physics, Botany and Zoology (or Biology) in an examination for a degree. A growing number of entrants already held University Degrees. At the end of the 1932–3 Session there were twenty students who possessed either a BA or a BSc Degree. During the 1933–4 Session, sixty-three students enrolled for the first time (Figure 7.8).

In a very important step towards a closer relationship with the University of Edinburgh, on 5 October 1934 the Order in Council was signed whereby the College was 'affiliated' to the University of Edinburgh (Bradley 1934).

During the 1934–5 Session, Bradley noted that 'the most important recent event in the history of veterinary science in Scotland' was the institution of a Research Board, consisting of representatives of the Animal Diseases Research Association, the College, the Department of Agriculture for Scotland and the National Veterinary Medical Association (Bradley 1935). It was the duty of the Board to co-ordinate and supervise Scottish veterinary research and foster a closer association of research and education. The Board reported that arrangements were in progress for members of the staff of the Animal Diseases Research Association to take some part in the teaching of veterinary students, with a view to linking as closely as possible veterinary teaching and research in Edinburgh.

During 1935–6 the academic status of the College physiologist, Henry Dryerre, was raised from part-time to that of a full-time member of the staff. His paper, with J. Russell Greig, describing 'The specific chemotherapy of milk fever by the parentral administration of calcium borogluconate' was judged a significant life-saving contribution for hypocalcaemic states in veterinary species.

Extension of the Summerhall infrastructure

At the Board meeting on 16 January 1929 it was reported:

> The Principal [Charnock Bradley had] indicated that the grounds and buildings on the south side of Hope Park Terrace, adjoining the College, could be purchased for a reasonable figure. It was agreed that such purchase would be very advantageous to the College, and it was resolved to approach the Department of Agriculture for Scotland for sanction to proceed with the proposal.

Further progress, however, was slow and it was not until 1 November 1929 that Charnock Bradley recorded 'the first interview with the architect, Constable, about plans for the building extension'. About six years were then to pass before he noted in his diary on 23 January 1936: 'a meeting to determine upon a Committee to make an appeal for funds for the extension of the College. "Extension" has been in the air for several years, but nothing has been done.' Later that year, the Chairman of the Board reported:

> When they decided to build twenty years ago on the present site they went carefully into the number of students who were likely to be in attendance during each year of study. Allowing for the prospective growth they had provided laboratories, lecture rooms, and a hospital, which they thought would be adequate for a considerable number of years. But the demand for veterinary workers, not only in this country, but in the tropical Dominions,

had grown so rapidly that their rooms were no longer anything like sufficient in size or capacity to give the proper training they desired to give to their students. (Beare 1936)

The introduction in 1930 of the six-month (October to March) University postgraduate Diploma in Tropical Veterinary Medicine and the extension in 1932 of the College's veterinary course to five years had placed additional demands on the available space (Figure 7.8) (Warwick and Macdonald 2011).

Funding for the extension was estimated at £40,000, for which a Government grant on the £ for £ basis of up to £20,000 from the Development Fund was offered. Charnock Bradley personally undertook fundraising for the College's share, tirelessly addressing letters ('begging' – his word) and writing envelopes. Appeals to the public for funds for the extension were frequently announced in the press (Warwick and Macdonald 2011). Construction began on the extension (eventually designed by architects Lorimer & Matthew FFRIBA) on 8–9 May 1937.

Charnock Bradley did not live to see his vision fulfilled. He died on 21 November 1937. Many tributes were paid to the services which he gave to science and to the College in particular (Greig 1939). He had striven for many years to improve veterinary education and to bring it into closer relationship with Medicine. He wanted the College's standard of veterinary education to be worthy of recognition and acceptance by the University of Edinburgh (Greig 1939).

Sir Arthur Olver appointed Principal

Following Charnock Bradley's death, Robert G. Linton was appointed as acting Principal. Sir Arthur Olver then assumed duty as administrative head of the College on 7 September 1938 (Figure 7.10); the Principal's Office had been divested of all teaching responsibility. He faced significant problems. War in Europe was looming again. Fresh action was urgently needed to raise funds for the College extension; only one portion of it, the Anatomy Block, had been completed. The teaching staff was very seriously depleted, owing to the impossibility of securing suitable lecturers at the very low rates of pay then offered; it sorely needed strengthening. At the same time the subordinate technical and laboratory personnel needed graded scales of pay corresponding to those being paid to those performing similar duties in Edinburgh University. In June 1939 Olver also commented that

they were faced with the teaching of 400 students, three times as many as the College was designed to accommodate originally, and with providing a

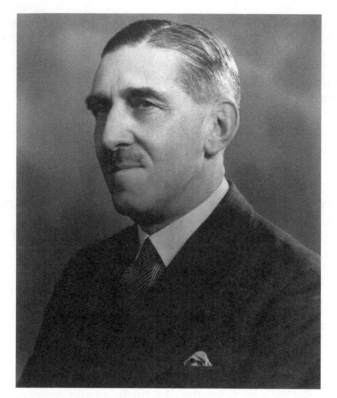

Figure 7.10 Professor Olver. Photographer: unknown.

course of training which was much longer – five years instead of four – and much more extensive than was the case in the past. (Olver, 1939a)

The very large student intakes in 1935, 1936 and 1937 (Figure 7.8) resulted in the intake numbers being restricted in 1938 and 1939 (Olver 1939b, 1940).

During the autumn of 1939, in accordance with the views Linton had earlier expressed in various venues, steps were taken to draw up a modified curriculum and timetable for the University degree of BSc in Veterinary Science and for the MRCVS course, to enable students to take the two courses concurrently, without overlapping. Principal Olver was fortunate in securing, from the Department of Agriculture for Scotland, a special grant to provide the very considerable number of up-to-date microscopes which were then sorely needed to make it possible to carry on the effective training of students (Olver 1945). Funding for the build-ing extension was found from various sources, and it was opened in 1940 (Figure 7.11).

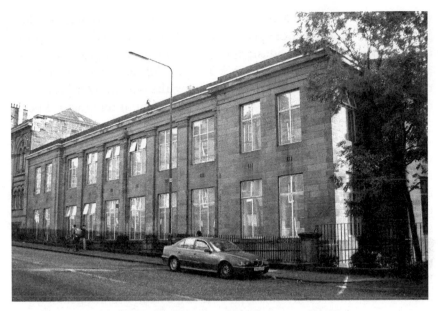

Figure 7.11 North extension of the College building on Hope Park Terrace. Photographer: Colin M. Warwick.

The Dick Vet during the Second World War

During the autumn of 1938, it had been decided that the College would not be evacuated in the event of hostilities. The alternative suggestion made early in 1939 was that arrangements should be made for the prompt evacuation of the students into the country on receipt of an Air Raid Precautions (ARP) warning. This was found to be impracticable. So, to provide satisfactory protection for all students, staff, clients and workmen likely to be at the College during an air raid (approximately five hundred people), it was necessary to incorporate within the air-raid shelter the existing students' smoke room, kitchen, cloakroom and lavatory as well as the old Officers Training Corps (OTC) office, armoury and miniature rifle range. All of these rooms were in the central and southern portion of the basement, the only place in the College where adequate protection could be provided. Initially, vertical 18 x 15 cm wooden posts were brought in to strengthen support of the basement ceilings. Windows were protected with old wooden piles and sandbagging (Olver 1939c). Later that summer of 1939, all the basement ceilings were covered with 23 x 8 cm timber on the flat supported by uprights of 15 x 13 cm and 18 x 15 cm timber. An improvised refectory, with luncheon room, snack bar, kitchen and scullery, was fitted up in the southern portion of the basement, staffed by 'a grand little lady who was called Mrs Dick by the students'. This accommodation and the old rifle range were permanently blacked out and fitted up for lectures, magic-lantern demonstrations, committee meetings and a certain amount of recreation up to 10 o'clock at night. All classrooms and lecture theatres had to be closed at 4 o'clock during the winter. War broke out on 3 September 1939. During that year a great deal of training had been carried out by the strong contingent of Dick College students (about 250) who had been enrolled in the Home Guard. The College contingent was under the administrative command of Thomas Grahame and was organised in sections to constitute a mobile reinforcing body in association with the Edinburgh University OTC. Reciprocal access given to the pitches on the University's recreation fields was of great benefit to the veterinary students (Olver 1939b).

At the request of the Deans of the Royal College of Surgeons and the Dental School, fifty-three of their students received instruction in Histology and Embryology at the Veterinary College at the beginning of the 1940 Summer Term. This type of arrangement was in operation for Physiology and Biochemistry from the beginning of the Autumn Term of Session 1940–1. During that session the opportunity arose to purchase Hope Park Church, which stood on the north corner of the site occupied by the College. It continued to be used by the Department of Health for Scotland for the storage of medical and surgical equipment and other material until the end of the war. The original sandbagging erected along the front of the College to provide air-raid protection had steadily deteriorated, and so it was removed. The sandbagging inside the courtyard remained (Figure 7.12). The College Home Guard Unit, involving all the students, continued to function very effectively during the session under the command of (now Major) Grahame and was recognised as one of the most highly trained Units in Edinburgh. Owing to war conditions, the amount of clinical material available at the College hospital was at first very much reduced. Later in the 1940–1 Session the number of horses increased considerably, but the numbers of small animal patients admitted to hospital remained comparatively small. This was inevitable because of the very large numbers of dogs and cats that were destroyed at the start of the war. The total number of students attending the College for the 1940–1 Session was 314. The composite curriculum fee that Session had risen to 33 guineas per Session of three terms. This included the Matriculation Fee, Athletic Club Fee, Curriculum Fee and all laboratory fees. An additional six graduates and occasional students and sixty-eight medical and dental students were under instruction at the College. The number of new veterinary entrants was therefore further restricted to forty-five (Olver 1941).

columbianum (with his right hand) – much to the delight of the class. Students of the 1960s also recall, with affectionate amusement, his rich Polish accent. (Personal communication, Barry Leek, grad. 1958)

The total number of Polish-based subjects made available to the final-year Polish students and graduates was thirteen. The number of lecture hours in the first trimester was twenty-six per week, in the second trimester twenty-three, and in the third trimester twenty-seven. The number of practical training hours per week in the first trimester was twenty-two, in the second twenty-two, and in the third thirty-two. Some of these lectures and practicals were given by Polish staff and others by College staff (Runge 1944). The Science of Veterinary Forensics and the Organisation of the Polish State Veterinary Services were taught by Polish lecturers.

The lecturers and examiners from the Dick Vet were:

Prof. A. Robertson on breeding and nutritional science
In 1945, Prof. G. F. Bodie on pharmacology
Prof. D. C. Matheson on bacteriology
Prof. T. Grahame on histology, embryology and anatomy
Dr R. G. Thin on physics

The Dick Vet final year curriculum (Calendar 1944) was listed as:

I. The principles and practice of veterinary medicine embracing general and contagious diseases and preventive medicine, clinical diagnostics, special therapeutics and case reporting, clinical parasitology and meat inspection.
II. The principles and practice of veterinary surgery embracing clinical diagnosis (including examinations for soundness) and case reporting; surgical and applied anatomy; operative surgery, including anaesthesia; obstetrics.

The requirements of the Royal (Dick) Veterinary College were very strict, both in terms of lecture and class attendance, and in the passing of exams (Calendar 1944). It was reported that, in general, Polish students studied diligently and obtained good exam grades. In addition to these lectures and practicals, they took part in three larger scientific trips to various breeding farms, experimental stations and meat-processing plants in Scotland and England, and had several clinical visits to outpatients (Runge 1944). All of the Diploma examinations were conducted in Polish by the Examination Committee composed of members of the EKASMW (Runge 1944; Terlecki 1989).

Graduates who passed all three groups of Diploma examinations – that is, sixteen examinations and three compulsory colloquiums – obtained

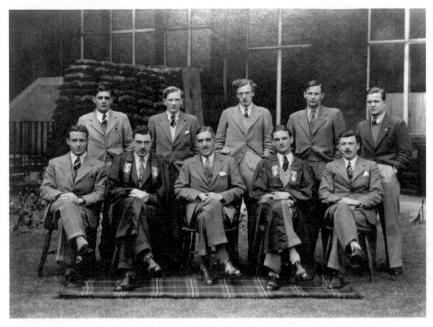

Figure 7.12 Photograph of the SRC representatives with Professor Olver in the Summerhall courtyard, Session 1940–1. Note the wartime sandbagging in place. Photographer: Richard Hood.

During Session 1941–2, apart from Home Guard and other Civil Defence activities, the teaching position continued to be abnormal. As before, large numbers of medical and dental students and a number of Polish Army Veterinarians (see chapter 8) were under training in addition to the now usual number of veterinary students. It had been anticipated that the numbers of students would be much reduced, but their numbers in the final years had increased and it was instead the numbers of staff that had been reduced due to war service. The most urgent needs at that time were firstly, a farm to be used as a field station for experimental work and for the practical training of students in pregnancy diagnosis and similar clinical work, and secondly, small-animal accommodation within the College itself. During the 1941 Christmas vacation, structural alterations were carried out in the basement and considerable additions were made to the kitchen equipment. These greatly facilitated the working of the refectory, and this improved amenity was much appreciated by the students. The total number of students attending the College for the 1941–2 Session was 271. In addition, fourteen graduates and occasional students and seventy-three medical and dental students were under instruction. The number of new entrants was forty-one (Olver 1942).

During Session 1942–3 there were 236 students studying for the MRCVS Diploma and of these ninety also took the University course for the BSc degree in Veterinary Science, much of the teaching of which was given in the College. In addition, eighty-two medical and dental students took classes in Physiology and Biochemistry, Histology and Embryology, and a few Polish students were admitted to the MRCVS classes under special arrangements with the Polish authorities. The number of new entrants for the MRCVS course in October 1942 was forty-nine. As a consequence of students volunteering for the fighting services, the total number of them taking the MRCVS course again suffered considerable reduction as the year went on. However, the numbers in some of the classes remained high because of the large numbers that had been admitted shortly before the beginning of the war. The refectory became more and more in demand and as such turned into an established feature of great importance to the health and wellbeing of the students; an average of 150 lunches, 60 tea meals and between 200 and 300 cups of tea or coffee were served daily. The recreation room also proved to be of great value in promoting social activities within the College, with the weekly dances becoming a regular feature. Dick Vet students continued to be intensively trained as a mobile civil defence unit, with fire-watching duties being carried out under a voluntary system in accordance with Government requirements. Despite the extra work involved in Home Guard and civil defence duties and the increase in teaching activities and research which had taken place in certain departments, the results of professional examinations did not suffer; in fact, they steadily improved. The total number of students attending the College for Session 1942–3 was 236. In addition, there were ten graduates and occasional students and eighty-two medical and dental students under instruction, as well as four Polish students (Olver 1943).

A very unfortunate accident, which shocked all staff and students at the College, occurred on the morning of 2 March 1943. A post-mortem examination of the incurably sick female elephant, Sundra, was due to be carried out at the Zoological Park on Corstorphine Hill. Colonel Sir Arthur Olver was in charge. Anaesthetising the animal proved impossible. During his professional and military life, Principal Olver, as a marksman, had previous experience of shooting elephants and game. Therefore, for safety, he had ordered the Elephant House to be cleared of onlookers. The .300 Browning rifle was loaded, and the safety catch was on. Sir Arthur was handed the gun with the muzzle pointing upwards. Without touching the trigger, he slipped the safety catch forward with his thumb and was astonished when it suddenly went off without the trigger being touched. Unknown to Olver, a group of four students had climbed up onto the flat roof over the entrance to watch the proceedings. One of these was hit in the chest and died. Eleven days later at Edinburgh Sheriff Court, an inquiry under the Fatal Accident Inquiry Act was led by Sheriff-Principal Fenton, KC. The likelihood of a defective rifle was confirmed by Detective Inspector William Lyall. After further evidence the enquiry concluded

> that death was caused by a gunshot wound on the chest, that Sir Arthur Olver was unaware of the presence of the deceased or anyone else on the roof, and, accordingly, no blame attached to him for the accident.

There were fifty-seven new entrants in October 1943 and of these, five were the first women admitted to the Dick Vet for the MRCVS course. Thirty students enrolled for the BSc (Vet.Sci.). In all there were 219 students studying for the MRCVS Diploma, of whom 19.6 per cent of the final year obtained First Class Honours. The greatly improved results obtained in Pathology also gave a clear indication that the prosecution of large-scale research in the College, in collaboration with outside bodies, had been very beneficial in stimulating interest and encouraging students to obtain a really sound understanding of the subject. In addition, there was the wartime training of ninety-six medical and dental students in preclinical subjects. Principal Olver, who believed in the principle of a healthy mind in a healthy body, suggested that '*Mens sana in corpore sano*' (A sound mind in a sound body) should be adopted as the official College motto (Olver 1944).

In the Clinical Practice, those few people unable to pay for animal treatment received equal services without charge (as had been the practice a hundred years earlier). All animals injured in street accidents, whose owners were unknown, were brought by the police for attention, and the Edinburgh Corporation was charged a nominal fee. Total Clinical Fee revenue for 1943–4 was £3,460, compared to £923 for the year 1918–19 (Olver 1944).

Session 1944–5 was the final one for Principal Olver, who had reached seventy. During 1944–5 there had been 223 Veterinary students, forty-seven of whom were male new entrants and five were female; thirty-four students matriculated onto the BSc (Vet.Sci.) course; four of the new entrants went into Second Year, one into Third Year and one into Fourth Year. In addition, there were the 116 medical and dental students, and fifty-one graduate and occasional students, including a Refresher Course. There had been a large increase in the number of applicants for the veterinary course and so the College Board of Governors decided to terminate from June 1946 the wartime provision of teaching for medical and dental students. Principal Olver agreed that one importance of a field station for a veterinary college might be due to the provision of a considerable amount of material for the training of veterinary students in clinical surgery and medicine, areas of expanded importance (Woods 2018). However, for him, the main advantage would be in enabling students to live at a farm and study the practice and scientific application of animal management, and the feeding and handling of various classes of livestock (Olver 1945).

The College was greatly indebted to the Carnegie Trustees, not only for their annual grant, but also for the special grants with which, from time to time, they assisted the College in obtaining necessary equipment for specific research which otherwise would have been beyond its resources.

Professor Matheson was appointed acting Principal from 9 October 1945. As anticipated, the number of new entrants in 1945–6 increased to sixty-six, with five of them women, three men entered Second Year, and one man entered into each of the third, fourth and final years. The total number of matriculated students was 265, which included old students returning from the forces during the Session (Matheson 1946). During that Session, Major Gavin Grey, of Portobello, presented the bust of his grandfather, Alexander Grey, to the College. Alexander Grey was the first qualified veterinary surgeon to practise in Scotland. The stone bust was carved by his son Edward Grey, also a veterinary surgeon, who took up sculpture as a hobby. It is believed that it was the example of Alexander Grey that inspired William Dick to go to London to study Veterinary Science and to obtain the Diploma (Matheson 1946). The current whereabouts of the bust is unknown.

The Westminster Government had instructed that 90 per cent of veterinary student places were to be given to those ex-service men and women and essential workers with the necessary preliminary education. The total number of matriculated students was 315, which included seventy-seven new entrants: fifty-two men and three women in First Year; eleven men into Second Year; five men into Third Year; one man into Fourth Year; and seven men into Final Year. Of the first-year places, forty-six were allotted to ex-service personnel and essential workers (whose average age was about twenty-four). The pass rate in their first professional examination in July 1947 was 82.2 per cent, compared with 56.7 per cent in the July 1946 cohort of students. As a consequence, the teachers were unanimous in testifying to the students' keenness to work and that it had been a pleasure to have had such a class (Mitchell 1947). The 1947 final year was the last all-male cohort of students (Figure 7.13) to have undertaken the complete course of veterinary training at the Dick Vet.

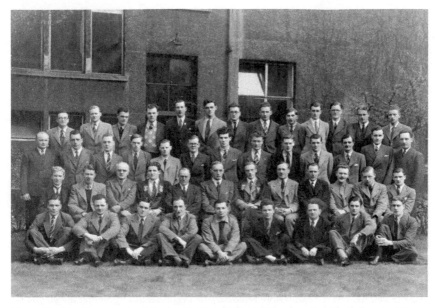

Figure 7.13 Photograph of the 1946–7 Final Year students and staff, the last year that only male students comprised the final year of studies. Photographer: Richard Hood.

References

Anonymous, 1914. Royal (Dick) Veterinary College. Marquis of Linlithgow to lay the Memorial Stone. *The Scotsman*, 21 July 1914, p. 6, col. 7.

Anonymous, 1917. Veterinary science teaching. Work of the Royal (Dick) College. Grant from the Scottish Agriculture Fund. *The Scotsman*, 9 July 1917, p. 3, col. 5.

Anonymous, 1922. War memorials. Royal (Dick) Veterinary College. New library inaugurated. *The Scotsman*, 14 June 1922, p. 7, col. 3.

Beare, T. H. 1936. Veterinary teaching. Edinburgh College extension. Appeal to public. Demand for veterinary workers. *The Scotsman*, 29 May 1936, p. 13, col. 4.

Board, 1927. Minutes of meeting of the Board of Management, held on Wednesday 20th of April 1927, p. 3. Archives of the Royal (Dick) School of Veterinary Studies, University of Edinburgh Centre for Research Collections - RDV3

Bradley, O. C. 1911. Opening of the Royal (Dick) Veterinary College. – Inaugural address: Veterinary Science and its relation to the community. *The Veterinary Journal*, 67, 742–9.

Bradley, O. C. 1920. *Royal (Dick) Veterinary College. Principal's report for session 1919–1920.* CRC, The University of Edinburgh.

Bradley, O. C. 1923. *History of the Edinburgh Veterinary College.* Edinburgh: Oliver & Boyd.

Bradley, O. C. 1924. *Royal (Dick) Veterinary College. Principal's report for session 1923–1924.* CRC, The University of Edinburgh.

Bradley, O. C. 1926. *Royal (Dick) Veterinary College. Principal's report for session 1925–1926.* CRC, The University of Edinburgh.

Bradley, O. C. 1928. *Royal (Dick) Veterinary College. Principal's report for session 1927–1928.* CRC, The University of Edinburgh.

Bradley, O. C. 1931. *Royal (Dick) Veterinary College. Principal's report for session 1930–1931.* CRC, The University of Edinburgh.

Bradley, O. C. 1934. Affiliation to the University. *The Centaur*, 3 (14), 6.

Bradley, O. C. 1935. *Royal (Dick) Veterinary College. Principal's report for session 1934–1935.* CRC, The University of Edinburgh.

Brook & Son, 1930. Royal (Dick) Veterinary College. Gift of a Silver Gilt Mace. *The Veterinary Record*, 52, 1206–7.

Calendar, 1911. *Royal (Dick) Veterinary College Edinburgh Calendar 1911–12.* Edinburgh: James Thin.

Cameron, W. M. 1930. The Alumnus Association. *The Centaur*, 1 (2), 9–11.

Doull, A. C. 1937. Personal tribute. *The Veterinary Record*, 49, 1549–50.

Greig, J. R. 1939. Obituary Notice: Orlando Charnock Bradley, M.D., D.Sc., F.R.C.V.S. *Proceedings of the Royal Society of Edinburgh*, 58, 254–7.

Lord Lyon, 1931. *Public Register of All Arms and Bearings in Scotland*, Vol. 29, Folio 59 of date 12 June 1931.

Macdonald, A. A., Warwick, C. M. and Johnston, W. T. 2005. Locating veterinary education in Edinburgh in the nineteenth century. *Book of the Old Edinburgh Club*, New Series, 6, 41–71. <era.ed.ac.uk/handle/1842/898/discover> (accessed 9 September 2022).

Matheson, D. C. 1946. *Royal (Dick) Veterinary College. Acting Principal's report for session 1945–1946.* CRC, The University of Edinburgh.

Mitchell, W. M. 1947. *Royal (Dick) Veterinary College. Principal's report for session 1946–1947.* CRC, The University of Edinburgh.

Mitchell, W. M. 1951. *Proposed new developments for the quinquennium 1952–57.* CRC, University of Edinburgh.

Olver, A. 1939a. Future of the profession. Veterinary Service. *The Scotsman*, 27 June 1939, p. 6, col. 5.

Olver, A. 1939b. *Royal (Dick) Veterinary College. Principal's report for session 1938–39.* CRC, The University of Edinburgh.

[Olver, A. 1939c.] *Memorandum on air raid protection measures carried out in the Royal (Dick) Veterinary College.* CRC, The University of Edinburgh.

Olver, A. 1940. *Royal (Dick) Veterinary College. Principal's report for session 1939–1940.* CRC, The University of Edinburgh.

Olver, A. 1941. *Royal (Dick) Veterinary College. Principal's report for session 1940–41.* CRC, The University of Edinburgh.

Olver, A. 1942. *Royal (Dick) Veterinary College. Principal's report for session 1941–1942.* CRC, The University of Edinburgh.

Olver, A. 1943. *Royal (Dick) Veterinary College. Principal's report for session 1942–1943.* CRC, The University of Edinburgh.

Olver, A. 1944. *Royal (Dick) Veterinary College. Principal's report for session 1943–44.* CRC, The University of Edinburgh.

Olver, A. 1945. *Royal (Dick) Veterinary College. Principal's report for session 1944–45.* CRC, The University of Edinburgh.

Rankine, J. 1917. Veterinary science teaching. Work of the Royal (Dick) College. *The Scotsman*, 9 July 1917, p. 3, col. 5.

Warwick, C. M. and Macdonald, A. A. 2010. The life of Professor Orlando Charnock Bradley, (1871–1937): Diary entries 1895–1923. Part 1. *Veterinary History*, 15 (3), 205–20. <era.ed.ac.uk/handle/1842/3643> (accessed 9 September 2022).

Warwick, C. M. and Macdonald, A. A. 2011. The life of Professor Orlando Charnock Bradley, (1871–1937): Building the Summerhall site. Part 2. *Veterinary History*, 15 (4), 309–34. <era.ed.ac.uk/handle/1842/4837> (accessed 9 September 2022).

Woods, A. 2018. Between Human and Veterinary Medicine: The History of Animals and Surgery. In T. Schlich (ed.), *Palgrave Handbook of the History of Surgery*. London: Palgrave Macmillan.

Chapter 8

The Polish Veterinary Faculty in Edinburgh (1943–8)

Alastair A. Macdonald, Maria Długołęcka-Graham and Colin M. Warwick

The creation of what became the Polish Veterinary Faculty in Edinburgh has a very different history from the formation of the three Veterinary Schools of Edinburgh that preceded it. Its staff and students were refugees from the Second World War, that started on 1 September 1939 with the German invasion of Poland (Davies 2015). It is therefore necessary to briefly describe those conditions and how it was that veterinary students and staff from Poland made their way to Scotland. After the Fall of France in June 1940, the Polish Army (including about forty veterinary surgeons) was evacuated to Britain. A small number of the individuals who studied at the Royal (Dick) Veterinary College will be taken as representative examples of the eighty students who attended the Polish Veterinary Faculty in Edinburgh.

Janina Sokołowska was born on 21 November 1914 in Lwów, Poland (Macdonald, Długołęcka-Graham, Knott, Hendrickx and Warwick 2023). In 1934 she applied for veterinary studies at the Veterinary Medicine Academy in Lwów and matriculated there on 5 December 1934 (Figure 8.1). By 18 March 1939 Janina had one year of study remaining to complete her veterinary training. However, these studies were disrupted by first the German and then the Red Army occupation of the city in September 1939.

Interestingly, Janina was not the only female student enrolled at the Polish Veterinary Faculty in Edinburgh. Ewa Missiuro, who was born on 24 November 1928, came to Britain after the outbreak of war. Her father was a doctor and medical scientist who came to Britain with the Polish Army and, as was the case with other army families, their spouses and children also sought refuge in Britain. Ewa completed her secondary education in Scotland in March 1945 and then commenced

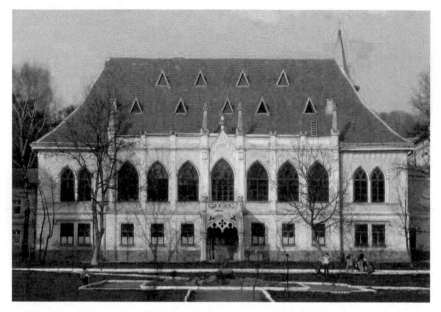

Figure 8.1 Veterinary Medicine Academy in Lwów, Poland pre-1940. Photographer: Jurij Skoblenko, CC BY-SA 2.0 <https://creativecommons.org/licenses/by-sa/2.0>, via Wikimedia Commons.

her veterinary studies at the Polish Veterinary Faculty (Macdonald et al. 2023).

Kazimierz Antoni Francizek Sołtowski was born on 27 February 1914. He also studied veterinary medicine at Lwów Academy of Veterinary Medicine, graduating from there in 1939. As required by Polish law, he immediately started national service in the Polish Army following graduation (Macdonald et al. 2023).

Mieczysław (Mietek) Jan de Sas Kropiwnicki was born 24 February 1912. He too studied veterinary medicine at Lwów Academy of Veterinary Medicine, completing his studies there in the spring of 1939 (Knott and Witkowski 2020).

Bronisław Zygadło was born into a Brzozowa Polish community in Chicago, USA in 1913 (Zygadło 2001). His mother returned to Poland with her two children in 1922, and in 1925 settled in Różniatów. Bronisław appears to have completed three years of study at Lwów Academy of Veterinary Medicine by September 1939 (Runge 1944).

Henryk Wincenty Hamerski was born on 22 February 1915. He matriculated in the Faculty of Veterinary Medicine at the Jósef Piłsudski University in Warsaw in 1933 and then from 1935 to 1939 he continued his studies at the Veterinary Medicine Academy in Lwów. By August

1939 he only needed to pass a further two exams to obtain his Diploma (Gąsiorowski 2003).

The Polish students' journeys to Edinburgh

Conditions in Lwów in September 1939 were chaotic. The German Army attacked the city from the west in mid-September and was then replaced by the Red Army invasion from the east several days later (Davies 2015). Lwów surrendered to the latter and all the Polish officers were arrested; most of them were subsequently murdered in 1940 in the Katyn Massacre (Andre 1954). In 1940 the civilians were put onto trains and sent first to Russia and then on to gulag camps in Kazakhstan and Uzbekistan as well as those in north, east and southern Siberia (Davies 2015). Zbigniew Doroszyński, another of the Polish Veterinary Faculty students, was captured by the Russians late in 1939, and was also transported to a Siberian gulag (Watkins 2014). Following the invasion of Russia by Germany in 1941, Marshal Josef Stalin was compelled to release the Poles held in captivity as he needed additional soldiers to fight the Nazis. Władysław Anders was tasked with forming those who were Polish soldiers into an army to fight the Germans (Davies 2015). Janina was notified she would join the Polish Army as a veterinarian. Under British leadership between 24 March and 5 April 1942, some 70,500 Poles were taken from prison camps and farms to Iran and then on to Iraq. A further 44,000 followed in July. The Polish refugees spent a year in the desert as part of 'Anders' Army', where they were issued with military equipment and received training (Davies 2015). From Iraq, some were sent to Palestine, to Egypt and then back to Palestine (Macdonald et al. 2023). After they arrived in Britain, many were moved to Scotland, where large numbers of other Poles had been gathered (Tomaszewski 1976).

In 1939 Kazimierz Sołtowski served in the Polish Army against the invading Germans (Anonymous 1979). He escaped to neutral Hungary, where he was interned. He later fled to Yugoslavia, Italy and, via France, to England (Severson 1952). A more detailed description of this escape route, taken by fellow Lwów veterinary student Mieczysław (Mietek) Jan de Sas Kropiwnicki, has recently been published (Knott & Witkowski 2021). Once in England, Kazimierz volunteered to join the British Colonial Forces and saw service in West Africa and Ghana from 1940 to 1942 (Severson 1952).

Bronisław Zygadło left Lwów with his veterinary student friend Mietek. He was captured and imprisoned near Tarnopol. Released unexpectedly, by mid-December 1939, he passed through the southern, snow-covered mountains into Hungary (Zygadło 2001). From Budapest, he travelled by train to Yugoslavia and via Italy managed to reach France and join the Polish forces in Paris. He fought in the brief battle of Narvik, Norway, in 1940, and returned to France as a second lieutenant. After the collapse of France he sailed to Portsmouth, arriving there on 23 June 1940. He, too, was one of about two hundred Polish soldiers who were seconded to the Royal West African Frontier Force and spent two years in West Africa (Zygadło 2001).

When war broke out, Henryk Hamerski was in Toruń, where he was working as a meat inspector in the town abattoir. Due to the proximity of the front line, he and his family left Toruń on 4 September 1939 as the city was being evacuated. He travelled to Warsaw, arriving on 10 September. He experienced the siege of the city and remained there until the Fall of Poland. In mid-October he journeyed from Warsaw back to Toruń by steamer, made contact with the Polish underground, and at the beginning of November cycled to Kraków using falsified papers. From there he crossed the southern border of Poland and reached the Polish Consulate in Bucharest on 6 December 1939. Then, with the help of a secret organisation, he crossed the Yugoslav border and made his way to Coëtquidan in France, where he was assigned to the 1st Division of the Polish Army. After the Fall of France on 20 June 1940, he was evacuated to Britain and served as an officer in the 2nd Artillery Regiment and Tank Division under General Maczek. He was drafted to the Polish Veterinary Study Unit at the Royal (Dick) Veterinary College in October 1943 (Gąsiorowski 2003).

Many of the prospective students and the qualified veterinarians who had come to France, passed through the camp at Carpiagne near Marseille (Preibisch 1986). They were then directed to Combourg in Brittany, where a Medical Training Centre had been established (Ruzyłło 1995). A veterinary service centre was organised as a part of it, under the aegis of Professor Dr Stanisław Runge, the former rector of the University of Poznań. Shortly thereafter, with the Fall of France, they were evacuated to Britain by 'Operation Aerial' (OR 1940; Worsfold 2022). Those who were appropriately trained, applied for and obtained leave from the Polish Army for one year to continue their veterinary studies at the Royal (Dick) Veterinary College.

Veterinary training in Edinburgh

There was a widespread desire to release fellow Polish veterinary colleagues from military camps and to launch training courses that would contribute to their professional preparation for a future return to Poland (Dowgiałło 1970; Preibisch 1986). Professor Runge, together with Lt Col Wroceński, persuaded the Polish military authorities to release veterinary surgeons from the army into British universities and other research centres. It was known by the Polish military that students of veterinary medicine from Lwów and Warsaw had been dispersed to various Polish military bases in Scotland (Jakubowski 1975). By November 1940, Dowgiałło (1970) reports that thirty-two Polish veterinary surgeons had received internships at the Royal (Dick) Veterinary College. Jerzy Preibisch recalled being one of a group of twelve of these Polish soldiers (Preibisch 1986). British graduates of the Dick Vet remembered being aware of Polish veterinary soldiers in the Dick Vet in 1940 (Denis F. Oliver, grad. 1942, personal communication). Edward Snalam (grad. 1943, personal communication) recalled that '2 or 3 Poles (in uniform) attend[ed] the College in [the] earlier years when I was in final year. Like their British student counterparts, they lived in private accommodation, so-called digs.' In Edinburgh, English was being taught to Polish soldiers in 1940 by Mrs McIntosh, Mrs Malcolm McLarty and others (Dowgiałło 1970). Some lessons were conducted in the army camps (Figure 8.2).

On 26 February 1941 the Principal of the Edinburgh Veterinary College, Sir Arthur Olver, reported to his Board of Management 'that a

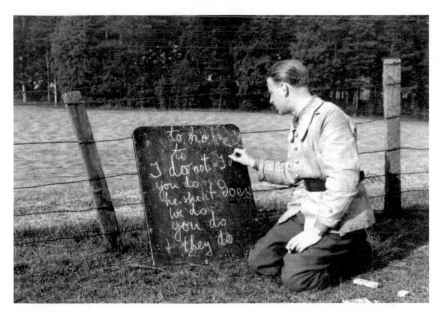

Figure 8.2 A Polish soldier learning English. Photographer: unknown. Private collection of Marian Długołęcki.

certain number of Polish officers were working in the various departments of the College. The hope was expressed that in the very near future certain classes might be conducted by Polish veterinary professors for any Polish students who might be in this country.' At the same meeting, 'Professor [Francis A. E.] Crew [a Board member] reported on the establishment of a Polish Faculty of Medicine in Edinburgh and expressed the hope that the Polish Government might establish a Polish Veterinary School here on similar lines.' On 13 November 1940 the University of Edinburgh Senatus Academicus approved the establishment of the Polish Medical School (PMS) (Wojcik and Bursary 2001).

During 1941 and 1942, nearly forty Polish veterinary surgeons were invited by Professor Olver and his staff to spend several months in the different laboratories and clinics of the Royal (Dick) Veterinary College, renewing those aspects of their contact with veterinary science which they had lost during their exile (Runge 1943).

Meanwhile, a group headed by Professor Runge had been busy with Superintendent-Inspector Major Rabagliati and Lt Col Wroceński of the Polish Army and others, creating the right conditions for veterinary students to obtain study leave from the army to continue their education and obtain a veterinary Diploma (Dowgiałło 1970; Preibisch 1986). The first indication of this surfaced on 1 December 1942 (RDVC Educ. 1942). The Education Committee of the Dick Vet

> considered a request by the Polish Military Veterinary Authorities that the privilege of studying and finishing their studies in the Royal (Dick) Veterinary College be granted to certain Polish veterinary students now resident in this country.
>
> The Principal [Sir Arthur Olver] stated that he understood that the number of students concerned was about eight, and it was agreed that facilities be granted to those students who would be obliged to pay the same fees as other veterinary students attending the College. The Polish authorities understood that these students would be examined by the College internal examiners and would be granted a certificate, if such was deemed justified. These students would not obtain the diploma of M.R.C.V.S. The question of the language difficulty was mentioned, but it was understood that this would not present any great difficulty.

A pencil addition to the 1941–2 Head of School's annual report already stated 'a number of Polish [students] have been under training'. Mieczysław (Mietek) Jan de Sas Kropiwnicki recorded that he had begun his veterinary studies in Edinburgh on 15 October 1942 (Knott and Witkowski 2021).

A Polish commission was appointed on 5 August 1943 to explore the possibility of establishing a veterinary study unit at the Royal (Dick)

Veterinary College in Edinburgh. The general internal organisation of the Commission of Academic Veterinary Medicine Studies was almost completely adapted from that pertaining to pre-war Polish university faculties.

A special meeting of the College Education Committee was held on 3 September 1943 and considered

> a letter from the Polish Board of Education enquiring whether the College would agree to accept a number of senior Polish students (in any case no more than 20–25), to give them access to the establishments and clinics of the College and facilitate the task of the Supervising Committee by giving it one or two rooms. (RDVC Educ. 1943)

The Principal was asked if he could make the necessary arrangements. Sir Arthur Older replied that,

> while the question of accommodation was a difficulty, he thought arrangements could be made. The meeting accordingly agreed to accede to the request but decided that an undertaking be obtained from the Polish Veterinary Committee, acting on the authority of the Polish Government, that none of the Polish students accepted under this arrangement will be permitted to take up any form of veterinary work in this country after the war. It was noted that the students would not be taking the RCVS diploma, and that the Polish Ministry of Education will be responsible for their fees. As it was necessary that the Department of Agriculture be informed of the position, a letter to the Department was to be drafted and submitted to the Chairman [Professor James Ritchie] in the first instance.

About one month later, the Department of Agriculture replied that it had no objection to the proposed arrangement. A letter was also submitted to the Polish Government (RDVC Board 1943).

After obtaining approval from the Royal College of Veterinary Surgeons and the Board of the Royal (Dick) Veterinary College, the Polish authorities were able to recommend nine students and ten veterinary alumni for the 1943–4 academic year (Runge 1944). A total of more than three times that number was later listed as having attended (Table 8.1).

The inauguration of the Edynburgu Komisję Akademickich Studiów Medycny Weterynaryjnej (EKASMW), the 'Polish Committee of Medical Veterinary Study in Edinburgh', took place in the Royal (Dick) Veterinary College at Summerhall on 13 September 1943. The President of Poland, Mr Władysław Raczkiewicz, General Janusz Głuchowski, the Commandant of the Training Brigade, the Rev. Prelate Zygmunt Kaczyński, the Polish Minister of Education and Professor Stanisław Runge, the senior Polish veterinary academic on the 'Committee', were welcomed to the College by Professor Sir Arthur Olver. The available

Table 8.1 Register of students who applied for admission to the Polish Department of Veterinary Medicine in Edinburgh. From: Ewidencja Studentow [Register of students]. Polish Institute and Sikorski Museum KOL. 459/7.

Jan Bernard	Mieczysław Kropiwnicki	Zenon Sobczak
Bruno Biliński	Jerzy Kruczkowski	Witold Sojka
Józef Buchta	Zdzisław Krynicki	Janina Sokołowska
Jerzy Buckiewicz	Wiesław Kubicki	Lesław Sokołowski
Tadeusz Cencora	Wacław Lisowski	Kazimierz Sołtowski
Stanisław Chmurowicz	Emil Mazurkiewicz	Henryk Stolarczyk
Alfred Chodkowski	Bronislaw Mendlowski	Jan Suzin
Zbigniew Doroszyński	Fabian Michałowski	Witold Świętkowski
Jerzy Drzewiecki	Stanisław Migocki	Juliusz Szandrowski
Tadeusz Dul (?)	Ewa Missiuro	Jan Tarała
Kazimierz Gargula	Mateusz Henryk Nitecki	Jerzy Wilhelm Thoma
T. Gąska	Stnisław Tadeusz Oleksy	Zdzisław Ulicki
Maurycy Gitter	Mieczysław Ostrowski	Władysław Uruski
Stefan Grzyremski	Tadeusz Piasecki	Adolf Michał Watrach
Feliks Gutowski	Edmund Rosadziński	Kazimierz Wojakiewicz
Henryk Hamerski	Julian Rostek	Stanisław Woźniakiewicz
Antoni Kiedziuch	Władysław Roziński	Tadeusz Zachorowski
Markus Koerner	Lesław Seredyński	Otton Henryk Zawodziński
Władysław Kosiewicz	Zbigniew Skowroński	Bronisław Zygadło
Aleksander Kosko	Daniel Słuszkiewicz	Alfred Stanisław Żebrowski
Feliks Marian Kozłowski	Kazimierz Snigocki	[Jana Cieślara – ID book]

Note: Jan Bernard selected to return to his army unit a relatively short time after starting veterinary training.

evidence indicates that Kazimierz Sołtowski, Bronisław Zygadło, Janina Sokołowska, Władysław Roziński and Mieczysław (Mietek) Jan de Sas Kropiwnicki had reached Edinburgh by the autumn of 1943; they were all photographed standing on the front steps of the College among the dignitaries (Figure 8.3).

Veterinary studies were to be conducted in accordance with the regulations in force in Poland before the war (Terlecki 1989). On the basis of an oral agreement with Sir Arthur Olver, Polish students could attend the Veterinary College lectures, and these classes were to be supplemented with Polish lectures and practicals in accordance with the Polish curriculum. Polish lecturers were assigned offices for their work and were permitted to use the clinics, laboratories and facilities of the College. Individual Polish departments were formed and had their own clinical equipment and laboratories, purchased from the Committee's budget. The Commission also had a small reference library which contained several dozen books. The Committee paid the College an annual fee of 33 guineas for each student (Preibisch 1986). The students and gradu-

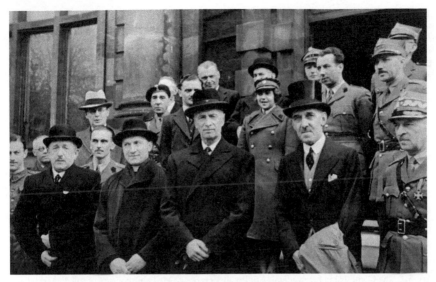

Figure 8.3 The opening of the Medical-Veterinary Study in Edinburgh (ASMW, soon to become the Polish Veterinary Faculty) on 13 September 1943. In the front row from left to right: Professor Stanisław Runge, Rev. Father Zygmunt Kaczyński (Minister of Education), President Władysław Raczkiewicz, Professor Sir Arthur Olver and General Janusz Głuchowski. From l to r, standing behind and seen, in uniform, between Professor Runge and Rev. Father Kaczyński, is Kazimierz Sołtowski. Standing directly behind him, with glasses and a trilby hat, is Lieutenant Vet. Dr Stanisław Mgłej. In the second row, from l to r, in civilian dress, between Rev. Father Kaczyński and slightly behind President Raczkiewicz, is Bronisław Zygadło; between President Raczkiewicz and Professor Olver is Janina Sokołowska; and behind Professor Olver, also in uniform, is Władysław Roziński. Between them, at the very back, is Mieczysław (Mietek) Jan de Sas Kropiwnicki. Photographer: unknown. Courtesy Michael Knott.

ates (*absolwenci*) became members of a Polish Society – the Veterinary Medicine Circle. Almost all of them also belonged to the British 'Students Union' (Anonymous 1946).

Edynburgu Komisję Akademickich Studiów Medycny Weterynaryjnej (EKASMW): 'Polish Committee of Medical Veterinary Study in Edinburgh'

A letter from the Minister of Religious Denominations and Public Enlightenment, Fr Zygmunt Kaczyński, dated 5 August 1943, established the Edynburgu Komisję Akademickich Studiów Medycny Weterynaryjnej (EKASMW), the 'Polish Committee of Medical Veterinary Study in Edinburgh' (Runge 1943; Mgłej 1955; Preibisch 1986). The members of this Committee in Edinburgh were: Professor Dr Stanisław Runge as dean,

Table 8.2   Decree of the President of the [Polish] Republic, 10 April 1945.

To the Committee for Academic Studies in Veterinary Medicine (Journal of Laws No. 4 of May 25, 1945, item 9).

Based on Article. 79 sec. (2) of the Constitutional Act reads as follows:

Art. 1.   A Commission for Academic Studies in Veterinary Medicine is established at the Royal (Dick) Veterinary College in Edinburgh.

Art. 2.   The Commission for Academic Studies in Veterinary Medicine has the powers of the faculty councils of Polish academic schools of veterinary medicine, as defined in the Act on Academic Schools of March 15, 1933 (Journal of Laws No. 1 of 1938, item 6), with the exception of conferring the degree of doctor and conducting habilitation proceedings.

Art. 3.   The task of the Committee for Academic Studies in Veterinary Medicine is to organize the studies of veterinary medicine at the Royal (Dick) Veterinary College in Edinburgh by adapting and supplementing these studies with the programs in force at academic universities of veterinary medicine in Poland.

Art. 4.   The Commission for Academic Studies in Veterinary Medicine may credit studies already completed by Polish youth at the Royal (Dick) Veterinary College in Edinburgh, if these studies were adapted and supplemented with the curricula in force at academic universities of veterinary medicine in Poland and issue diplomas of a veterinary doctor in place of the previous certificates.

Art. 5.   The Commission for Academic Studies in Veterinary Medicine consists of full and associate professors and associate professors of Polish academic schools of veterinary medicine residing in the United Kingdom, appointed by the President of the Republic on the motion of the Minister of Religious Denominations and Public Enlightenment.

Art. 6.   The Commission for Academic Studies in Veterinary Medicine elects a chairman from among its members for a period of one year, whose powers correspond to those of the dean of a Polish academic school.

Art. 7.   This decree is in force for the duration of exceptional circumstances caused by the war and shall become invalid on the date specified by the ordinance of the Council of Ministers.

Art. 8.   The implementation of this decree is entrusted to the Minister for Religious Denominations and Public Enlightenment.

Art. 9.   This decree shall come into force on the day of its promulgation.

President of the Republic: Wł. Raczkiewicz
Prime Minister: T. Arciszewski
Head of the Ministry of W. R. i O. P.: W. Folkierski

Professors Bolesław Gutowski, Józef Kulczycki and Tadeusz Ołbrycht, and associate professor Dr Stanisław Mgłej.

The first academic year for the Polish staff and students at the Royal (Dick) Veterinary College was officially opened on 11 October 1943. It was attended by Fr Kaczyński and the Director of the National Culture Fund, Dr Jan Hulewicz. The Dean of the Polish Medical Faculty in Edinburgh, Professor Dr Antoni Jurasz, together with the professors of the Polish Medical Faculty and the Principal of the Royal (Dick) Veterinary College, Sir Arthur Olver, with a group of professors and assistants, also participated. Fourteen students, mostly senior students or graduates from the Academy of Veterinary Medicine in Lwów and the Veterinary Faculty at the Józef Piłsudski University in Warsaw, enrolled (Runge 1944; Preibisch 1986).

A review of activities in the academic year 1943–4 carried out from 30 August to 6 October 1944 by an employee of the Supreme Audit Office, NIK (Najwyższa Izba Kontroli), revealed an important administrative problem. The EKASMW that had so far been established in Edinburgh was a 'Study Unit' in line with the requirements for a Higher Education School, but without its status or that of a duly constituted Faculty. Action to remedy the situation was taken swiftly; in November 1944 the Polish Board of Education in London changed the name of the Polish Committee of Medical Veterinary Study to the Polish Veterinary Faculty (Olver 1944; Anonymous 1944b). This had been the name in common use at the Edinburgh Veterinary College since 1943. The issuing of a Government decree on 10 April 1945 (Table 8.2) gave the Polish Veterinary Faculty the appropriate powers (Preibisch 1986).

The chairmen of the Edinburgh Academic Studies of the Veterinary Medicine Committee (EKASMW), who sequentially acted as Deans, were:

Prof. S. Runge from September 1943 to 31 January 1946
Prof. B. Gutowski from 1 February 1946 to 30 September 1946
Dr Mgłej from 1 January 1947 until the closure of the Faculty on 1 October 1948

Their deputies were:

Prof. T. Olbrycht from September 1943 to 30 April 1946
Dr S. Mgłej from 1 May 1946 to 31 December 1946

The secretariat was run by Dr S. Mgłej from September 1943 to 1948

Polish teaching and examining responsibilities

Prof. Stanisław Runge taught pathology, morbid anatomy, gynaecology and veterinary forensic science from September 1943 to January 1946, examining in those subjects as well as obstetrics and pharmacology. He presided over the Diploma examinations.

Prof. Tadeusz Ołbrycht, from the Academy of Veterinary Medicine in Lwów, taught animal breeding, genetics and nutrition, with farm visits, from September 1943 until April 1946, examining in these and other aspects of agriculture.

Prof. Józef Kulczycki, from the Józef Piłsudski University in Warsaw, taught surgery, ophthalmology and topographic anatomy from September 1943 to September 1946. He examined in these subjects as well as the clinical introduction to surgical diseases.

Dr Bolesław Gutowski, from the Józef Piłsudski University in Warsaw, taught animal physiology and physiological chemistry from May 1944 to December 1946.

Prof. Mirosław Ramułt, from the Jagiellonian University, Kraków, taught biology and protozoa, with particular emphasis on the pathogenic aspects, from January 1944 to September 1948.

Dr Stanisław Mgłej from the Academy of Veterinary Medicine in Lwów taught, from 1 September 1943, internal and infectious diseases of animals, internal medicine, with visits to outpatients, and organisation of the state veterinary service and public health. He was also responsible for the Polish Faculty until 1 October 1948.

Dr Alfred Ginsberg lectured and examined on food and utility products of animal origin from September 1943 to September 1948, with visits to slaughterhouses. He graduated MRCVS in 1946.

Dr Jerzy Witold Preibisch lectured and conducted farm-visit practicals on dairy hygiene from January 1944 until December 1946, and practicals in animal physiology from April 1945 until December 1946.

Dr Dominik Jastrzembski conducted classes in histopathology for veterinary graduates in the 1943–4 academic year.

Dr Józef Dowgiałło ran blood-test practicals for veterinary graduates in the 1943–4 academic year.

Dr Zdzisław Krynicki was a junior assistant for descriptive anatomy during the 1945–6 academic year. He graduated MRCVS in 1947.

Dr Marian Soltys gave a series of lectures on bacteriology and serology in the third semesters of academic years 1943–4 and 1944–5 for students repeating examinations. He examined in microbiology.

Czesław Rayski was initially one of the students, who graduated MRCVS in 1946. He became a lecturer in parasitology, made his home in Edinburgh, went on to gain a PhD and continued to teach parasitology until the 1960s:

> He was remembered by students for being ambidextrous – taking great delight in standing in the middle of the blackboard and writing very legibly but in different styles, e.g. Oesophagostomum (with his left hand)

certificates confirming the completion of the prescribed five years of study. Having passed all examinations and compulsory Diploma examinations, they were awarded the degree and title of a veterinary doctor. They also had the right to replace the Edinburgh-gained certificate with an original certificate of veterinary doctor, issued by one of the Polish university veterinary schools after returning to Poland. Following completion of their studies, all graduates were obliged to undergo a three- to six-month postgraduate internship in a veterinary experimental facility or at a private veterinary clinic (Runge 1944; Anonymous 1946; Terlecki 1989).

The organisation of studies for the Polish students in their first to fourth years was conducted mainly by British lecturers according to the MRCVS programme (Runge 1944). Some lectures were delivered in Polish by staff of the Polish Veterinary Faculty (SRC 1944). All students in these earlier years were examined in English by the College staff and progress to the following year of study depended on the results of those exams (Runge 1944). A notification of the result of each examination was kept by the student and entered into both the Polish Faculty (ASMW) examination directory and the student's ID book. After completing the fourth year of studies, the student had to complete one year or two trimesters of studies with the Polish Faculty staff before obtaining a certificate of discharge and acquiring the right to take the Diploma examinations before the EKASMW (Runge 1944).

Polish commemorative plaque unveiled

During that first year of study, a special ceremony was held on 14 April 1944 in the College Hall. The Government of the Republic of Poland had funded a commemorative marble plaque, designed by Andrew Dods, the acting head of the Edinburgh College of Art, and this was presented to the College by the members of the Polish Committee of Medical-Veterinary Study in Edinburgh and the Polish students (Figure 8.4a). It states:

> This plaque was erected to commemorate the centenary of the Royal College of Veterinary Surgeons in the year 1944. It was presented to pay homage to the Royal (Dick) Veterinary College, Edinburgh, Scotland as a token of the deep gratitude of all the exiled Polish Professors of Veterinary Science, Veterinary Surgeons and students who were working here during the war.

The plaque was unveiled by His Excellency the President of the Polish Republic, Władysław Raczkiewicz (Figure 8.4b), supported by the Polish Minister of Education and the Commander-in-Chief of the Polish Forces in Great Britain.

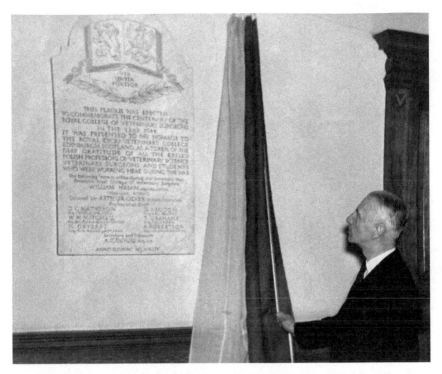

Figure 8.4 The unveiling, by His Excellency the President of the Polish Republic, Władysław Raczkiewicz on 14 April 1944, of the commemorative marble plaque designed by Andrew Dods and presented to the Royal (Dick) Veterinary College by the members of the Polish Committee of Medical-Veterinary Study in Edinburgh and the Polish students. Photographer: unknown. Courtesy Michael Knott.

On 5 June 1944 the Principal intimated to the College Council that the Polish Committee of Medical Veterinary Study desired their first-, second- and third-year students to sit a professional examination, to be conducted by the respective Royal (Dick) Veterinary College Professors. If considered Proficient, each Polish student would receive a certificate to that effect, which would entitle him or her admission to the following year. Professors would conduct the examinations of their students and would be remunerated on the same scale as the RCVS examiners. The meeting expressed satisfaction with the proposals.

A scientific meeting of Polish veterinary surgeons and students was held from 27 to 29 July 1944 at the Dick Vet (Figure 8.5). Janina, Kazimierz, Bronisław and Mietek attended (Macdonald et al. 2023).

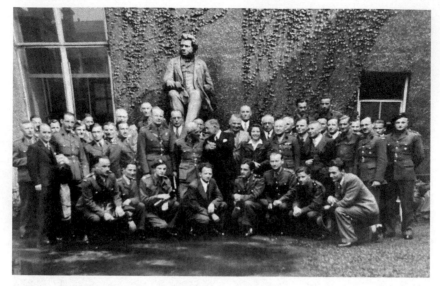

Figure 8.5   Photograph, taken on the north side of the courtyard of the Royal (Dick) Veterinary College, of those Polish veterinary surgeons and students who attended a Polish scientific meeting, 27–9 July 1944. Janina Sokołowska is clearly seen as the only woman, with Bronisław Zygadło crouched down in front of her. Kazimierz Sołtowski is the tall figure, standing fifth from the left of the group. The tallest person in the second row, just to the left of the William Dick statue, is Mieczysław (Mietek) Jan de Sas Kropiwnicki. Photographer: unknown. Courtesy Michael Knott.

Polish veterinary diplomas awarded

In the summer of 1944 it was reported that four students had both completed their studies (Table 8.3) and received their diplomas (Preibisch 1986). As previously indicated, all graduates were obliged to undergo a three- to six-month postgraduate internship at a veterinary experimental facility or in an EKASMW-approved private veterinary clinic (Runge 1944).

In his annual report for 1944–5, Sir Arthur Olver reported that sixteen Polish students had been under training in the Polish Veterinary Faculty during that year (Olver 1945). Two second-year students returned to Polish army duties that semester, one due to poor academic results, the other, Jan Bernad, due to a stronger attachment to his military unit (Runge 1944). On 17 July 1945 a request from the Dean of the Polish Veterinary Faculty was made to the Board of Management. He asked for the teaching arrangements whereby Polish students were admitted to various years of study in the College to continue for another year; this was agreed to (RDVC 1).

Table 8.3 Polish students who obtained the Polish Veterinary Diploma and the dates these were later reported to have been awarded (Preibisch 1986).

Mieczysław Ostrowski	14 July 1944
Henryk Wincenty Hamerski	17 July 1944
Mieczysław Jan Sas-Kropiwnicki	27 July 1944
Bronisław Mendłowski	15 August 1944
Wacław Lisowski	19 January 1945
Markus Koerner	10 April 1945
Otton Henryk Zawodziński	10 April 1945
Wladyslaw Rozinski	5 May 1945
Zdzisław Krynicki = John Stanley Kay	26 June 1945
Bronisław Zygadło	27 June 1945
Leszek Seredyński	10 July 1945
Andrzej Franciszek Wiernek	24 July 1945
Zbigniew Wincenty Doroszyński	16 August 1945
Janina Maria Sokołowska	24 August 1945
Kazimierz Sołtowski	6 October 1945
Lucjan Wlaziński	22 November 1945
Stefan Przyrembel	30 November 1945
Jósef Zdzisław Ulicki	20 December 1945
Adolf Michal Watrach	31 May 1946
Alfred Stanislaw Zebrowski	18 July 1946
Jerzy Buckiwicz	22 July 1946
Teodor Mościsker	31 November 1946
Zygmunt Modełski	1 February 1947

The students who received their diplomas in 1945 were listed (Table 8.3). Thus, Janina Maria Sokołowska (Figure 8.6) was the first woman ever to have completed her veterinary studies (Figure 8.7) at the Royal (Dick) Veterinary College (Runge 1944; Mgłej 1955; Preibisch 1986; Macdonald et al. 2023). Further details of the life of Janina Maria Sokołowska have recently been published elsewhere (Macdonald et al. 2023).

Post-war developments

On 8 May 1945 war in Europe officially ended. Six weeks later the process of demobbing the troops began (Allport 2009). However, war continued in East Asia, and it was not until 2 September 1945 that the Second World War finally ended. Later that year the process of demobbing the troops based in Asia and South-east Asia began. The Dick Vet had already estimated the numbers of demobbed former students returning to the College to be 15 (first year), 33 (second year), 24 (third year), 11 (fourth year) and 5 (fifth year), totalling 88 ex-soldiers (Anonymous 1944a).

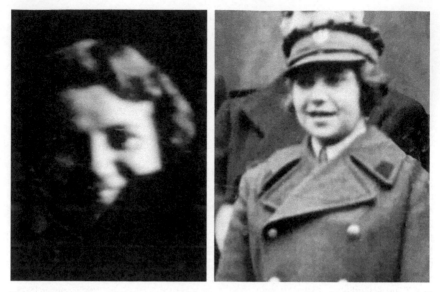

Figure 8.6 Janina Sokołowska, 1944, photographed inside Summerhall and on the front steps of Summerhall. Photographers: unknown. Courtesy Michael Knott.

In the spring of 1945 Sir Arthur Olver retired. He was replaced by Professor D. C. Matheson as acting Principal from October 1945 to September 1946, when Professor A. Mitchell took over (RDVC 1). It was the latter who served notice, following instruction received from the British Government, that the agreement with the Polish Veterinary School would not be renewed after the 1945–6 session.

By 18 October 1945 the College Council considered that the position that had arisen, particularly in the first year through the large influx of Polish students in addition to the returning demobbed British soldiers, was unsustainable. As some of the members of the Selection Committee which had interviewed prospective British students were unaware that there was the possibility of an influx of Polish students, the Secretary read communications which had passed between the Polish Veterinary Medical Faculty and the College. From this correspondence it was gathered that there was a possible entry of 20–25 Polish students into the first year and 25–30 into the other four years. In view of the information given to them, the Board of Management agreed to the request of the Polish Medical Veterinary Faculty that such numbers could be admitted for the year 1945–6 (RDVC 1). In the event, eighteen Polish students studied during the 1945–6 Session, Ewa Missiuro being one of them (Missiuro 1945; Matheson 1946).

On 18 March 1946 Professor Matheson read a letter from Professor Gutowski requesting the College re-admit the following year the

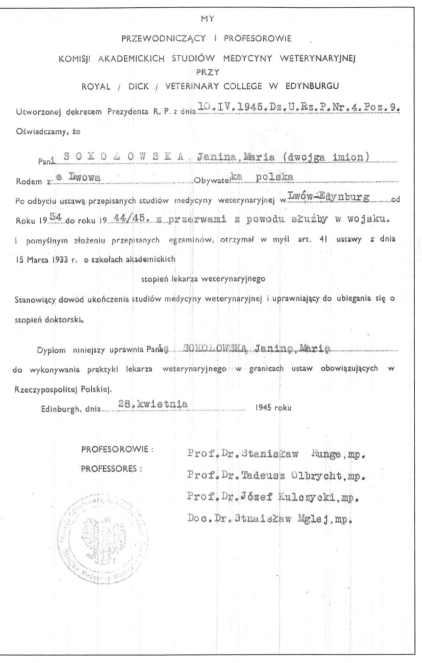

MY

PRZEWODNICZĄCY I PROFESOROWIE

KOMISJI AKADEMICKICH STUDIÓW MEDYCYNY WETERYNARYJNEJ
PRZY
ROYAL / DICK / VETERINARY COLLEGE W EDYNBURGU

Utworzonej dekretem Prezydenta R. P. z dnia 10.IV.1945.Dz.U.Rz.P.Nr.4.Poz.9.

Oświadczamy, że

Pani S O K O Ł O W S K A Janina,Maria (dwoja imion)

Rodem z e Lwowa Obywatelka polska

Po odbyciu ustawą przepisanych studiów medycyny weterynaryjnej w Lwów-Edynburg od

Roku 19 34 do roku 19 44/45. z przerwami z powodu służby w wojsku.

I pomyślnym złożeniu przepisanych egzaminów, otrzymał w myśl art. 41 ustawy z dnia

15 Marca 1933 r. o szkołach akademickich

stopień lekarza weterynaryjnego

Stanowiący dowód ukończenia studiów medycyny weterynaryjnej i uprawniający do ubiegania się o

stopień doktorski.

Dyplom niniejszy uprawnia Panią SOKOLOWSKA Janinę,Marię

do wykonywania praktyki lekarza weterynaryjnego w granicach ustaw obowiązujących w

Rzeczypospolitej Polskiej.

Edinburgh, dnia 28.kwietnia 1945 roku

PROFESOROWIE :
PROFESSORES :

Prof.Dr.Stanisław Runge,mp.

Prof.Dr.Tadeusz Olbrycht,mp.

Prof.Dr.Józef Kulczycki,mp.

Doc.Dr.Stnaisław Mglej,mp.

Figure 8.7 The diploma, signed on 28 April 1945 by professors of the Polish Veterinary Faculty in Edinburgh, certifying that Janina Maria Sokołowska had passed the prescribed exams and was now qualified to practise as a veterinarian in the limits of the statutes applicable in the Polish Republic. (Polish Institute and Sikorski Museum, Kol.459/8.)

twenty-five Polish students presently attending the College. The request was referred to the Board of Management for its consideration (RDVC 1).

In March 1946 Professor Runge, who had vacated his position as Dean of the Polish Faculty of Veterinary Science, expressed his thanks to the College authorities for all the consideration and kindness shown to him and his colleagues during their stay in the College (RDVC 1). Relations between the Commission and the College were said to have been perfect from the very beginning of co-operation until the summer of 1946, the year after the retirement of the Principal, Sir Arthur Olver, who had been a great friend of the Poles. In the spring of 1945 Olver had been decorated by Professor Władysław Folkierski, the Minister of Religious Denominations and Public Enlightenment, with the Commander's Cross of the Order of Polonia Restituta, and at the same time Mr Alexander Campbell Doull, Secretary and Treasurer of the College, had been decorated with the Officer's Cross of that Order (Preibisch 1986).

Dr Ginsberg had approached Professor Matheson before 3 June 1946 on behalf of eleven Polish graduates who desired to take the final-year classes plus one subject in the fourth year for the Diploma of the RCVS. This request was remitted to the Selection Committee and clinical teachers to decide which of the graduates should be admitted to the College (RDVC 1).

The lectures and practical classes conducted by the Polish Veterinary Faculty were suspended at the end of the 1945–6 academic year. The students who received their Diploma in 1946 are listed in Table 8.3. At that time there were still thirteen students awaiting admission to the second year of their studies, seven to their third year, two to their fourth year and two to their fifth year, a total of twenty-four students. As a result of the efforts of the Council of the Polish Veterinary Faculty, all senior students, from the third, fourth and final years, were admitted to the Royal (Dick) Veterinary College as its own students. Several second-year students were also admitted individually, including Maurycy Gitter (Table 8.4). However, the remaining students were forced to interrupt their studies (Preibisch 1986).

The Polish Faculty was given notice of termination of the use of college premises and had to leave the College at the end of April 1947. On 11 December 1946 Principal Mitchell reported to the Board of Management that the Polish Veterinary Faculty was in the progress of closing down, and that the Polish students who were in the first and second years would discontinue their studies as from 13 December; Ewa Missiuro was one of these. Regarding students in the third, fourth and fifth years who were

Table 8.4 Polish Army veterinary staff and students of the Polish Veterinary Faculty in Edinburgh, showing the year they became Members of the Royal College of Veterinary Surgeons (MRCVS) and the qualifications held (from the Register of the RCVS).

Year	Name	Qualifications
1942	Izrael Zlotnik	BVSc (Warsaw); MRCVS; PhD (Edin)
1946	Hieronim Cembrowicz	BVSc (Warsaw); MRCVS; PhD (Cantab)
	Alfred Chodkowski	Dr.Med.Vet. (Lwów); MRCVS
	Karol Chodnik	MRCVS; PhD (Edin)
	Alfred Ginsberg	Dr.Med.Vet. (Lwów); MRCVS; PhD (Edin)
	Dominik Jastrzebski	MRCVS
	Czeslaw Rayski	MRCVS; PhD (Edin)
	Mieczyslaw Reichert	Dr.Med.Vet. (Lwów); MRCVS
	Olgierd Rymaszewski	MRCVS; MD (Pol.Sch.Med.Edin)
	Wladyslaw Uruski	MRCVS
1947	Tadeusz Cencora	MRCVS
	Wincenty Zbigniew Doroszynski	MRCVS
	Tadeusz Podhaniuk	MRCVS
	Mieczysław Jan Sas Kropiwnicki	MRCVS*
	Zdzisław Krynicki = John S. Kay	MRCVS
	Bronislaw Mendlowski	MRCVS
	Stanislaw Michna	MRCVS
	G.A.Sziland = George Alexander Linton	MRCVS; BSc (Reading); DVM (Michigan)
1948	Kazimierz Stanisław Roszek	MRCVS
	Adolf Michal Watrach	MRCVS
1949	Emil Sluszkiewicz	MRCVS
	Otton Henryk Zawodziński	MRCVS*
1950	Witold Joseph Sojka	MRCVS
	Jan Tarala	MRCVS
1951	Zbigniew Josef Kazimierz Skowronski	MRCVS
	Maurycy Gitter	MRCVS
1953	Jerry Wilhelm Thoma	MRCVS

* MRCVS examination taken in Glasgow.

not taking the ordinary Diploma course, requests had been received that the RCVS might admit such students to the regular MRCVS course, but this was a matter for the RCVS authorities (RDVC 1). The last student to receive a Polish veterinary Diploma, in 1947, was Zygmunt Modelski (Table 8.3). From that time until its final decommissioning at the end of 1948, the seat of the Polish Veterinary Faculty was at 2 Brandon Street, Edinburgh (Figure 8.8; Preibisch 1986).

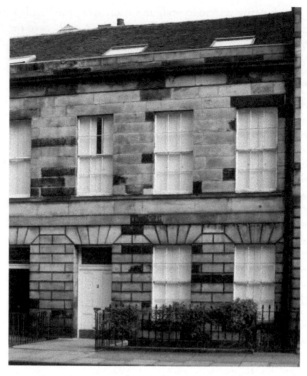

Figure 8.8 No. 2 Brandon Street, Edinburgh, where the Polish Veterinary Faculty decommissioned in 1948. Photographer: Colin M. Warwick.

Achievements of the Edinburgh Polish Veterinary Faculty

In total, sixty-three students and graduates were named as having enrolled in the Polish Veterinary Faculty (Table 8.1). Of those listed, eighteen received Polish diplomas as veterinary doctors (Table 8.3). An additional five students, not listed in Table 8.1, also received diplomas. Fifteen of the twenty-three Polish Diploma students were granted permission to sit for Membership of the Royal College of Veterinary Surgeons (MRCVS). Six succeeded, four graduating from the Royal (Dick) Veterinary College and two from the Glasgow Veterinary College (Watkins 2014; 2022). Two Polish Diploma recipients, Henryk Hamerski and Olgierd Rymaszewski, went on to study medicine and graduated from the Polish Medical School (Jakubowski 1975). Rymaszewski also received his MRCVS (Table 8.4). On 11 March 1947 Professor Mitchell read the names of nineteen Polish students who had been granted permission by the Royal College of Veterinary Surgeons to enter the Diploma Course of study at the College. Eight of these subsequently graduated MRCVS (Watkins

2014). A total of twenty-seven staff and students of the Polish Veterinary Faculty obtained MRCVS (Table 8.4). Thus, the total number of graduating and non-graduating students of the Polish Veterinary Faculty was 63 + 5 + 12 = 80, plus Alfred Ginsberg and Czeslaw Rayski who were on the Polish Veterinary Faculty staff (Tables 8.1, 8.3, 8.4).

Many of the Polish staff returned to university teaching positions in Poland. Several remained in Edinburgh or went to New Zealand. Some of the newly qualified veterinarians went to Africa, while others remained in Britain and most emigrated to North America (Millak 1962; Preibisch 1991; Watkins 2014; Knott and Witkowski 2021; Macdonald et al. 2023).

References

Allport, A. 2009. *Demobbed: Coming Home After the Second World War*. London: Yale University Press.

Andre, J. 1954. Woman is ex-Polish officer: Siberia is a fuzzy nightmare. *Minneapolis Sunday Tribune*, 12 April 1954, p. 19.

Anonymous, 1944a. *Post war rehabilitation. Undated, between 8 and 13 July 1944*. College Council Minutes. CRC, University of Edinburgh, RDV 34.

Anonymous, 1944b. *Polish Board of Education. Minutes of Wednesday 22nd November, 1944*. Board of Management 1940–1951. CRC, University of Edinburgh, RDV 4.

Anonymous, 1946. *Weterynaryjna medycyna studia w Wielki Britanii* (Veterinary Medicine studies in Great Britain), *Lekarz Wojskowy (Journal of the Polish Army Medical Corps)*, 37 (2–3), 204. [Comment: This article reported data that did not seem to entirely match more detailed information found elsewhere: viz, In the academic year 1944/45, there were 13 students and 9 graduates . . . , all of whom obtained their veterinary diplomas. In academic year 1945/46, 27 students and 3 graduates (absolwentów) pursued their studies.]

Anonymous, 1979. *A collection of historical sketches and family histories*. Benson, MN: Swift County Historical Society, 123.

Calendar, 1944. *Royal (Dick) Veterinary College Edinburgh Calendar 1944–45*. Edinburgh: James Thin.

Davies, N. 2015. *Trail of hope: The Anders Army, an odyssey across three continents*. Oxford: Osprey Publishing.

Dowgiallo, J. 1970. Polscy lekarze weterynarii w II wojnie światowej na terenie Francji I Wielkiej Brytanii w latach 1940–1945. [Polish veterinarians in World War II in France and Great Britain in 1940–1945.] *Życie Weterynaryjne*, 45, 307–8.

Gąsiorowski, J. 2003. *Losy absolwentów Polskiego Wydziału Lekarskiego w Edynburgu* [The fates of the graduates of the Polish School of Medicine], PhD thesis, Wydziału Lekarskiego Pomorskiej Akademii Medycznej [Faculty of Medicine of the Pomeranian Medical Academy], Szczecin, 121–2.

Jakubowski, S. 1975. Polskie studia weterynaryjne w w Edynburgu 1943–1948. [Polish Veterinary Studies in Edinburgh 1943–1948.] *Medycyna Weterynaryjna*, 31 (9), 569–70.

Knott, M. and Witkowski, M. 2021. Dr Mieczysław Jan de Sas Kropiwnicki (1912-1971): The first Polish veterinarian to perform a caesarean section on a brood mare. *Medycyna Weterynaryjna*, 77 (2), 106–10.

Macdonald, A. A., Długołęcka-Graham, M., Knott, M., Hendrickx, C. and Warwick, C. M. 2023. Janina Maria Sokołowska (1945): the first woman veterinary surgeon from the Royal (Dick) Veterinary College, Edinburgh. *Veterinary History*, 21 (3), 287–310.

Matheson, D. C. 1946. *Annual Report 1945–1946*. Royal (Dick) Veterinary College Annual reports, CRC, Edinburgh University Library.

Mgłej, S. 1955. Komisia Akademickich Studiów Medycyny Weterynaryjnej w Edinburgu (1943–1948). *Nauka Polska Na Obczyznie* 1, 44–9.

Millak, K. 1962. Z zagranicznej weterynarii: lekarze weterynaryjni pochodzący z Polski w Stanach Zjednoczonych i Kanadzie. [From foreign veterinarians: veterinary doctors from Poland in the United States and Canada.] *Medycyny Weterynaryjnej*, 18, 238–41.

Missiuro, E. 1945. *Manuscript letter of application to Stanisław Runge, Chairman of the Academic Board of Veterinary Studies at the Royal (Dick) Veterinary College in Edinburgh*. Ewidencja Studentow/Student Records, Polish Institute and Sikorski Museum KOL 459/7.

Olver, A. 1944. *Letter to Prof. Stan. Runge, 23rd November 1944*. Polish Institute and Sikorski Museum KOL 459/3.

Olver, A. 1945. *Annual Report 1944–1945*. CRC, University of Edinburgh.

OR, 1940. 'Operation Aerial'. <en.wikipedia.org/wiki/Operation_Aerial> (accessed 11 September 2022).

Preibisch, J. 1986. Polska uczelnia weterynaryjna w Szkocji. [Polish Veterinary University in Scotland.] *Życie Weterynaryjne*, 61 (1), 23–8.

Preibisch, 1991. Personal communication (to A.A.M.).

RDVC 1. *Board of Management Minutes, 1940–1951*. CRC, University of Edinburgh, RDV 3.

RDVC Board 1943. *5th October 1943*. Minutes of the Board [of Management], 1940–1951. CRC, University of Edinburgh, RDV3.

RDVC Educ., 1942. *1st December 1942*. Minutes of the Education Committee, Royal (Dick) Veterinary College, CRC, University of Edinburgh, RDV5.

RDVC Educ., 1943. *3rd September 1943*. Minutes of Special Meeting of the Education Committee. Royal (Dick) Veterinary College, CRC, University of Edinburgh, RDV5.

Runge, S. 1943. Polish committee for veterinary education. *The Veterinary Record*, 55, 427.

Runge, S. 1944. *Sprawozdanie z działalnoáci komisji akademickich studion medycyny weterynarijnej przy Royal (Dick) Veterinary College – Edinburgu za rok akad, 1943* (od październik do paździemilca). [Report on the activities of the Academic Committee of Veterinary Medicine Study at the Royal (Dick) Veterinary College – Edinburgh for the academic year, 1943 (from October to October)]. KOL. 459/1.

Ruzyłło, E. 1995. Centrum Wyszkolenia Sanitarnego Wojska Polskiego we Francji. *Archiwum Historii I Filozofii medycyny*, 58 (2), 104–14.

Severson, H. 1952. Polish woman veterinarian finds U.S. worth struggle. *Winona (Minnesota) Daily News*, 20 May 1952.

SRC, 1944. *15th February 1944*. Royal (Dick) Veterinary College SRC minute book 3, 1941 to 1952. CRC, University of Edinburgh, RDV 6.

Terlecki, R. 1989. Komisja Akademickich Studiów Medycyny Weterynaryjnej W Edynburgu 1943–1948. [Commission for Academic Studies in Veterinary Medicine, Edinburgh 1943–1948.] *Roczniki Nauk Społecznych*, 17 (2), 41–7.

Tomaszewski, W. 1976. *Na Szkockiej Ziemi* [On Scottish Soil], London: White Eagle Press.

Watkins, P. 2014. The Polish committee of Medical-veterinary study in Great Britain. *Veterinary History*, 17 (2), 168–83.

Watkins, P. 2022. Fortunes of War. *Veterinary History*, 22 (2), 209–29.

Wojcik, W. A. and Bursary, M.-S. 2001. Time in context – the Polish School of Medicine and Paderewski Polish Hospital in Edinburgh 1941 to 1949. *Proceedings of the Royal College of Physicians of Edinburgh*, 31, 69–76.

Worsfold, D. 2022. *Operation Aerial: Churchill's second miracle of deliverance*. Oxford: Casemate.

Zygadlo, M. 2001. *Lying Down with Dogs: A personal portrait of a Polish exile*, Aberdour: Inyx Publishing.

Chapter 9

The Dick Vet Embodied within the University (1947–69)

William M. Mitchell appointed Principal

Professor William M. Mitchell was appointed Principal from 1 October 1946 (Figure 9.1). By arrangement with the Principal of the East of Scotland College of Agriculture, during the 1946–7 Session sixty-nine Agriculture students attended for classes in veterinary hygiene in the Department of Veterinary Hygiene and Animal Husbandry, where there were facilities for practical demonstrations.

The post-war period for the Dick Vet was characterised by a series of substantial changes. Mitchell had to deal with these. Initially attempts were made to reconstruct some elements of the pre-war patterns of life. Staff were seeking to return to an earlier sense of 'normality', either from war duties or from the pressures of heavy additional wartime teaching responsibilities. It was not to be. 'Change' continued. Accommodating ex-servicemen who were returning to their veterinary studies meant that accepting school-leavers into the College was no longer possible. The number of applications from ex-service men and women for admission in October 1947 was, like the previous year, more than the total number of places available in the College (Mitchell 1947). Following careful selection based on qualifications and interview, of the sixty places available, fifty-three male places went to ex-servicemen or essential workers, and one each to a colonial scholar, a Chinese student and a student classified as medically exempt from service. Two of the four women students were ex-service and the other two were ordinary students. The average age of entrants in 1947 was about twenty-two. The total number of matriculated veterinary students in the College was 315.

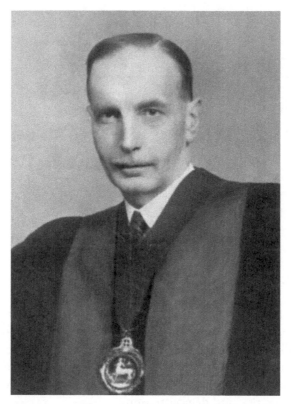

Figure 9.1   William Mitchell. Photographer: unknown London photographer.

The first women Dick Vet graduates

Nineteen forty-eight was the first year that women had completed five years of veterinary studies and were included in the list of Dick Vet graduates. They were Ann C. Preston, Marjorie E. Millar, Elizabeth A. Copland and Elizabeth A. Y. Caird (Figure 9.2). Marjorie E. Clarkson (née Millar), recalling her early days at the Dick Vet, wrote, 'I do remember that we four women students did feel rather strange among so many men who I think regarded us somewhat as curiosities.' After 1946 there had been a much more serious and hard-working atmosphere in the College due to the presence of returning military personnel either starting or returning to continue their studies: 'they were of course more mature and determined to pass exams'. After her graduation she married, had a family and worked in small-animal practice until 1975, after which she was occupied with locum and part-time work.

The following year, 325 veterinary students were in attendance, of

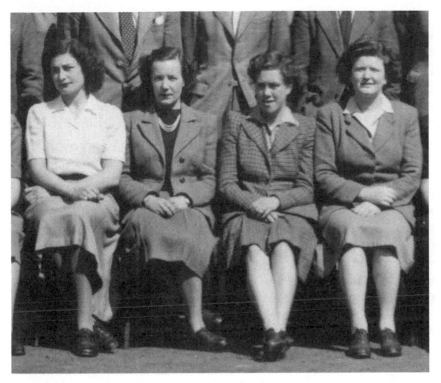

Figure 9.2 The first four women to complete five years of undergraduate veterinary studies at the Dick Vet: Left to right: Ann C. Preston, Marjorie E. Millar, Elizabeth A. Copland, Elizabeth A. Y. Caird. Photographer: E .R. Yerbury & Sons, Edinburgh.

whom fifty-one men and four women were newly admitted students. Once again, added to these were ninety-five Agriculture students who attended for instruction in veterinary hygiene (Mitchell 1948).

Further radical change in the appearance for the foreseeable future of veterinary education was detailed in the two reports of the Government-appointed Committee on Veterinary Education, the so-called Loveday Committee (MAF 1938, 1944). These reports stressed the need in Britain and its overseas colonies for larger numbers of more adequately trained veterinary practitioners. They emphasised that it was essential that veterinary colleges should become integral parts of their neighbouring universities. They also stressed that these universities should then become responsible for veterinary education and research, and for the institution of degrees which would be accepted as registrable qualifications for membership of the Royal College of Veterinary Surgeons.

Loss of 'institutional memory'

Long-established administrative and educational cultures within the College and the University were going to have to change. One early indication of this starting to happen was the loss of institutional memory personified by the departure of Alexander C. Doull, CA, the Secretary and Treasurer of the College; he relinquished his appointment for health reasons on 28 February 1948. His part-time replacement, Eric G. S. Melvin, CA, was appointed Secretary and Treasurer on 1 March 1948. Another example was Donald C. Matheson, the Professor of Pathology and Bacteriology, who retired at the end of September 1946. He returned in the spring of 1947 to fill the vacancy in the Pathology Department caused by the resignation of David McFarlane, the Senior Lecturer. As no suitable person could be found to fill McFarlane's post, Matheson continued to serve the College in his usual conscientious way until his sudden death in his laboratory on 8 March 1948.

It now became clear that the earlier decision of the College's Board of Management to hold in abeyance the filling of the Professorial Chairs in Physiology, Pathology and Bacteriology, when integration of the College with the University appeared to be about to take place, had greatly diminished the efficiency of these departments. Steps were taken in 1948 to fill the vacant chair in the Department of Pathology, but as no guarantee about the future status of the post could be given, the submitted applications were withdrawn. The ongoing uncertainty about the future after the University assumed responsibility for veterinary education also caused a lot of unrest among all grades of the veterinary staff. An additional cause for unrest, more particularly among the Senior and Junior Lecturers, was the unequal payment treatment meted out to the staff of the Royal (Dick) Veterinary College compared to the staff of the Royal Veterinary College in London. Veterinary teaching posts were no longer attractive. In every other branch of veterinary professional life, the financial rewards were greater than the veterinary colleges could offer. The professional staff in the veterinary colleges came last as far as remuneration was concerned when compared with general practitioners, and the veterinary staff of the various Government departments, ministries, research institutions and commercial firms (Mitchell 1949).

Until something concrete was decided regarding their future status and financial prospects, it was feared there would be further staff losses that the Dick Vet could ill afford. It was also said that unless the University of Edinburgh was prepared to make provision for sufficient senior posts, which need not be filled until men of sufficient calibre became available, young men of ability would not embark on a career which offered only limited possibilities for future advancement compared with other professions (Mitchell 1949). Following representation to them, the urgency of this need to build for the future was appreciated by the Department of Agriculture for Scotland; six posts as Demonstrators were offered to the Dick Vet at very short notice in 1948. These posts, at £400 per annum, were intended to attract young graduates, not so much by money but by offering them the opportunity to improve their education along specialised lines. At the same time, they would obtain experience in a wider field of their chosen subject by taking some part in the general teaching of undergraduates. Men who had been among the best students in their year took up these positions and helped infuse new life into the Dick Vet (Mitchell 1949).

Post-war reconstruction at Summerhall

The temporary structural modifications made to create Summerhall's wartime facilities and their subsequent heavy physical usage by large cohorts of medical, dental, agriculture, Polish and veterinary students, together with the relative lack of resources during wartime for routine building maintenance, meant that the plumbing, heating, lighting and other structural elements of the College estate required attention (Mitchell 1947). Consequently, during 1947–8 the staff and students at the College had to work under conditions of great discomfort due to the upheaval associated with the complete renewal of these facilities. The Refectory in the basement of the College was reconstructed during the Easter vacation, the three rooms previously used being converted into one large dining hall. Quicker service was thereby provided, and seating was increased to provide for two hundred at one time. Repairs were also made to the external fabric of the College, with the replacement of many of the metal window frames and the completion of all the outside paintwork. To overcome the necessity of duplicating classes, the laboratories in the Physiology, Pathology and Bacteriology departments were converted from thirty-eight- to fifty-place laboratories. That completed, the interior decoration proceeded during the vacation periods over the next two years. By 1950 all the roofs had been completely overhauled and the defective harling work on the outside walls repaired. The demolition and removal of Hope Park United Free Church had been completed in May 1949 and the site was levelled (Figures 6.9 and 9.3).

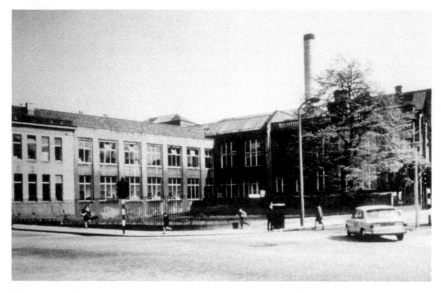

Figure 9.3 Space on the north-west corner after the demolition and removal of Hope Park United Free Church. Photographer: unknown.

The Field Station

The Loveday Committee had also recommended very strongly that field stations should be established and attached to every centre of veterinary education in the country (MAF 1944). The land in the vicinity of the Bush House (Figure 9.4) was already under consideration by William Mitchell when Sir Stephen Watson, Professor of Agriculture and Rural Economy of the University of Edinburgh and Principal of the East of Scotland College of Agriculture, approached him with his compatible ideas about developing a centre of 'Rural Economy' on the Bush & Dryden Estate. The University acquired the land in 1947. An area within the estate of about 175 acres around the Bush Home Farm and Easter Bush Farm and certain fields within the policies of Bush House (Plate 9.1) was selected for the use of the Dick Vet. The advantage of proximity to Bush House was the anticipation of permanent veterinary teaching and research buildings and a students' hostel that might eventually be built there.

The next step in the formation of a Field Station took place in November 1949, when the College obtained possession of the farm buildings of Easter Bush Farm and 16 hectares of adjacent land. The adjacent Bush Home Farm buildings and the remainder of the land were due to be acquired in November 1950, but with the approval of the Board of

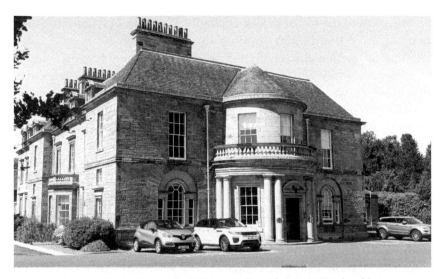

Figure 9.4 Bush House, Bush estate. Photographer: Alastair A. Macdonald.

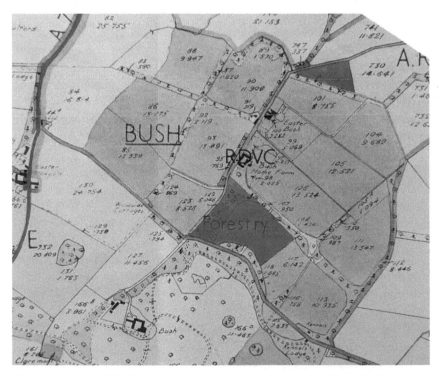

Plate 9.1 Map of R(D)VC land round Bush Farm. Image: Adapted from Ingham, A.G. 1947.

Management of the Estate an area of about 31 hectares of Easter Howgate land was taken over in May 1950 on the understanding that an equivalent amount of land already allotted on the Bush Home Farm would be relinquished. By this arrangement a more compact area of land around the farm buildings was achieved. The dairy stock, non-pedigree Ayrshire type, belonging to the outgoing tenant was taken over on entry and the poorer animals sold to reduce their number to thirty cows. By taking over an already formed herd, Easter Bush Farm immediately became available as a teaching farm for the College's Department of Veterinary Hygiene and Preventive Medicine. Two breeding sows, one workhorse and eight riding horses were added to the stock. The Clinical Department made regular use of the dairy herd for pregnancy diagnosis work at all stages of gestation. The riding horses were used for the instruction of preclinical students in animal management (Mitchell 1950).

During Session 1949–50 a total of 312 veterinary students were in attendance. Male intake was again largely ex-servicemen (forty-seven), together with five men from overseas and one man medically unfit for service. Four women were admitted. The number of agriculture students who attended instruction in veterinary hygiene was 106. Twenty-seven of the College students had the BSc (Vet.Sci.) degree conferred upon them (Mitchell 1950). However, during that Session the staffing problem continued to be difficult. Applications following advertisement of vacant lectureship posts were confined to members of the staff already holding junior appointments within the College. The position in the Department of Physiology was particularly serious. The Head of the department, Frederick J. Elliott, had only a technical assistant to help him. It had been impossible to attract lecturers in biochemistry and biophysics. Although the promotion of junior staff stabilised the teaching position to some extent, at the end of the year the total number of staff vacancies (eleven) remained the same as in 1948–9 (Mitchell 1950).

Veterinary College embodiment within the University of Edinburgh

A University Committee met on 20 and 31 January 1949 to consider the position of the School of Veterinary Medicine within the University (Mackie 1949). It had gathered information from informal discussions between representatives of the University, the Royal (Dick) Veterinary College, the Department of Agriculture for Scotland, and the Inter-Departmental Committee for Grants for Veterinary Education concerning the whole question. This included how the integration of veterinary teaching with university teaching, and the institution of a registrable degree in veterinary medicine and surgery might take place. Incorporation had been agreed in principle, possible methods of integration had been considered, and the view had been expressed that veterinary education should be closely aligned with medical education, particularly in the early stages of the curriculum. However, during the discussions in January 1949, the main problems, from the University point of view, appeared to be associated with (a) the creation of University Chairs in veterinary subjects, (b) the additional responsibilities which would be placed on the Heads of certain established University departments and (c) the geographical location of accommodation for the teaching of veterinary students (Mackie 1949). The Committee also expressed concern about the proposed transfer to the University staff of veterinary teachers who had held professorial status in the College without giving them 'Associate Professorship' status. The complexity of the considerable reorganisation that the Committee foresaw prompted them to suggest that the new degree course should not be introduced before October 1952.

It was subsequently reported that the Medical Faculty agreed that the veterinary degree should be awarded in the Faculty of Medicine and that the curriculum and examination for the degree should be under the administration of a Board of Veterinary Studies. The then current BSc (Vet.Sci.) degree should be discontinued, and veterinary students wishing to combine a science degree with a veterinary qualification should take a degree in Pure Science. The Faculty of Medicine was requested to proceed without delay to plan the curriculum for the proposed degree in Veterinary Medicine and Surgery. It was made clear to the Faculty that the title of 'Associate Professorship' was not available within the University of Edinburgh.

On 14 June 1950 the Senatus Academicus instituted an eight-member interim Board of Veterinary Studies in the Faculty of Medicine, comprising four members (including Professor Francis A. E. Crew from the Dick Vet Board) from Medicine and four members from the Dick Vet (Crew 1950a). Secretaries and lawyers were in attendance. It was agreed, following written advice from the Lord Lyon King at Arms, that the phrase 'embodiment of the College within the University' should be used, and 'to associate the name of "Dick" with the Veterinary School within the University, retaining, if possible, the designation "Royal"'.

Later that year, on 29 November, the memorial plaque to O. Charnock Bradley (Figure 9.5), installed on the left side of the entrance hall of the College, was unveiled by Mr W. Nairn in the presence of many alumni and others (Jennings 1951). The small plate on the memorial read:

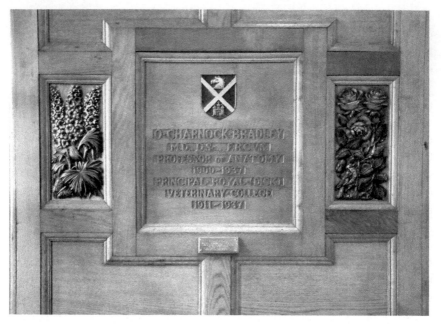

Figure 9.5   O. Charnock Bradley Memorial Plaque decorated with delphiniums, roses, a goldfinch and a butterfly. Photographer: Colin M. Warwick.

> This Memorial has been placed here to honour the name of Dr O. Charnock Bradley and to record the esteem and affection with which he was regarded by his students, his colleagues and all those who were associated with him.

Also that year, the gift of pictures offered to the Dick Vet in 1946 by Miss E. B. Barclay of 17 Coates Crescent, Edinburgh, had been received. They consisted of the sketch by Turner, five paintings, a pen-and-ink drawing and two prints (Crew 1950b).

On 9 May 1951 the Senatus gave approval to the proposal for an Ordinance instituting degrees of Veterinary Medicine and Surgery and Relative Regulations (Senatus 1951). On 10 May 1951, Royal Assent was given to the University of Edinburgh (Royal (Dick) Veterinary College) Order Confirmation Act, which provided for the dissolution of the Veterinary College and for its embodiment within the University of Edinburgh, effective from 1 April 1951 (Confirmation 1951). Later that summer, on 16 August, a letter was sent from the Secretary of the University, Charles H. Stewart, to the Dean of the Faculty of Medicine and copied to William M. Mitchell, the Head of the Veterinary College, intimating 'that His Majesty [George VI] has been graciously pleased to approve the continued use of the title "Royal" by the Department of Veterinary Studies of the University'. His Majesty's pleasure was intimated to the Faculty of Medicine and to the Veterinary College (Medicine 1951), as well as to the University Court at their first meeting in October that year; the Department would accordingly be known as The Royal (Dick) School of Veterinary Studies (Dalling 1951; Macdonald 2013).

On 22 October 1951 the Court of the University of Edinburgh made an Ordinance, No. 282 (Edinburgh No. 92): [Institution of Degrees in Veterinary Medicine and Surgery and Relative Regulations], and as a consequence of due procedure, on the 10th of March 1952, Her Majesty Queen Elizabeth gave her approval (Court, 1952). Subsequently the University Court promoted ordinances for the institution of three University Chairs, in Veterinary Surgery, Veterinary Medicine and Veterinary Hygiene and Preventive Medicine. The 1952 register from the RCVS listed the Dick Vet as 'The Royal (Dick) School of Veterinary Studies, University of Edinburgh' (Anonymous 1952).

The entry of the College into the University was celebrated by a Garden Party at the Bush preceding a dance in the McEwan Hall. At the same time there was an exhibition in Summerhall of various books and articles of veterinary historical interest (Anonymous 1951a). In May 1951 the Dick Vet Association members gathered in Summerhall to mark its embodiment within the University. After refreshments, an impromptu concert was held (Jennings 1951).

Thereafter, the Veterinary School functioned as a constituent part of the Faculty of Medicine for over a decade. The composite Curriculum Fee, listed in the last Royal (Dick) Veterinary College Calendar 1951–2, was £35 13s. for each of the three terms.

At 3 pm on Tuesday, 27 November 1951 there was a War Memorial unveiling ceremony (Anonymous 1951b). The Memorial was unveiled by Mrs Steele, widow of Alastair P. Steele (Matthews et al. 2015, 2016). The now designated Director of Veterinary Education, William M. Mitchell, asked the Principal of the University of Edinburgh, Sir Edward V. Appleton, to accept custody of the Memorial (Figure 9.6).

A listing of the proposed new building developments for 1952–7 was drawn up by Mitchell. The first priority was given to the new building at the Field Station on the Bush Estate (Mitchell 1951).

Curiously, and somewhat unexpectedly, some of the data for the initial years of the incorporation of the Veterinary College within the University of Edinburgh have been rather difficult to access. The detailed history of the embodiment of the R(D)VC within Edinburgh University's Faculty of Medicine must therefore await a much more complete availability of the relevant documentation. Part of the problem of access may be because the administration of the Veterinary School, during the initial approximately ten-year period, was carried out by four main groups: (1) the Secretary,

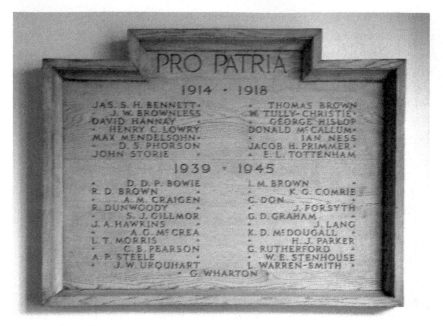

PRO PATRIA

1914 · 1918

JAS. S. H. BENNETT·   · THOMAS BROWN
· J. W. BROWNLESS   W. TULLY-CHRISTIE·
DAVID HANNAY   ·   · GEORGE HISLOP
· HENRY C. LOWRY   DONALD M'CALLUM·
MAX MENDELSOHN·   ·   IAN NESS
· D. S. PHORSON   JACOB H. PRIMMER·
JOHN STORIE   ·   · E. L. TOTTENHAM

1939 · 1945

·   D. D. P. BOWIE   I. M. BROWN   ·
R. D. BROWN   ·   ·   K. G. COMRIE
·   A. M. CRAIGEN   C. DON   ·
R. DUNWOODY   ·   ·   J. FORSYTH
·   S. J. GILLMOR   G. D. GRAHAM   ·
J. A. HAWKINS   ·   ·   J. LANG
·   A. G. M'CREA   K. D. M'DOUGALL   ·
L. T. MORRIS   ·   ·   H. J. PARKER
·   C. B. PEARSON   G. RUTHERFORD   ·
A. P. STEELE   ·   ·   W. E. STENHOUSE
·   J. W. URQUHART   L. WARREN-SMITH   ·
·   G. WHARTON   ·

Figure 9.6   War memorial in 1951. Photographer: Colin M. Warwick.

Accountant and other officers of the University's General Administration at Old College, (2) a section of administration in the Veterinary School, (3) the Faculty of Medicine office, and (4) the Director of Veterinary Education and his private secretary at Summerhall (Robertson 1957). For example, from April 1951 until December 1953 the arrangements for the organisation and administration of the new School of Veterinary Studies were described as 'somewhat ill-defined'; not until November 1952 were the five non-professorial Heads of the veterinary departments and one other Senior Lecturer in the School appointed to the Board of Veterinary Studies, and were thus able to obtain direct representation on matters relating to the courses qualifying for the degrees of BVM&S. and DVM&S (Beattie 1957). The membership of the Board of Veterinary Studies also included five professors from the Faculty of Medicine, the Reader in Botany, the Dean of the Faculty of Medicine and the Principal *ex officio* (Anonymous 1957). Following review of this situation, the Heads of the veterinary departments were informed in December 1953 of a number of the University Court's decisions, which then formed the basis for the administration and organisation of the Veterinary School during the subsequent three years. It was said that subsequent experience of these arrangements did not meet the needs of the School (Alexander 1957; Beattie 1957).

The combining of two organisations with long and largely independent histories was never going to be an easy process. Any expectation that it might be smooth and trouble-free was quite unrealistic. Although some of the procedures chosen to bring the Royal (Dick) Veterinary College into the much older University of Edinburgh may have recognised several of the difficulties of such an organisational 'transplant', others were over-looked. The management of both the University and the College had decided that the Faculty of Medicine was the most appropriate adminis-trative 'home' for the College. However, the failure to immediately create a Faculty of Veterinary Medicine came as something of a shock to many in the outside veterinary world.

The changeover of the College to a more or less subordinate position was said to have caused 'the loss of something indefinable' among the College staff. As an example of this, in December 1953 the University Court decided that the duties of the Director of Veterinary Education 'should be defined simply as those of Director of Studies for students proceeding to Veterinary Degrees or Diplomas in the Faculty of Medicine and as Convenor of the Board of Veterinary Studies under the Faculty of Medicine' (Court 1953). The main administrative body of the Veterinary School, the Board of Veterinary Studies, met only spasmodically and was not allowed to handle the veterinary matters it could well have done. The Convenor of the Board of Studies had been appointed by the Senate and was not elected by members of the Board. Veterinary departmental Heads, who were not members of the Medical Faculty, had to conduct their deal-ings with the Medical Faculty through a third party. Business discussed at the Medical Faculty affecting the Veterinary School was not transmitted to the non-professorial Heads of veterinary departments except unofficially.

On 7 October 1952 thirty-one male and five female students had embarked upon the new five-year BVM&S course run by the University of Edinburgh. The following year, thirty-nine male students and another five women were enrolled.

On 14 December 1953 a Veterinary School Committee was approved by the University Court to review, co-ordinate and facilitate such Veterinary School activities as were not dealt with by the Faculty of Medicine and were outwith the responsibility of the individual Heads of departments. Its membership consisted of the Veterinary School members of the Veterinary Board of Studies plus other members as the University Court may from time to time decide. The duties of the Committee were to supervise the administration of the Veterinary School library, Reading Rooms and the Refectory, to supervise the redecorations and maintenance of the general fabric of the School, to consider and report on any matters referred to it by the Senatus or University Court or any of its Committees, and to discuss other non-educational matters relating or incident to the activities of the Veterinary School. However, the Veterinary School was inadequately represented – by the three professorial clinicians – on the Faculty of Medicine; there was no veterinary representation from the pre-clinical staff.

It seems that many of the problems affecting the Veterinary School never reached the Veterinary Board of Studies. This subsequently led to the formation of a Special University Committee on the future organisation and administration of the Royal (Dick) School of Veterinary Studies. In May 1957 it reported to Senate, and on 10 July 1957 their Report was approved:

> The School's Board of Veterinary Studies, which was responsible for advising Senate, through the Faculty of Medicine, on matters relating to veterinary education, had met at irregular and infrequent intervals and had not fulfilled the objectives for which it was instituted. Business other than of an academic nature had been dealt with by the Veterinary School Committee, instituted in 1953, and only had Dick Vet staff on it. The Chairman was elected annually, but this office was not held and had never been held by the Director of Veterinary Education. The Special Committee were of the opinion that creation of a Veterinary Faculty, by concentrating general academic and administrative responsibility on a Dean, would improve the conduct of veterinary business, and should be regarded as the ultimate objective of a reorganisation of the then present system. (Senatus 1957)

This Special University Committee recommended to the University Court that:

> (1) The board of veterinary studies should be reconstituted to include the remaining Senior lecturers in the School and those Readers and Lecturers in Medical and Scientific Departments with special responsibility for teaching veterinary students. The Board should be required to meet on a prescribed number of occasions during the academic year. With a view to the eventual institution of a Veterinary Faculty, the Board should be given power and encouraged to discuss and decide those matters which more usually fall within the province of a Faculty rather than a Board of Studies.
> (2) There should be a Director of the Veterinary School, whose standing should be that of Assistant Dean of the Faculty of Medicine with special responsibility for veterinary affairs. His appointment should lie in the Medical Faculty on the annual nomination of the Board of Veterinary Studies, of which he should be the Convenor. He should be responsible for the general co-ordination of the School's activities, and should be given every opportunity to obtain experience through membership of Committees, especially those in which veterinary business is discussed.
> (3) The Veterinary School Committee and its sub-committees should be dissolved.
> (4) The Administration Officer in the School should work under the immediate instruction of the Director, in control of the day-to-day administration of the School. The Veterinary Office should be a self-contained service for the School.

(5) The Faculty of Medicine should be invited to consider the possibility of appointing to its membership one or more of the non-professorial heads of Veterinary Departments.

Alexander Robertson appointed Director of Veterinary Education

William Mitchell retired in 1957 and the following year Professor Alexander Robertson was appointed the next Director of Veterinary Education (Figure 9.7). Under his chairmanship the working of the initial BVM&S curriculum was reviewed that year and improvements introduced. From 1 October 1958 the curriculum arrangements were:

First Year: Chemistry; Physics; Biology; Veterinary Anatomy; Practical Animal Management.
First Professional Examination: Physics (March); Chemistry; Biology (June). (Resit Examination in September).
Second Year and Autumn Term Third Year: Anatomy, including Histology and Embryology; Physiology; Biochemistry.

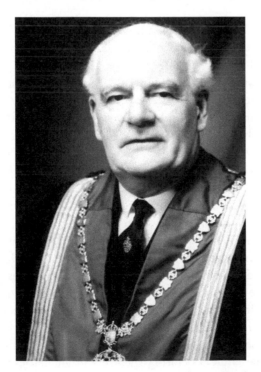

Figure 9.7 Sir Alexander Robertson. Photographer: unknown London photographer.

Second Professional Examination: (December). (Resit Examination in March): Veterinary Anatomy, Histology and Embryology; Veterinary Physiology and Biochemistry.

Third Year, Spring and Summer terms: Genetics; Applied Physiology; Veterinary Hygiene, Dietetics and Animal Husbandry; Veterinary Pharmacology.

Third Professional Examination: (June). (Resit Examination in September): Pharmacology; Hygiene (including Dietetics and Animal Husbandry).

Fourth Year: Veterinary Pathology; Veterinary Bacteriology; Veterinary Parasitology. Meat Inspection: Introducing Veterinary Medicine and Veterinary Surgery: Clinical Medicine and Surgery.

Fourth Professional Examination (June). (Resit examination in September): Veterinary Pathology; Bacteriology; Parasitology.

Fifth Year: Veterinary Medicine; Veterinary Surgery; Veterinary Preventative and State Medicine; Meat Inspection; Veterinary Obstetrics; Clinical Medicine and Surgery.

Final Professional Examination (June). (Resit examination in November): Veterinary Medicine; Veterinary Surgery; Veterinary Preventative and State Medicine; Veterinary Obstetrics.

In accordance with the recommendations of the Loveday Committee, the School admitted approximately fifty students annually to the BVM&S course (Figure 9.8).

The Veterinary School had not pressed for the construction of the Field Station during 1952–7 because it was felt desirable to await until 1956, at the end of the period of transition from the former MRCVS curriculum to the new BVM&S curriculum. Alan Reiach and Partners were appointed to be the architects (Anonymous 1964; Figure 9.9). The University's Development Committee proposed that the finances for the construction should be applied for in 1958, and the University Grants Committee delayed the start of phase one until 1959 (Figure 9.10). Work on the construction of phase two started in 1961.

The visiting RCVS inspectors felt that the 1958 revised curriculum simplified and improved the BVM&S course (Sumner 1959). It reduced the time allotted to some preclinical subjects and was designed to make the best possible use of the facilities at the new Field Station. Most of the final-year teaching was to be undertaken there, as well as tuition of earlier years in animal management and animal husbandry. However, in Summerhall, the visiting RCVS inspectors found that the facilities for the small-animal clinic, operating theatre and ancillaries were far below the desirable standard (Sumner 1959). Prior to about 1950, most of

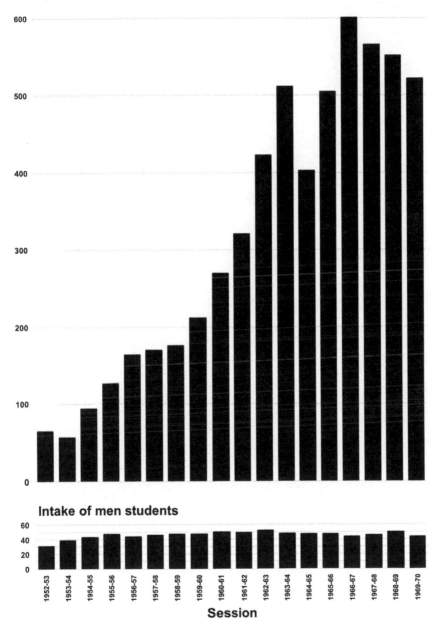

Figure 9.8 Graph of men applicants and BVM&S male student intake, 1952–69.

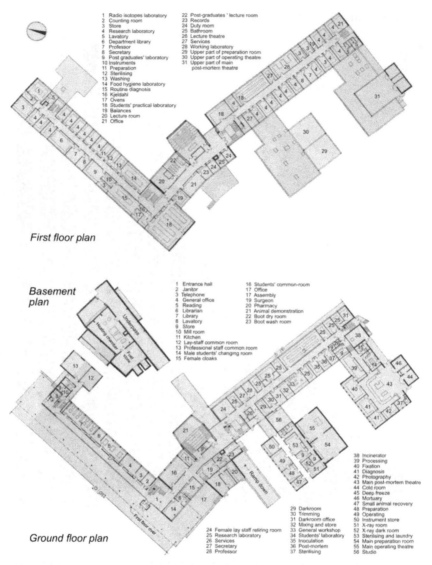

Figure 9.9 Architect's drawings (Alan Reiach and Partners) of the proposed buildings at Easter Bush. Image: adapted from [Reiach, A. 1964] *The Architects' Journal*, 139, 1311–24.

the training of veterinary graduates had been in preparation for mixed general practice, where they would be treating a variety of domestic animals; a special emphasis had been placed on the diseases of the horse. The treatment of companion animals (dogs, cats, small mammals and birds) was beginning to occupy a larger proportion of professional time (Gardiner 2014).

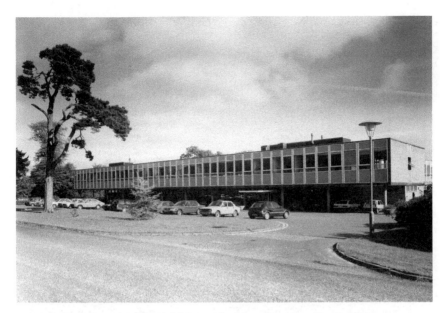

Figure 9.10   Frontage of the Field Station building. Photographer: Bob Munro.

The inspectors also noted a shortage of suitably trained technical staff, that the Medical School Professor of Physiology was in charge of Veterinary Physiology at Summerhall and that Veterinary Biochemistry was part of the University Department of Biochemistry. Class certificates (in Physiology and Biochemistry) were required to certify that the student had achieved a sufficient number of attendances and had 'duly performed the work of the class' in order to be granted permission to be examined (Sumner 1959). In the spring of 1962 Ainsley Iggo was appointed Professor of Veterinary Physiology and a significant infusion of new life of international quality resulted (Anonymous 1962). The final year of the revised BVM&S curriculum came into operation during the 1962–3 Session. The Field Station on the Bush Estate opened, and a proportion of the final-year teaching was transferred there (Figure 9.11a and b). A new sectional class timetable provided the fifth-year students with increased opportunities for clinical and pathological study of individual cases of disease (Robertson 1963).

Faculty of Veterinary Medicine and Surgery established

In April 1962 the Faculty of Medicine gave consideration to a report concerning the establishment of a Faculty of Veterinary Medicine and Surgery at an appropriate time within the quinquennium 1962–7, and

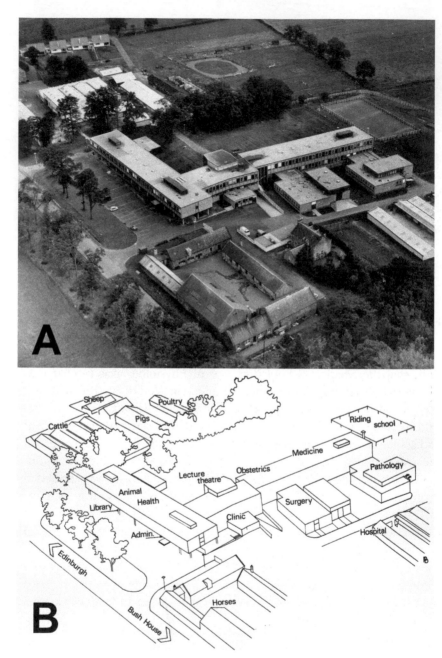

Figure 9.11 A. Aerial view of the Field Station. Photographer: unknown, attributed to A. Reiach, architects; B. Key to the Field Station buildings.

the recommendation was supported (Medicine 1962). Because of the work of the Northumberland Committee (MAFF 1964), for a decade (1964–74) significant capital investment was obtained for new buildings at Summerhall for both large- and small-animal facilities, as well as for postgraduate education and research. In May 1964 a report from the Board of Veterinary Studies was circulated to the Faculty of Medicine. Its recommendation, that a Faculty of Veterinary Medicine be formed with effect from 1 October 1964, was approved for transmission to the Senatus Academicus and the University Court (Medicine 1964). At its meeting on 15 June 1964 the University Court approved the proposal that the Royal (Dick) School of Veterinary Studies should begin to operate administratively as a Faculty with effect from 1 July 1964 (Court 1964). Alexander Robertson was appointed Dean of the Faculty of Veterinary Medicine and the following Chairs were assigned to the Faculty: Animal Health, Veterinary Anatomy, Veterinary Medicine, Veterinary Pathology, Veterinary Physiology and Veterinary Surgery. A new teaching timetable for the BVM&S degree was published in the 1964–5 Calendar. This was amended slightly for Session 1965–6.

The RCVS visit in 1964 commented that there was a need for further accommodation at Summerhall to facilitate the teaching of pre-clinical and para-clinical subjects and to enable extension of research to be carried out (Dalling 1966). The accommodation for research was very inadequate. In 1965, during the British Veterinary Association (BVA) congress in Edinburgh, a plaque was put on the wall in White Horse Close to commemorate the birthplace of William Dick. Cast by Henshaws, it was unveiled by Mr Oliver, the President of the BVA that year (Figure 9.12).

Student intake

The intake of male students from 1954 to 1963 had largely stabilised around an average of forty-seven (Figure 9.8). During that period, however, there had been more than a quadrupling of male applications. Although the intake of women over the same period averaged about five, the numbers in the last four years had edged above that (Figure 9.13). However, there had been a ten-fold increase in the number of women making applications to enter the Dick Vet. At the Veterinary Faculty meeting on 12 October 1965, it was agreed that, for a variety of reasons, the annual intake of female students should not exceed ten women. A limit of 10 per cent was mentioned as a suitable average, which would reduce this figure to five or six. One year later, at the Veterinary

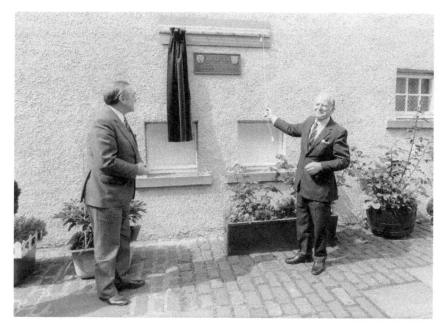

Figure 9.12 Unveiling of the White Horse Close plaque by Denis Oliver, with the Principal of the University, Sir John Burnet, in attendance. Photographer: Fiona Manson.

Faculty meeting on 11 October 1966, there was again some discussion as to whether or not the intake of women students should be restricted (Faculty minute No. 119 of 12 October 1965) or indeed whether applicants should be considered on merit alone, regardless of sex. In response to an enquiry from Professor Iggo, the Dean (Robertson) said that he had no information on any national policy on this question. Factors to be considered included: (a) Acceptance of male applicants to the exclusion of better-qualified women applicants: (b) Exclusion of male applicants in favour of women who may not even enter or may remain only for a few years in the profession: (c) Adequate hostel, common room and other facilities for women students if relatively large numbers were admitted. The Dean said that it was open to Faculty to reconsider the recommendation (Minute No. 119) that 'intake of women students should not exceed ten'. (Note: Intake of women students 1960 to 1963; average 6.5: 1964; 10; 1965; 9: 1966; 10.) At the Faculty meeting on 7 October 1969 the attention of Faculty was called to the relative increase in numbers of women applicants in recent years (Figure 9.13) and it was suggested that, on these grounds, there might be a case for an increase in the intake of women students. However, there was no strong support for this suggestion and Faculty agreed to maintain the present arrangements under which the Selection Board aimed at restricting intake of women students

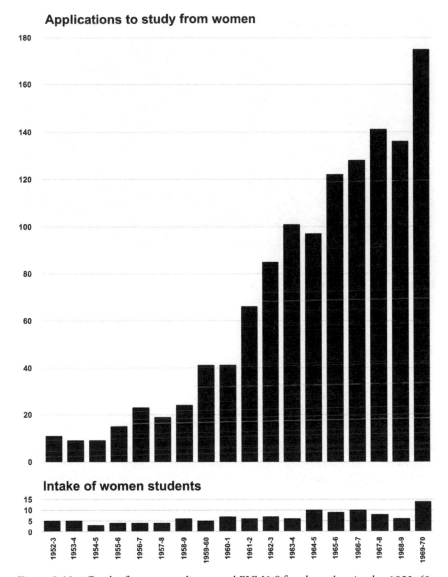

Figure 9.13 Graph of women applicants and BVM&S female student intake, 1952–69.

each year to a maximum of ten. Somewhat ironically, in October that year the student intake was forty-four males and fourteen females (Figures 9.8, 9.13). The numbers graduating in 1969 were forty-one men and six women (Figure 9.14).

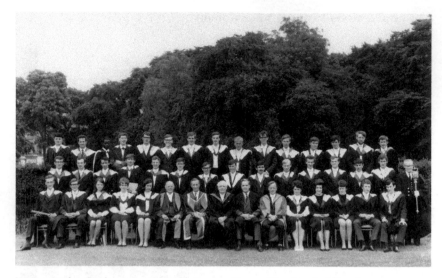

Figure 9.14 Graduation 1969, with Servitor Jimmy Morrison holding the mace. Photograph attributed to Ken Thomson.

References

Alexander, F. 1957. Organisation and administration of the Royal (Dick) School of Veterinary Studies. Memorandum. CRC, University of Edinburgh, EUA INI/ADS/SEC/B. L.04/3/3/5 Box 96 of 211.

Anonymous, 1951a. Comment by the horse above the clinical yard. *The Centaur*, 16 (1), 16–19.

Anonymous, 1951b. *University of Edinburgh Royal Dick School of Veterinary Studies War Memorial unveiling ceremony.* CRC, The University of Edinburgh.

Anonymous, 1952. *The veterinary surgeons acts 1881–1948 the register of veterinary surgeons and the supplementary veterinary register 1952.* London: Royal College of Veterinary Surgeons, 437.

Anonymous, 1957. *May 1957 Report of the special Committee on the future organisation and administration of the Royal (Dick) School of Veterinary Studies.* CRC, University of Edinburgh. EUA INI/ADS/SEC/B. L.04/3/3/5 Box 196 of 211.

Anonymous, 1962. Professor Ainsley Iggo, M.Agr.Sc., B.Sc., Ph.D. *The Centaur*, 25 (1), 6–7.

Anonymous, 1964. Veterinary Field Station. *The Architects' Journal*, 139, 1311–24.

Beattie, 1957. A memorandum to the members of the Special Committee of the University Court. Organisation + Admin (1). CRC, University of Edinburgh, EUA INI/ADS/SEC/B. L.04/3/3/5 Box 96 of 211.

Confirmation, 1951. *University of Edinburgh (Royal (Dick) Veterinary College) Order Confirmation Act, 1951. 14 & 15 Geo. 6 Ch xiv; 'Affiliation of the Veterinary College'.* CRC, University of Edinburgh, EUA INII ADS/SEC/ N(II - 1948–1953).

Court, 1952. [Institution of Degrees in Veterinary Medicine and Surgery and Relative Regulations.] *The Court of the University of Edinburgh, 22nd October 1951, ordinance No. 282 (Edinburgh No. 92).*

Court, 1953. *Letter from the Secretary to the University dated 21st of December 1953.* R(D) SVS Archives, CRC, University of Edinburgh.

Court, 1964. *Court Minutes 15 June 1964; Minute of the meeting of the Faculty of Medicine held on 19th June 1964, minute 313.* CRC, University of Edinburgh, EUH INI/ACU/MED/1.

Crew, F. A. E. 1950a. *Minutes of a meeting of representatives of the Royal (Dick) Veterinary College and the University held in the University Court Room, Old College on Wednesday 5th July 1950, at 9.30.* CRC, University of Edinburgh.

Crew, F. A. E. 1950b. *Gift of pictures. Minute of meeting of the Board of Management held on Tuesday, 18th July 1950, at 2.30p.m.* CRC, University of Edinburgh. Minutes of the Board of Management, 1940–51.

Dalling, T. 1951. Foreword. *The Centaur,* 16 (1), 4–5.

Dalling, T. 1966. *University of Edinburgh 1964. Report of Visitors appointed by the Council of the Royal College of Veterinary Surgeons.* London.

Gardiner, A. 2014. The 'Dangerous' Women of Animal Welfare: How British Veterinary Medicine Went to the Dogs. *Social History of Medicine,* 27 (3), 466–87.

Ingham, A. G. 1947. *Preliminary report on proposed development of the estates of Bush, Boghall & Dryden for agricultural research & education.* Edinburgh.

Jennings, S. 1951. Honorary secretary's report. Royal (Dick) Alumnus Association. *The Centaur,* 16 (1), 51–2.

Macdonald, A. A. 2013. The Royal (Dick) School of Veterinary Studies: what's in a name. *Veterinary History,* 17 (1), 33–65.

Mackie, T. J. 1949. *University of Edinburgh Faculty of Medicine. Report.* CRC, University of Edinburgh. Box 2 TD, Vol. II 1948–53.

MAF, 1938. *Report of the Committee on Veterinary Education in Great Britain.* Ministry of Agriculture and Fisheries, HMSO.

MAF, 1944. *Second Report of the Committee on Veterinary education in Great Britain.* Ministry of Agriculture and Fisheries, HMSO, cmd 6517.

MAFF, 1964. *Report of the Departmental Committee of Inquiry into Recruitment for the Veterinary Profession.* HMSO, cmd 2430.

Matthews, P. K., Macdonald, A. A. and Warwick C. M. 2015. The Royal (Dick) Veterinary College contingent of the Officers Training Corps. *Veterinary History,* 18, 5–27. <era.ed.ac.uk/handle/1842/14176> (accessed 11 September 2022).

Matthews, P. K., Warwick C. M. and Macdonald, A. A. 2016. The War Memorial and Roll-of-Honour of the Royal (Dick) School of Veterinary Studies. *Veterinary History,* 18, 117–64. <era.ed.ac.uk/handle/1842/14209> (accessed 11 September 2022).

Medicine, 1951. *Minute of the Meeting of the Faculty of Medicine held on 5 October, 1951, minute 3684.* CRC, University of Edinburgh, EUA LNIIACUIMED/1; Archives of the Royal (Dick) School of Veterinary Studies, The University of Edinburgh, CRC – correspondence.

Medicine, 1962. *Minute of Meeting of the Faculty of Medicine held on 20th April 1962. Minute 176.* CRC, University of Edinburgh, EUA INV/ACU/MED/1.

Medicine, 1964. *Minute of the meeting of the Faculty of Medicine held on 22nd May 1964. Minute 273.* CRC, University of Edinburgh, EUH INI/ACU/MED/1.

Mitchell, W. 1947. *Royal (Dick) Veterinary College. Principal's Report for session 1946–1947.* CRC, The University of Edinburgh.

Mitchell, W. 1948. *Royal (Dick) Veterinary College. Principal's Report for session 1947–1948.* CRC, The University of Edinburgh.

Mitchell, W. 1949. *Royal (Dick) Veterinary College. Principal's Report for session 1948–1949.* CRC, The University of Edinburgh.

Mitchell, W. 1950. *Royal (Dick) Veterinary College. Principal's Report for session 1949–1950.* CRC, The University of Edinburgh.

Reiach, A. 1964. Veterinary field station at Roslin. Edinburgh. Building study ([97]). *The Architects' Journal,* 139, 1311–24.

Robertson, A. 1957. Memorandum. CRC, University of Edinburgh, EUA INI/ADS/SEC/B. L.04/3/3/5 Box 96 of 211.

Robertson, A. 1963. Report to the Dean of the Faculty of Medicine Royal (Dick) School of Veterinary Studies Session 1962/1963. *The Centaur*, 26 (1), 5–9.

Senatus, 1951. *Proposals for an Ordinance instituting Degrees in Veterinary Medicine and Surgery and Relative Regulations.* Senatus Academicus signed Minutes 11, October 1949–August 1951, 522–9.

Senatus, 1957. *Appendix I. Report of the special committee on the future organisation and administration of the Royal (Dick) School of Veterinary Studies. May 1957.* Senatus Academicus signed Minutes 14, October 1955 to July 1957, 766–7.

Sumner, H. 1959. *Veterinary Surgeons Act, 1948. University of Edinburgh. Report of Visitors appointed by the Council of the Royal College of Veterinary Surgeons.* London.

Chapter 10

The Centre for Tropical Veterinary Medicine (1970–2005)

Tropical Veterinary Medicine teaching established

We must now step back in time to find the beginnings of the university team that was established to concentrate solely on the postgraduate training of veterinary medicine, and to specifically focus on the research and delivery of veterinary information relevant to tropical and subtropical parts of the world. The embryonic development of the Centre for Tropical Veterinary Medicine can be said to have begun in 1928 (Bradley 1928). According to Charnock Bradley's diary entry of 5 December 1928, 'Then to the university to see Lorrain Smith about a suggested (by T. W. M. Cameron) course of Tropical Veterinary Medicine.'

In June 1930 the Court of Edinburgh University agreed to institute a Diploma in Tropical Veterinary Medicine, DTVM (Univ.Edin.). Its initiators were O. Charnock Bradley, Principal of the Royal (Dick) Veterinary College, and James Lorrain Smith, the Dean of the University's Faculty of Medicine. The course for this Diploma, which would be held partly at the University and partly at the R(D)VC, would occupy six months (October to March) and would commence that year (Anonymous 1930a). It was noted that many graduates of the College were already occupying responsible and important veterinary posts in East and South Africa (Anonymous 1930b).

The institution of this Diploma was considered by the Principal of the Dick Vet to have been the most important development that took place in the preceding twelve months (Bradley 1930). The Lovat Committee (Anonymous 1929) had recommended a postgraduate course for newly appointed Colonial Veterinary Officers, refresher courses for Veterinary Officers on leave in Britain, and that scholarships (ten) should be given to encourage suitable students to join the colonial veterinary service. It had also recommended that a school of tropical veterinary medicine should be established. Bradley (1930) indicated that 'they had already all the machinery that was necessary for a properly equipped and thoroughly efficient school of tropical veterinary medicine in Edinburgh'. The Edinburgh Veterinary College had its newly constructed building, suitably trained and experienced staff and appropriate professional links to tropical environments.

> The curriculum consisted of two parts; Part I was held in the Autumn Term and comprised 120 hours of entomology and parasitology, 75 hours of bacteriology, and 20 hours of lectures and demonstrations on special subjects. Part II was taken in the Spring Term and consisted of 80 hours of parasitology and entomology, 10 hours of personal hygiene in the tropics, 20 hours of meat and milk production, 50 hours on feeding of animals in the tropics, 20 hours on breeding of animals, 40 hours of epizootiology, and 20 hours of lectures and demonstrations on special subjects. The division of the curriculum was to enable candidates to interrupt their course, return to their tropical station, and take Part II while on their next home leave. Although it was anticipated that most applicants for the course would be British serving officers, 77% of the successful candidates were overseas veterinarians. The inclusive fee for either Part was £15-15-0d (£15.75). Instruction was provided by the Professors and staff of the University Departments of Natural History and Bacteriology in Part I and by the University Professors of Natural History and Genetics in Part II together with the Professors of Veterinary Hygiene and Animal Husbandry at the Veterinary College. (Scott and Smith 1996)

The DTVM course was not taught during the Second World War because home leave for Colonial Officers for educational purposes had been stopped for its duration. It was resuscitated in 1954 on the initiative of Alexander Robertson, the then Professor of Animal Health in the Royal (Dick) Veterinary College. He convinced the College, the University and the Colonial Office that a refresher course for colonial veterinary officers was viable and was required. He was also far-sighted enough to anticipate the demand for further postgraduate training by veterinary graduates from the universities of the newly independent and developing countries. Teaching restarted in October 1955, with Archie W. Chalmers as the Course Director (Figure 10.1). The previous two-part curriculum was followed for the first two years, but thereafter was gradually expanded to cover more material. The course was enlarged further in 1962 and, in 1964, it was extended to cover the whole academic year. It was designed to provide a comprehensive training for overseas veterinarians, particularly those aiming at the senior ranks of field services. The demand for places did indeed exceed forecast expectations and four new teaching posts, for staff with tropical experience, were created in the early 1960s. In this way, in 1962, an unofficial Tropical Unit came into being within the College's Department of Animal Health. It initially comprised four lecturers, two technicians and a 'technical librarian' post. This unit was financed by an annual grant from the Ministry of Overseas Development (ODM) (Robertson 1972a). By 1967 this unit had become so large that the ODM agreed to provide funding for the establishment of a 'Centre' which would be concerned with postgraduate training, research and documentation in Tropical Veterinary Medicine, together with technical assistance in that field in developing countries (Robertson 1972b). A recurrent grant for five years was secured from the ODM to cover the staffing and maintenance of the teaching and documentation activities of the Centre. The first published issue of *Tropical Animal Health and Production* was edited in the department and issued by Edinburgh University Press in August 1969 (Hunter 1998). Prior to the establishment of the Centre, the University of Edinburgh had trained approximately fifteen students per year from forty-four countries (Robertson 1972b). The total number trained in Tropical Veterinary Medicine was 229.

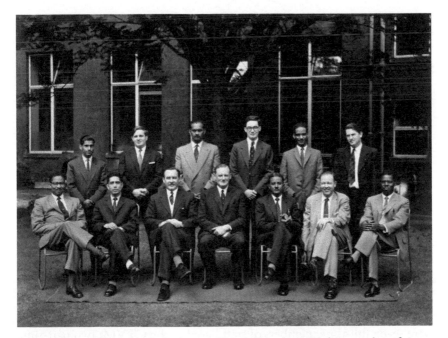

Figure 10.1 Group of 1961 Diploma in Tropical Veterinary Medicine students from India, Malaya, Southern Rhodesia, Sudan, Tanganyika, British Guiana, Nigeria and Paraguay together with Archie W. Chalmers (centre) in Summerhall. Photographer: E. R. Yerbury & Sons.

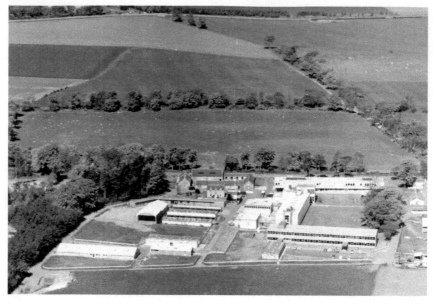

Figure 10.2 Aerial view from the south-west taken in 1971 of CTVM (bottom right with cars parked outside). Photographer: unknown, attributed to A. Reiach, architects.

The Centre for Tropical Veterinary Medicine

On 20 November 1970 the Centre for Tropical Veterinary Medicine (CTVM) was officially opened by the University Chancellor, the Duke of Edinburgh. It occupied a newly constructed wing adjacent to the existing 1960s buildings at Easter Bush (Figure 10.2). Later that year the Overseas Development Administration (ODA) funded the Chair in Tropical Animal Health for five years. A commemorative mural was painted on the wall near the library by Dr Jack K. H. Wilde, the Head of Protozoology at CTVM (Plate 10.1). The University created a Department of Tropical Animal Health in the Faculty of Veterinary Medicine and on 1 November 1971 transferred to it the staff concerned with the Centre's teaching activities in tropical veterinary medicine along with its research, documentation, administration and technical assistance work (Robertson 1972b). Alex Robertson was appointed to the newly created Professorship of Tropical Animal Health; he was made the first Director of the CTVM and was awarded a knighthood. At the time there were seven full-time members of staff based at the CTVM, two part-time and one permanently based overseas. There were seven research fellows and ten research Associates. The role of Librarian was performed by Bill Beaton (Sewell 1996). The library was largely financed by the ODA but

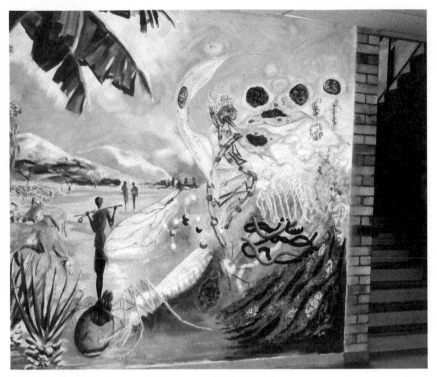

Plate 10.1   Ground-floor mural, painted by Dr Jack K. H. Wilde, and stair to lecture room. Photographer: Bob Munro.

was closely associated with and serviced by the University Library as part of the Veterinary Faculty Library. In 1970–1 the CTVM matriculated fifteen students onto the single Diploma course of Tropical Veterinary Medicine (TVM). There were also two students taking the newly created Tropical Laboratory Orientation course. During the second year of this course, 1971–2, there were twenty Diploma students (Robertson 1972b). A total of nineteen students matriculated for a PhD and two students for an MSc degree.

The functions of the Centre agreed by the University Court and the ODA included:

(a) The provision of facilities for continuing and if necessary expanding instruction in the principles and practice of tropical veterinary medicine for individuals or groups intending to proceed overseas under arrangements made by the Administration; and for overseas students taking the University's Diploma Course in Tropical Veterinary Medicine or such other advanced courses as may be considered desirable.

(b) The provision of research training on problems related to tropical veterinary medicine for British and overseas postgraduate students under the supervision of staff who are familiar with the background to these problems.

(c) The maintenance of a group of senior staff with knowledge of and an active and continuing interest in tropical veterinary matters who will participate in the teaching and research activities of the Centre, who will supervise the activities of research workers, and who will be competent and will be encouraged as occasion arises to organise and supervise research projects carried out in appropriate institutions in developing countries.

(d) The deployment of staff from the Centre, as occasion arises and circumstances permit, to take temporary posts in overseas Universities and other institutions pending the appointment of nationals or expatriates to these posts.

Short 'Briefing Courses', lasting one to four weeks, were organised to meet the specific requirements of individual veterinary officers, usually recruited for overseas assignments by the ODA. In 1970–1 five such courses were organised and the following year there were seven (Robertson 1972b). These were later developed into Personal Training Plans, a concept pioneered by the Centre and actively taken up elsewhere in the University. Staff were already in demand for consultancies and teaching assignments overseas, a role which in no way diminished in subsequent years (Sewell 1996).

The broadly based TVM course had been designed for the training of senior veterinary field officers. In 1972 it was supplemented by the three-month-long orientation course to teach British veterinarians how to run diagnostic laboratories in developing countries. This amalgamated course was then further upgraded in 1974 to a twelve-month MSc course in Tropical Veterinary Science (TVS) (Scott and Smith 1996). Up to that date only veterinarians were admitted to the CTVM. It was soon recognised that graduates in other disciplines could also be trained, specifically in the many and varied skills required for the husbandry and production of animals in the tropics. There was therefore a need to widen and deepen the CTVM training base. In 1974 the Diploma/MSc course in Tropical Animal Production and Health (TAPH) was introduced and the first MSc (TAPH) students graduated in November 1975. It became the most sought-after course of the three on offer (Scott and Smith 1996). Shortly afterwards, in 1977, the other two courses adopted this format, whereby Diploma students were admitted whose basic qualifications did not allow direct admission to an MSc course, with the possibility of being transferred to the latter if their performance proved of sufficient merit. The MSc students continued for another three months beyond the three teaching terms, during which time they prepared and presented a dissertation on their additional work (Robertson 1978). The transfer to the CTVM in 1977 of much of the teaching in TAPH that had previously been conducted in the College of Agriculture created a serious accommodation problem. This was somewhat relieved by the acquisition of three Portakabins which also provided much-needed additional office and storage space (Robertson 1978; Brocklesby 1979). In 1977–8 there were forty-eight postgraduate students, forty-one Diploma/MSc and seven PhD students. Twenty PhD students graduated that year (Robertson 1978). During the first nine years (1970–9) there were 254 students from fifty-nine countries taking these Diploma/MSc courses and twenty-six PhD graduates (CTVM Annual Reports 1971–9). The bulk of the funding support for the CTVM during those years came from the ODA, with the British Council funding studentships for many of those from overseas (Taylor 1996). Sir Alexander Robertson retired as Director of CTVM in 1978 and David Brocklesby was appointed its Director (Brocklesby 1979).

The expansion plans proposed in 1977 for additional accommodation for both teaching and research (Robertson 1977) were unable to go ahead due to Government cuts in public expenditure. Further cuts in funding made it impossible to replace staff who had decided to leave (Brocklesby 1980), and in 1981 the ODA withdrew its support for the teaching activities of the Centre (Brocklesby 1981). Emergency funding had to be found for teaching staff. The staff were placed on annual one-year contracts (Brocklesby 1981). No Tropical Veterinary Medicine course was run in 1980–1, although the other two courses did run (Anonymous 1980, 1981; Scott and Smith 1996). It was made clear that for the Diploma/MSc courses to continue after 1980 the fee revenue had to completely cover the costs. The Tuition Fee for the TVM and TAPH courses was therefore raised to £5,000, and to £6,000 for the TVS course. It was also necessary to increase student numbers from about thirty-five to fifty and to increase the proportion of overseas students. During the teaching-free 1980–1 session the TVM course was revamped to change the bias more towards epidemiology and the control of livestock disease. It was redesigned to provide postgraduate training for veterinary officers working in the middle and upper ranks of the field services in tropical countries whose functions were to plan and implement disease control measures on a regional and national scale (Anonymous 1981; Brocklesby 1982). In 1981 some forty-seven students enrolled for the three CTVM courses and forty were from overseas. In response, the University now offered two-year contracts (Brocklesby 1982). In 1982–3 the University gave all those teaching a contract until

1986. The University also took over the Chair in Tropical Animal Health (Brocklesby 1983). The ODA research funding returned to a three-year cycle (from an annual cycle). Student recruitment was maintained, with forty-seven students attending in 1982–3, of whom thirty-nine were from overseas (Brocklesby 1983). The total number of Diploma and MSc students enrolled between 1970–1 and 1982–3 was 432. The TVM courses were taken by 195 students, the TVS courses attracted seventy-eight students, and 159 students had enrolled in the TAPH courses. Throughout those years the students represented seventy-four countries from around the world. In addition, five students gained MPhil degrees and thirty-eight graduated PhD.

Research activities

During the initial decade of its existence the emphasis of the research being carried out at the CTVM was on adaptive and strategic research programmes targeted at developing countries (Taylor 1996). Much of this was field-based. It fell broadly into four categories: Protozoology, Helminthology, Microbiology and Animal Husbandry. These were the mainstays of research at the CTVM (Taylor 1996). In 1989 the ODA requested that the Centre should manage the animal health programme not only within the CTVM but in a number of other British universities and research institutes (Sewell 1991a). In the 1990s the research staff were increasingly spending much of their time in the tropics, in a wide range of countries, but notably in research institutes in Mexico, Malawi, Ghana, Kenya, Nepal, Colombia, Morocco, Tunisia, Turkey, India, Tanzania and Indonesia (Sewell 1991a, 1996). Many of the research students were working in associated institutes or were spending most of their time in their home countries on 'home and away' research projects for degrees.

Protozoology

The tsetse-transmitted trypanosomes *Trypanosoma brucei*, *T. congolense* and *T. vivax* were restricted to Africa, where they had been responsible for the exclusion of livestock from large areas of land which had the potential of supporting cattle and other ruminants (Boid et al. 1996). It was felt that no other animal disease had had such an influence on cattle distribution and in preventing the intensification of livestock production. At the CTVM in the 1970s and early 1980s, research work on antigenic variation of the trypanosomes concentrated on *T. gambiense* and *T. congolense* (Boid et al. 1996). Cultivation of the infective organisms was a major area of trypanosomosis research at the CTVM. Advances were made in tissue culture, developing to the cultivation of the entire life cycle of *T. congolense*. These culture facilities, and access to trypanosome stocks from a wide geographical area and links with field sites, made the CTVM an ideal environment for the development and adaptation of tests to measure the sensitivity of trypanosomes to trypanocidal drugs in the laboratory (Boid et al. 1996).

Helminthology

The objective of the research into helminths at the CTVM was to increase animal productivity. Helminth diseases occurred in many of the less developed and tropical countries, causing death, poor weight gains, condemnation and downgrading of carcasses (Harrison, Hammond and Sewell 1996). The research work was broadly based and involved studies into cestodes, trematodes and nematodes. Studies in the tropics and sub-tropics were conducted in collaboration with workers from various countries in Africa, Asia and Latin America. Much of the work of the helminthology section took the classical approach. First, a problem in the field was identified, if necessary, a solution in the laboratory was devised and then the solution was tested in the field prior to its implementation on a wider scale (Harrison, Hammond and Sewell 1996). The ODA funded research on the cattle and human tapeworm *Taenia saginata* and the closely related pork and human tapeworm, *T. solium*. Their presence in a population was an indicator of poor general standards of public health and sanitation (Harrison and Sewell 1990). Initially, development of a vaccine against cestodes was considered the most feasible approach, but a lot of research was required to find the appropriate immunological targets (Harrison, Hammond and Sewell 1996).

The *Fasciola hepatica* infection of goats and buffaloes provided a very appropriate model system that was extensively used by the CTVM to investigate the host–parasite relationship of this trematode infection. Initial studies were mainly concerned with the pathogenesis of the disease in domestic livestock. These were extended to research on *F. gigantica* in buffalo calves (Harrison, Hammond and Sewell 1996). Studies of parasitic nematodes formed a smaller part of the research programme than those on platyhelminthes.

Microbiology

The microbiology section at the CTVM examined six bacterial, eighteen viral and five ricketsial infections, but was best known for its research into cattle plague (rinderpest), orf in sheep, bovine dermatophilosis and granulocytic cytoecetes (Ehrlichia) infections of ruminants, horses and man (Scott 1996). The absence of 100 per cent containment facilities in the UK meant that the study of these organisms was carried out overseas. It was forcefully pointed out in 1988 that since 1977 at least thirty-four major animal plagues had erupted and that seven of these episodes involved organisms that were previously unknown; most of them were viruses and these events dramatically emphasised the importance of veterinary virology as a subject for research and teaching (Scott 1988; Brocklesby 1988).

Animal husbandry

The research programme on draught animals was first mooted at the CTVM in 1976, 'and was met with a certain amount of incredulity' (Pearson, Laurence and Smith 1996). However, at that time, draught animals provided the farm power in many developing countries. They derived their energy sources from local rather than imported expensive materials. In addition, the farm equipment required could be made by local blacksmiths. There was a huge gap in the available knowledge of the nutrition and the physiology of the working animal. The questions asked included: How did diseases affect work output? Did different types and species of draught animals have different ways of working? Were some better than others in certain situations? In what experimental ways could these questions be addressed and answered? The invention, design and manufacture of appropriate equipment and measuring instruments at the CTVM was seen as central to the draught animal research programme, and guidelines on their application and the wider aspects of research methodology were then published (Pearson, Laurence and Smith 1996). Most of the research was funded by the ODA.

Non-graduating courses, conferences and publications

Through Tropag, a University of Edinburgh agency, consultancy missions in 1982–3 were undertaken in Kenya, Burma, Sri Lanka, the Philippines, Costa Rica, Oman, Somalia and Uganda. The ODA contracted research at the CTVM through Tropag and provided administrative staff support in the CTVM office (Brocklesby 1983). Courses in tropical agriculture and rural development became a feature of the Tropag consultants in the 1980s (Figure 10.3). Two CTVM Tropag courses in Agricultural Extension Technology in the Tropics were run in 1987, along with the fifth Tropag course on Recent Developments in Animal Nutrition and their Application to Tropical Countries (Figure 10.3). By 1988 a third annual Tropag course on Recent Advances in Tropical Animal Health was held and attracted twenty-two participants (Figure 10.3), as was one on Draught Animal Technology attended by thirteen participants from Africa and Asia (Brocklesby 1987). This pattern of teaching continued up until the early 1990s. At the beginning of April 1991, the third course on Draught Animal Technology was held. It ran for ten weeks. The overall objective was to train extension workers and others in techniques that would enable them to encourage farmers to boost agricultural production and improve standards of living while using the minimum of imported resources. The previous year a ten-day workshop for senior staff involved in policymaking, planning and evaluation of draught animal technology programmes in (sub)tropical countries had been hosted by the CTVM and held, from 2 to 12 April, jointly with colleagues in the Larenstein International Agricultural College in Deventer, the Netherlands. In the first week of September 1990 a three-day colloquium on Donkeys, Mules and Horses in Tropical Agricultural Development had been jointly organised by the CTVM and the Edinburgh School of Agriculture. The seventh annual intensive short CTVM course in Recent Advances and Current Concepts in Tropical Veterinary Medicine was again fully subscribed and held from 6 to 17 April 1992 (Smith 1993). It was run again in 1993. In 1993 four CTVM staff conducted a four-day course on Tropical Veterinary Medicine and Animal Production for 170 students and veterinarians, most of whom were from Spain, at the Veterinary Faculty of the Independent University of Barcelona (Smith 1993).

On a larger scale, a series of five international conferences dealing with various aspects of tropical animal production and diseases were organised and the proceedings published by CTVM:

Smith, A. J. (ed.). 1976. *Beef cattle production in developing countries: Proceedings of the Conference held in Edinburgh from the 1st to 6th September 1974 organised by the Centre for Tropical Veterinary Medicine.* Roslin: University of Edinburgh, Centre for Tropical Veterinary Medicine.

Wilde, J. K. H. (ed.). 1978. *Tick-borne diseases and their vectors. Proceedings of an international conference held in Edinburgh from the*

Table 10.1 The Tropical Agriculturalist series of fifteen inexpensive handbooks produced for the CTVM by the staff and colleagues.

Series Editor: Dr Anthony J. Smith
Published by CTA-Macmillan. Price: £6 15s.
This series of inexpensive but up-to-date handbooks in English and French have been written for personnel requiring information on livestock in the tropics at a non-professional level. All are in straightforward, nontechnical language complemented by photographs, illustrations and tables. Organisations in African, Caribbean and Pacific countries may be able to obtain free copies from the CTA, POB 380, 6700 AJ Wageningen, The Netherlands.

Poultry	1990	Anthony J. Smith
Pigs	1991	David Holness
Sheep	1991	Ruth Gatenby & J. M. Humbert
Rabbits	1991	Denis Fielding & G. Matheron
Ruminant nutrition	1992	John Chesworth
Dairying	1993	Richard Matthewman
Beef	1993	Anthony J. Smith
Animal Breeding	1994	Gerald Wiener
Animal Health. Vol. 1	1994	Archie Hunter
Animal Health, Vol. 2	1996	Archie Hunter & Prof. Uilenberg
Goats	1995	Mike Steel
Animal Production Systems	1995	R. Trevor Wilson
Camels	1998	R. Trevor Wilson
Donkeys	1998	Denis Fielding, Patrick Krause & Erik Vall
Tilapia	1998	J. Arrignon & M. W. Dickson

27th September to the 1st October 1976, organised by the Centre for Tropical Veterinary Medicine. Edinburgh: Edinburgh University Press.
Smith, A. J. and Gunn, R. G. (eds). 1981. *Intensive animal production in developing countries. Proceedings of a symposium organised by the British Society of Animal Production and held at Harrogate in November 1979.* Thames Ditton: British Society of Animal Production.
Smith, A. J. (ed.). 1985. *Milk production in developing countries. Proceedings of the Conference [Strategies for Dairy Development] held in Edinburgh from the 2nd to the 6th of April 1984, organised by the Centre for Tropical Veterinary Medicine.* Edinburgh: University of Edinburgh Press.
Hunter, A. G. (ed.). 1991. *Biotechnology in livestock in developing countries: proceedings of Biotechnology 1989, an International Conference on the Application of Biotechnology to Livestock in Developing Countries, held in the University of Edinburgh from 4th to 8th September 1989, organised by the staff of the Centre for Tropical Veterinary Medicine.* Edinburgh: Centre for Tropical Veterinary Medicine.

Other tropical handbooks were edited by Robertson (1976, 1984) and by Sewell and Brocklesby (1990). In addition, during the 1990s a series of fifteen low-priced books were produced by CTVM staff on animal production in the tropics for international distribution (Table 10.1).

ANNOUNCEMENTS

TWO TROPAG COURSES IN AGRICULTURAL EXTENSION TECHNOLOGY IN THE TROPICS

The first from 1 July to 10 September 1987
(with optional Induction Unit from 9 to 30 June 1987) and the second from 7 October to 17 December 1987

The main objectives of the courses are to develop an understanding of potential barriers to change in rural communities, to equip participants with the expertise needed to communicate effectively for the promotion of agricultural development in tropical countries and to motivate them to train colleagues in their own country.

Course curriculum – the curriculum covers the principal components of extension practice:
– Identifying the needs of farmers
– Identifying techniques appropriate for particular situations
– The management of available extension resources
– The evaluation of results of extension programmes.

Reply to Dr A. J. Smith, Centre for Tropical Veterinary Medicine, University of Edinburgh, Easter Bush, Roslin, Midlothian, EH25 9RG, Scotland.

FIFTH TROPAG COURSE ON RECENT DEVELOPMENTS IN ANIMAL NUTRITION AND THEIR APPLICATION TO TROPICAL COUNTRIES

The fifth course in Animal Nutrition in the Tropics will be held at Edinburgh University in September, 1987.

The objective will be to review recent developments in the nutrition of farm animals and to consider possible applications of these developments to the feeding of farm animals in the tropics. The course is designed for a wide variety of persons including advisors, consultants, postgraduate students and teachers. The dates for the course are: September 10 to 25, 1987.

The course is being organised by Mr R. Matthewman, Centre for Tropical Veterinary Medicine, University of Edinburgh, Easter Bush, Roslin, Midlothian, EH25 9RG, Scotland.

TROPAG COURSE ON RECENT ADVANCES IN TROPICAL ANIMAL HEALTH

The course will be held at the University of Edinburgh's CTVM from 4 to 15 April, 1988 and is designed specifically for veterinarians. The objectives of the course are to review recent advances in animal health in the tropics and to consider the implications of these advances in the organisation of animal health programmes and animal production.

The course is being organised by Mr A. G. Hunter and Dr J. A. Hammond of the CTVM. For further details please write to Mr A. G. Hunter, Centre for Tropical Veterinary Medicine, University of Edinburgh, Easter Bush, Roslin, Midlothian, EH25 9RG, Scotland.

Figure 10.3 Announcement in 1987 of two additional CTVM courses, from *Tropical Animal Health and Production*, 19, 127.

Draught Animal News was published as a newsletter from 1989 to 2009 by Ann Pearson. It was circulated twice a year as a printed volume. The index and all the volumes are available on the internet: <https://www.vet.ed.ac.uk/ctvm/Research/DAPR/draught%20

animal%20news/danindex.htm> (accessed 26 February 2022). The journal was funded by the UK Department for International Development (DFID) for the first fifteen years. However, in 2005 DFID changed the focus of its funding for research and development, and the journal's financial support ended. The journal contained studies, reports and practical tips concerning the management and use of working animals – cattle, buffalo, equines, camels and so on – plus notices of events, presentation of new publications, bibliographical references as well as questions and comments from readers. It was valued worldwide as a platform for the exchange of information and ideas. Publication continued with charity support for four more years but ceased in 2009 on financial grounds (Figure 10.4): <http://www.draughtanimalnews.org/index.php/en/about-dan> (accessed 26 February 2022).

Diploma and MSc teaching (1981–91)

Between 1981 and 1985 the CTVM matriculated 47–50 students into the Diploma/MSc courses each year. In 1984–5 it welcomed fifty-one students from twenty-one countries to study on the three Diploma/MSc courses (Brocklesby 1985). Three years later Brocklesby (1988) reported that the forty-nine-student intake that year represented thirty countries. However, in 1986 and 1988 student numbers dropped to forty-three and forty-two respectively. It was recognised that the numbers of students for any one course fluctuated from year to year, mainly due to variations in the availability of finance, particularly from governmental sources (Sewell 1996). The annual Diploma/MSc student intake remained relatively high between 1988–9 and 1991–2 (Figure 10.5) and was reported to be 47, 47, 47, 56 (Smith 1991). It was also reported that a total of 917 students had graduated from the CTVM courses since 1970, when the Centre opened. A new development in 1991 was the two-year 'hybrid' MPhil course, during which nine months were spent studying a coursework programme in any of the three Diploma options followed by a dissertation prepared after fifteen months of research investigation (Smith 1991). Between 1984 and 1994 thirty-two students graduated PhD.

The arson attack

'Disaster' struck on the night of 26–7 November 1991. Animal rights activists broke into the CTVM and lit three petrol-fuelled fires. Had the

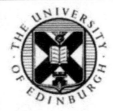

DRAUGHT ANIMAL NEWS

No. 47

December 2009

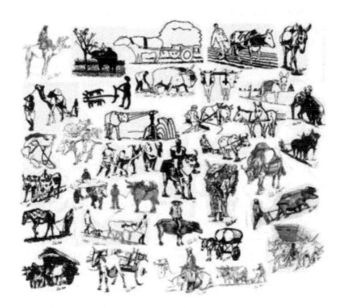

Produced by:
Centre for Tropical Veterinary Medicine, University of Edinburgh

Personally sponsored by:
Pit Schlecter

Figure 10.4 Front cover of Vol. 47 of *Draught Animal News* (2009) showing a selection of the draught animal drawings by Archie 'Picasso' Hunter.

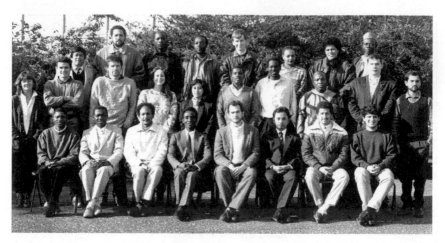

Figure 10.5 Group of 1991–2 Tropical Animal Production and Health students from nineteen countries at Easter Bush. Photographer: Bob Munro.

flames not been detected soon after they began, the Centre would probably have been destroyed. As it was, the arsonists succeeded in burning many of the administrative records and a considerable amount of teaching material, some of which was irreplaceable. Luckily, very little research data was lost. Most of that was duplicated elsewhere. Teaching recommenced on the day after the fire and all essential administrative and research functions were maintained (Sewell 1991b, 1993; Anonymous 1993). However, the main lecture theatre, the TVS teaching laboratory, the library and the canteen were all badly affected by the fire. Work began immediately to bring order from the chaos. Temporary teaching and research laboratory accommodation was found nearby, and repairs and restoration began rapidly. It was not until four months later that all the remaining books were cleaned and reshelved in the newly redecorated library. Around 1,500 items were either lost or damaged in the fire. Many were rapidly replaced by generous donations and new purchases. Copies of unpublished documents were sought and found. All the staff moved back into their offices in November 1992 (Smith 1994).

The attack prompted a public explanation of the relevance of undertaking teaching and research on tropical veterinary medicine in Edinburgh (Sewell 1991b). The primary aim of the Centre was

> to provide a wider, global view of the ways in which disease and inappropriate management cause economic loss and suffering to the animals and of the means by which these defects can be remedied. We do this for a small but important group of graduate students. Most of these have been selected by their own governments, who see the value of a small cadre of veterinarians and animal production experts with a wider knowledge of animal diseases

and production methods than can be given by in-country undergraduate or postgraduate training. Other students, who come from the developed world, including the United Kingdom and the European Community, are intending to make a career in assisting the development of tropical and sub-tropical agriculture. Some of the latter are self-funding, others are funded by their employers, which include both governmental and international organisations. (Sewell 1991b)

The Centre provided access to excellent local facilities and expertise, staff with extensive tropical experience and research interests, and 'the opportunity of sharing knowledge between students drawn from a wide range of countries and backgrounds, including new graduates in veterinary science or animal production and students who have years of field experience in widely differing climatic, sociological and economic circumstances' (Sewell 1991b). The research undertaken at the Centre was all directed for the control, treatment or alleviation of major diseases or causes of dysfunction in tropical livestock.

Research adaptation

But times were changing for research. The Centre had to accept the challenge of meeting both the ODA's requirements for a greater concentration of adaptive research and the needs of the University and Faculty for research which would enhance their reputations in the Government-inspired Research Assessment Exercises. It had to do so while seeking research funding from wider sources than hitherto and, in particular, expanding the collaboration which already existed with colleagues of similar interests in other European countries (Sewell 1996). By the early to mid-1990s the pattern of research at the CTVM had begun to take into account the changing emphases of many of the funding agencies. The traditional areas of expertise continued but the important developments in quantitative epidemiology, genetics and biotechnology were addressed. This expertise was built up in-house and frequently through collaboration with other institutions in the UK, the EU and increasingly the developing countries (Taylor 1996). Additional money was supplied in the late 1980s and 1990s from the European Community and the Royal Society in London to support some of the overseas work. This was carried out in collaboration with local institutions in Costa Rica, Colombia, Nepal, Indonesia, Nigeria, Morocco, Niger, The Gambia, Ethiopia, Zimbabwe and Chile (Pearson, Laurence and Smith 1996). Financial support could still be obtained from the Animal Health Programme of the ODA and the INCO-DC programme of the European Union. The Wellcome Trust continued to provide innovative schemes to promote all aspects of human and animal health (Taylor 1996). However, the message was becoming clear. Many European agencies were now focused on wealth creation within the European Union. Research into tropical animal health had become more difficult to sustain. It required increased political support from those countries where the diseases were endemic.

In the late 1980s trypanosomosis research at the CTVM had turned towards *T. evansi* and cultures of this organism were initiated. These grew in suspension culture, and as a consequence of biochemical developments it became possible to initiate cultures free from other living organisms. This enabled stocks from Africa, Asia and South America to be maintained indefinitely. Their use in research focused upon drug resistance, the development of drug assays, the screening of potential drugs and investigations of the mechanisms of drug resistance (Boid et al. 1996). Rapid and inexpensive methods for testing the sensitivity and resistance to drugs were developed at the CTVM and the value of these assays were both laboratory- and field-tested to show proven success (Boid et al. 1996). Subsequent work focused on the application of these assays for epidemiological studies assessing the extent of the problem of drug resistance in the field, the screening of new trypanocidal agents and the monitoring of the drug sensitivities of isolates during experiments. Further understanding came about following experiments at a DNA level.

Rinderpest was radically reduced but not eradicated from India or equatorial Africa following the international mass vaccination campaigns in the 1950s and 1960s. It flared up again from residual foci and the CTVM was invited to participate in the effort to contain and eradicate it in India and South-east Asia. In 1987 the Microbiology Section of the CTVM was also allocated the task of assessing the rinderpest diagnostic facilities in African countries, thirty-four of which participated in the Pan-African Rinderpest Campaign (Scott 1996). This collaborative international effort was effective. Rinderpest was officially eradicated from the world in 2010.

CTVM attention and expertise were then directed towards a further tropical scourge. More than 99 per cent of all human deaths from the viral disease rabies (*Rabies lyssavirus*) occur in the developing world. Domestic dogs are largely responsible for its transmission to humans. Quantitative prediction of the human mortality, disability and economic burden of rabies in Africa and Asia indicated almost 20,000 deaths in India and about 1.1 million patients receiving post-exposure treatment (Knobel et al. 2005). Vaccination of domestic dogs against rabies was most cost-effective in the medium to long term, with costs typically recouped within five to ten years. Expansion of this research interest to wildlife veterinary medicine culminated in exploration of rabies reservoir dynamics in the Serengeti ecosystem in north-west Tanzania (Lembo et al. 2008).

Postgraduate teaching (1991–2002)

In 1991–2 the CTVM accommodated fifty-six MSc students, of whom six were British and the rest drawn from around the world (Sewell 1996). However, in each of the following three years the numbers fell, with only thirty-two students having enrolled for the 1994–5 Session (Smith 1994). By 1995 it had become clear that the focus of the main funding agencies was changing. Since it opened in 1970, more than 1,100 postgraduate students from 108 countries had graduated from the CTVM (Figure 10.6). Most of them had come from Africa and the impact these students were having in their own countries was now considerable. Nevertheless, a number of adjustments had to be introduced into the teaching practices of the CTVM. The modularisation of the three established MSc courses, the introduction of a fourth in 1995 and the further introduction of two new interdisciplinary MSc courses in 1996 and 1997 were ways in which the Centre responded to this challenge (Table 10.2). These six modular MSc courses could be spread over a maximum of five years. The expectation was that they would attract individuals for MSc training from governments and institutions not normally able to release individuals for a twelve-month academic year. It was also thought that the option

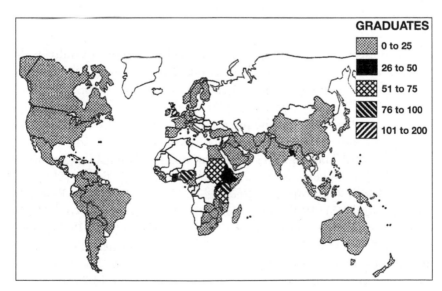

GRADUATES

0 to 25
26 to 50
51 to 75
76 to 100
101 to 200

Figure 10.6 Worldwide distribution of CTVM graduates, 1970–95.

Table 10.2 Postgraduate courses available from the CTVM in 1997.

UNIVERSITY OF EDINBURGH CENTRE FOR TROPICAL VETERINARY MEDICINE DIPLOMA/MSc/MPhil POSTGRADUATE COURSES
The following postgraduate courses available at the CTVM comprise a series of training modules. Each course has mandatory core modules coupled with optional modules on a wide range of topics thus ensuring maximum flexibility in designing a programme of studies that best suit students' needs.
Tropical Veterinary Medicine. This course provides postgraduate training in the evaluation and management of disease control and animal health programmes. It is targeted at veterinarians working in developing countries who have responsibility for disease control, herd health, veterinary public health, disease surveys, epidemiological investigations, planning, management and policy formulation.
Tropical Veterinary Science. This course is aimed at veterinarians concerned with the laboratory diagnosis and investigation of animal disease, particularly in developing countries. The course gives an in-depth training in the theory and practice of diagnostic techniques relevant to the main diagnostic disciplines (microbiology, helminthology, vector-borne disease, immunology, haematology and biochemistry) coupled with optional modules in allied disciplines relevant to disease investigation.
Veterinary Laboratory Science. This course provides training in the laboratory diagnosis and investigation of animal disease. It is open to veterinarians and non-veterinarians and provides an ideal opportunity for training in modern investigation approaches to animal disease, including recent developments in immunological and molecular biological methods.
Tropical Animal Production and Health. This course is designed to meet the needs and in-service training requirements of a wide range of animal-related occupations. Former graduates are now working in livestock extension, planning, policy formulation, disease control, livestock and project management, consultancy, education, training and many other posts with livestock components.
Sustainable Rural Development in the Tropics. The modules available for this course are designed to provide students training on the sustainable provision of food and a reasonable standard of living in the less developed parts of the tropics and subtropics; one of the major problems currently confronting the world.
International Animal and Crop Production. This course is designed to meet the needs and in-service training requirements of persons working in all aspects of tropical agriculture.

of spreading studies over several years might be attractive to individuals working away from home for long periods. In addition, modularisation paved the way for bilingual MSc courses with the CTVM's sister institute, CIRAD-EMVT in Montpellier (Taylor 1996). An additional example of the CTVM's flexibility was the provision of shorter courses. These could be by taking individual MSc degree modules or by extending the Centre's unique Personal Training Plans and Continual Professional Development courses for UK and overseas veterinarians (Sewell 1996; Taylor 1996).

The British Government's Renewable Natural Resources Research Strategy (RNRRS), 1995–2005, came into operation on 1 April 1995. It exerted a considerable influence over the Animal Health Programme throughout that year. Available funds declined, and further falls were predicted. This situation also flagged up a lack of long-term career structure for young people in livestock development and animal health in the developing world. Young scientists in the UK and elsewhere in the developed world were warned not to expect long-term support for work in developing countries in the tropics even though there was still a need there for innovative concepts and their implementation (Brown 1995). The reduction in funding being provided to the ODA and its effect on the aid programme was disconcerting and the long-term career prospects of scientists committed to the ODA's strategic/adaptive research programme were identified as 'not good' (Brown 1995). In 1997 advertisements for the six CTVM courses on offer were placed in international journals (Table 10.2). Despite the reportedly healthy number of 'eager applicants' for CTVM courses in 1996 (Sewell 1996), in the later 1990s the demand for places fell as the authorities in most tropical countries decided that their home universities could supply their needs (Sewell 2013). Although data for the numbers who matriculated after 1995 are no longer available, it is clear from the numbers who graduated with MSc degrees from CTVM courses that there was a progressive decline; 27 students graduated MSc in 1995, 14 with MSc in 1998, 12 with MSc in 2000 and 7 with MSc in 2002. These numbers also correspond to the decline in the course options offered to students from 1998–9 to 2001–2, when, finally, only the Diploma/MSc in Tropical Animal Production and Health was offered. None of the Tropical Diploma/MSc courses were advertised in the University Calendar for Session 2002–3. The effect of the withdrawal of British development aid for residential international students was clear. The total number of students who graduated from studies at the CTVM was 1,158, representing 109 countries (Plate 10.2).

The training situation was investigated at an Animal Health and Production (AHP) sponsored workshop, held in Naivasha, Kenya in October 2005. The participants recognised the need for flexible learning opportunities which enabled students to remain in their home environments and continue working. There was a demand for flexible courses delivered through distance-learning formats and a strong but largely unmet demand for 'continuing professional development' (CPD) opportunities (DFID 2006). Participants saw the power of e-learning approaches such as those based on virtual patients. The existence of strong political support for greater use of information and communication technology (ICT) among governments, regional bodies, donors and commercial service providers was noted (DFID 2006).

At a follow-up workshop, also sponsored by AHP, held in Entebbe in March 2006, an umbrella body of sub-Saharan African veterinary institutions, from Ethiopia, Kenya, Uganda, Tanzania, Zambia, Zimbabwe, South Africa, Malawi and Sudan, joined to form the new African Universities Veterinary e-Learning Consortium (AUVEC) to help strengthen the African animal health sector (DFID 2006). Both the African Virtual University and

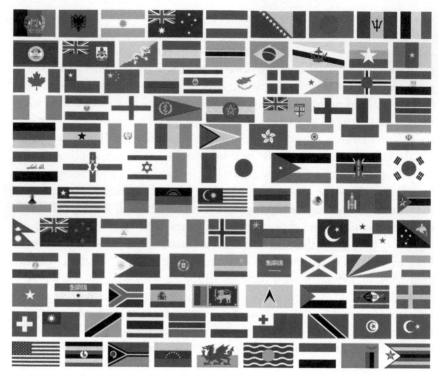

Plate 10.2 Flags of the 109 countries whose postgraduate students graduated at the CTVM. Image: Alastair A. Macdonald.

the University of Edinburgh played key support roles in building the infrastructure needed by the consortium and sharing knowledge and expertise to develop world-class e-learning. The e-learning courses could be updated much more easily and cheaply than conventional courses. Spearheaded by the CTVM, they worked to develop and deliver the online MSc in International Animal Health, which began matriculating students in 2006. A two-week summer school in Uganda provided students and teaching staff with an opportunity for face-to-face interaction (Fitzpatrick 2006; DFID 2006; Anonymous 2007). However, the restructuring of the University undertaken during 2002–3 meant that the Veterinary Faculty was reorganised, and all clinical staff were assimilated into Veterinary Clinical Studies. The CTVM ceased to function as such by 2005.

References

Anonymous, 1929. The position of veterinary education and service [Lovat Report]. *Nature*, 123, 269–70.

Anonymous, 1930a. Veterinary Diploma. Edinburgh University course. First in Britain. *The Scotsman*, 2 June 1930, p. 14, col. 3.

Anonymous, 1930b. Veterinary service. Recruits wanted in colonies. Royal (Dick) College. *The Scotsman*, 3 July 1930, p. 7, col. 2.

Anonymous, 1980. Teaching. *CTVM Annual Report 1979–1980*, 8.

Anonymous, 1981. Teaching. *CTVM Annual Report 1980–1981*, 8.

Anonymous, 1993. The CTVM fire. *Dick Vet News*, 5, 12–13.

Anonymous, 2007. Dick Vet leads online education in International Animal Health. *Dick Vet News*, 18, 8.

Boid, R., Hunter, A. G., Jones, T. W., Ross, C. A., Sutherland, D. and Luckins, A. G. 1996. Trypanosomosis research at the Centre for Tropical Veterinary Medicine (CTVM) 1970 to 1995. *Tropical Animal Health and Production*, 28, 5–22.

Bradley, O. C. 1928. *Diary entry, 5th December. Vol. 8*. Archives Royal (Dick) School of Veterinary Studies, CRC, The University of Edinburgh.

Bradley, O. C. 1930. Edinburgh's lead in tropical training. *The Scotsman*, 3 July 1930, p. 7, cols 2–3.

Brocklesby, D. W. 1979. Director's report. *CTVM Annual Report 1978–1979*, 7–8.

Brocklesby, D. W. 1980. Director's report. *CTVM Annual Report 1979–1980*, 7.

Brocklesby, D. W. 1981. Director's report. *CTVM Annual Report 1980–1981*, 7.

Brocklesby, D. W. 1982. Director's report. *CTVM Annual Report 1981–1982*, 7.

Brocklesby, D. W. 1983. Director's report. *CTVM Annual Report 1982–1983*, 7.

Brocklesby, D. W. 1985. Director's report. *CTVM Annual Report 1984–1985*, 7

Brocklesby, D. W. 1987. Director's report. *CTVM Annual Report 1986–1987*, i–ii.

Brocklesby, D. W. 1988. Director's report. *CTVM Annual Report 1987–1988*, i–ii.

Brown, C. G. D. 1995. ODA/NRRD Animal Health Programme Annual Report 1995. *CTVM Annual Report 1995*, 3–14.

DFID, 2006. *AHP Annual Report, 2005–2006*, 35–6. <assets.publishing.service.gov.uk /media/57a08c3ced915d622c0011ff/AHP_Annual_Report_2005-06.pdf > (accessed 11 September 2022).

Fitzpatrick, J. 2006. Online training for vets in Africa. *The Veterinary Record*, 159, 3.

Harrison, L. J. S., Hammond, J. A. and Sewell, M. M. H. 1996. Studies on helminthosis at the Centre for Tropical Veterinary Medicine (CTVM). *Tropical Animal Health and Production*, 28, 23–39.

Harrison, L. J. S. and Sewell, M. M. H. 1990. The zoonotic taeniae of Africa. In: C. N. L. MacPherson and P. S. Craig (eds). *Parasitic helminths and zoonoses in Africa*. London: Unwin Hyman, 54–82.

Hunter, A. 1998. Editorial comment. *Tropical Animal Health and Production*, 30, 1.

Knobel, D. L., Cleaveland, S., Coleman, P. G., Fèvre, E. M., Meltzer, M. I., Miranda, M. E. G., Shaw, A., Zinsstag, J. and Meslin, F.-X. 2005. Re-evaluating the burden of rabies in Africa and Asia. *Bulletin of the World Health Organisation*, 83, 360–8.

Lembo, T., Hampson, K., Haydon, D. T., Craft, M., Dobson, A., Dushoff, J., Ernest, E., Hoare, R., Kaare, M., Mlengeya, T., Mentzel, C. and Cleaveland, S. 2008. Exploring reservoir dynamics: a case study of rabies in the Serengeti ecosystem. *Journal of Applied Animal Health and Production*, 45, 1246–57.

Pearson, R. A., Lawrence, P. R. and Smith, A. J. 1996. The Centre for Tropical Veterinary Medicine (CTVM) pulling its weight in the field of draught animal research. *Tropical Animal Health and Production*, 28, 49–59.

Robertson, A. 1972a. Introduction. *CTVM Annual Report 1970–1972*, i.

Robertson, A. 1972b. Activities of the Centre. *CTVM Annual Report 1970–1972*, 7 & appendix.

Robertson, A. (ed.) 1976. *Handbook on animal diseases in the tropics*. 3rd edition. London: British Veterinary Association.

Robertson, A. 1977. Director's report. *CTVM Annual Report 1976–1977*, 7.

Robertson, A. 1978. Director's report. *CTVM Annual Report 1977–1978*, 7.

Robertson, A. (ed.). 1984. *Handbook of tropical veterinary laboratory diagnosis*. Edinburgh: Centre for Tropical Veterinary Medicine.

Scott, G. R. 1988. Microbiology section. *CTVM Annual Report 1987–88*, 12.

Scott, G. R. 1996. Microbiological research at the Centre for Tropical Veterinary Medicine (CTVM). *Tropical Animal Health and Production*, 28, 40–8.

Scott, G. R. and Smith, A. J. 1996. Technology transfer in tropical animal health and production at the Centre for Tropical Veterinary Medicine (CTVM). *Tropical Animal Health and Production*, 28, 60–6.

Sewell, M. M. H. 1991a. Director's report. *CTVM Annual Report 1989–90*, 1–3.

Sewell, M. M. H. 1991b. Director's report. *CTVM Annual Report 1991*, 1–3.

Sewell, M. M. H. 1993. Director's Review of 1992. *CTVM Annual Report 1992*, 1–2.

Sewell, M. M. H. 1996. Teaching and research at the CTVM – the first 25 years. *Tropical Animal Health and Production*, 28, 1–2.

Sewell, M. H. H. 2013. Dr John Arthur Hammond, D.V.S.M., D.T.V.M., D.A.P.&E., M.R.C.V.S., 1925–2013. *Tropical Animal Health and Production*, 45, 1459–60.

Sewell, M. M. H. and Brocklesby, D. W. (eds). 1990. *Handbook on animal diseases in the tropics*. 4th revised edition. London: Baillière Tindall.

Smith, A. J. 1991. Activities of the Centre. Teaching Report. *CTVM Annual Report 1991*, 4–5.

Smith, A. J. 1993. Teaching report. *CTVM Annual Report 1992*, 3.

Smith, A. J. 1994. Teaching report. *CTVM Annual Report 1993–1994*, 2–7.

Taylor, D. 1996. The CTVM: the next 25 years. *Tropical Animal Health and Production*, 28, 2–4.

Chapter 11

The Royal (Dick) School of Veterinary Studies (1970–2003)

Veterinary Faculty adaptations and developments

The available evidence suggests that after the Royal (Dick) School of Veterinary Studies became an established Veterinary Faculty within the University of Edinburgh it took on a new and different lease of life. Most obviously there was a significant change in internal administrative culture. In place of the settled continuity of relatively long leadership shown in previous decades there came three decades of fluctuations caused by relatively frequently changes in deanship – different men from differing academic backgrounds and professional cultures were sequentially allocated responsibility as Head of School; there were eleven changes in deanship between 1970 and 2003. This can be compared to five changes in Principal of College/Head of School in the preceding thirty-three years, and the continuity of two Principals of College during the forty-two years before that. Externally driven events also had a significant impact. However, the 'continuity factor' for the Dick Vet over this period turned out to be the need to renew, rebuild, modify and then finally replace the available teaching space at Summerhall. This was required to accommodate the teaching demands of the curriculum, the research needs of the staff, the improvements to the small-animal clinic, and latterly, to provide space for an over 75 per cent increase in student intake that took place between 1988 and 2003 (Figure 11.1).

As a direct consequence of the work of the Northumberland Committee (MAFF 1964), from 1962 to 1974 a significant capital investment was made available to the Veterinary Faculty. Planning for the rebuilding of the north-west corner 'church site' began in the spring of 1967 (Figure 9.3). The coal bunkers on the 'church site' and the old coal-fired heating plant

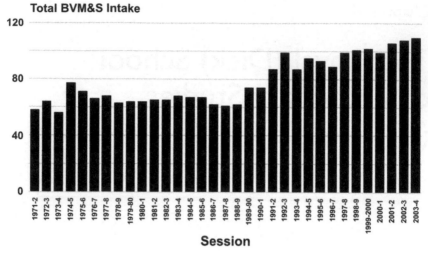

Figure 11.1   Total undergraduate (BVM&S) student intake, 1971–2003.

were removed. The old chimney in the courtyard was demolished and replaced with a lift to serve all five floors of the main building. The fumes from the replacement oil-fired boilers vented through a new 36.5-metre-high chimney that took only seven days to erect. A seven-storey tower was constructed on the corner site (Figure 11.2). Veterinary Biochemistry occupied the ground- and first-floor levels, with the remainder of the tower given over to accommodation for Veterinary Pathology. Large teaching laboratories were placed on the ground-floor and second-floor levels. Accommodation for small laboratory animals was placed in the basement. The Evelyn Head Lecture Theatre, seating eighty-six people, was also placed at basement level in the link between the new tower and the main building (Anonymous 1971).

The second phase of construction work faced Summerhall Square and involved building the four-storey Small Animal Clinic and the Wellcome Research Facility (Figure 11.3). An X-ray suite and expanded teaching and research capabilities were provided for the Small Animal Clinic on the ground and first floors. On the upper two floors were laboratory and small-animal accommodation rooms for the Wellcome unit and the Veterinary Physiology Department. A bridge linked the first floor of this new build-ing to the existing first-floor surgical accommodation in the middle of the Veterinary School courtyard (Anonymous 1971). The buildings were completed in 1972.

Dr Frank Alexander was awarded a personal Chair in Veterinary Pharmacology and was appointed Dean of the Veterinary Faculty from 1970 to 1974 (Figure 11.4). His department became the first professorial

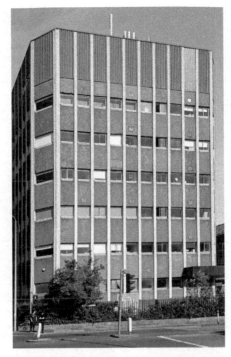

Figure 11.2 Tower building on the north-west corner of the Summerhall Veterinary School site. Photographer: Alastair A. Macdonald.

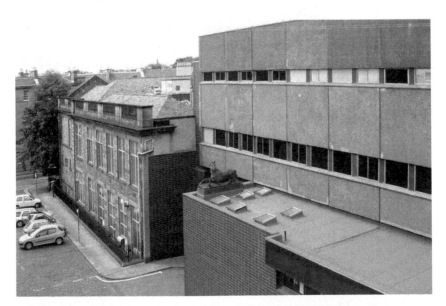

Figure 11.3 Wellcome (upper) and small-animal clinic (lower) buildings on Summerhall Square, with original masonry of the Dick Vet beyond. Photographer: Colin M. Warwick.

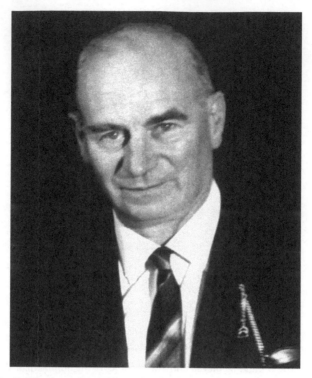

Figure 11.4 Frank Alexander. Photographer: unknown.

department of Veterinary Pharmacology in the UK. The BVM&S curriculum, having been significantly revised for a third time in 1969–71, was introduced in October 1971. It had been noted in the Veterinary Faculty minutes of 13 October 1970 that because the situation was sufficiently exceptional due to the planned introduction of this new curriculum, it had not been possible to accept any first-year students into Session 1970–1. However, seventeen students, including six women, had obtained qualifications which permitted their direct acceptance into the second year. Faculty decided that from 1971 onwards the Selection Board would continue to aim to restrict to ten the annual intake of women students (the total number of women students in the school to equal fifty-five). However, this policy was abandoned in 1974 (Figure 11.5a).

The Senatus Minutes recorded that the subjects of study for the BVM&S degree in 1971–2 would include: Anatomy, Physiology, Biochemistry (including Chemistry), Animal Management, Animal Husbandry (including Nutrition and Breeding), Genetics, Statistics, Microbiology, Pathology, Parasitology, Pharmacology and General Therapeutics, Medicine, Surgery, Obstetrics, Reproduction, Animal Health, Meat Inspection and Jurisprudence (Senatus 1970). In 1972 the MSc Neurobiology degree was

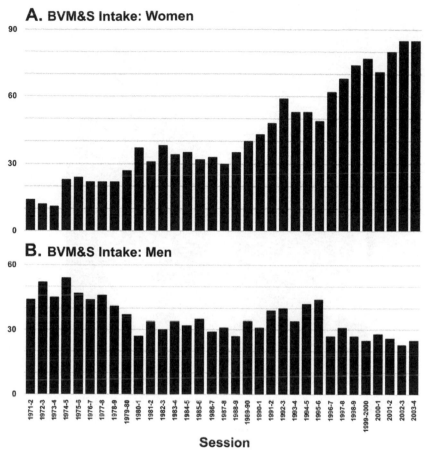

Figure 11.5 A. Graph of women BVM&S numbers, 1971–2001. B. Graph of men BVM&S numbers, 1971–2001.

instituted at the Dick Vet. This was the first of what was to become a series of Masters degrees that developed thereafter.

Undergraduate intake fluctuated slightly around sixty for the first three years of the new curriculum and then increased abruptly in 1974 from fifty-six to seventy-seven, causing some staff anxiety (Faculty 1973). At the same Faculty meeting it was decided to phase out, from 1974, the student Regent Scheme, which had been running for about two decades, and replace it with the appointment of five staff Directors of Studies. Meanwhile, University finances were such at that time that a savings target of 3.5 per cent of the 1973–4 expenditure was expected of Faculties (Letter 1974).

Ainsley Iggo, the Mary Dick Professor of Veterinary Physiology, was elected Dean from 1974 until 1977 (Figure 11.6a). By that time the effects

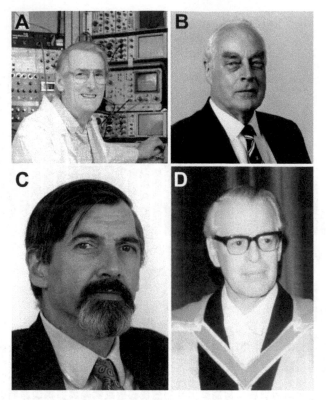

Figure 11.6 A. Ainsley Iggo. Photographer: Colin M. Warwick; B. Ian Beattie. Photographer: Kenny Thompson; C. Keith Dyce. Photographer: Kenny Thompson; D. James Baxter. Photographer: Kenny Thompson.

of the new curriculum had extended into the fourth-year courses and students were being taught in the new large-animal post-mortem room at the Bush for the first time. Special arrangements were made in Veterinary Medicine to provide the full course of practical and theoretical study for the last final year of six students who were following the old curriculum. No final-year medals were awarded in Session 1974–5.

The final-year Veterinary Medicine class of 1975–6 was the first to have undertaken the new BVM&S curriculum. The new arrangement, which largely allocated lectures to the afternoon, provided four hours each morning for other forms of clinical instruction. This generally commenced with a small-group discussion based on disease syndromes, differential diagnoses, transparencies of common conditions, therapeutics and the like. This was followed by clinical casework with small groups of students and included the programme of tutorials on cases with individual students. The last part of one morning each week was set aside for a student presentation of a case report for small-group discussion. The rapid post-war expansion in small-animal ownership had a direct impact on the balance of coursework being taught (Swabe 1998; Gardiner 2014).

In Veterinary Surgery the agreed departmental policy to improve and extend each student's training in practical clinical procedures met with problems due to the increased teaching load and a lack of staff. In order to give small-group clinical teaching to the final-year students, the fourth-year instruction groups had to be whole- or half-class groups.

Ian Stuart Beattie, the Director of Applied Veterinary Pathology, became Dean from 1977 to 1980 (Figure 11.6b). On 10 May 1978 approval was given by Senate for the BSc (Vet.Sci.) degree to be intercalated in the BVM&S degree. Although the student intake figures ranged between sixty-one and sixty-eight from 1977 until 1988 (Figure 11.1), the proportion of women in the intake increased from 33 per cent in 1977 to 56 per cent in 1988. A survey in the United States had shown that there was no difference in wastage between male and female veterinary graduates; nor was there any evidence so far to suggest that women were not being smoothly assimilated into the veterinary profession (Anonymous 1978). Early in 1980 it was agreed by Faculty that the fees for overseas and second-degree students would be raised from £1,165 to £3,000 per year for BVM&S Years 1 and 2, and to £5,000 per year for BVM&S Years 3, 4 and 5 (Faculty 1980). The latter figure when converted to 2022 values was £19,716.

It was on the petition of Beattie, as 'Dean of the Royal (Dick) School of Veterinary Studies, Faculty of Veterinary Medicine in the University of Edinburgh', that the Royal Lyon King of Arms, on 19 December 1977, awarded a second Coat of Arms (Plate 11.1) in the name of the Royal (Dick) School of Veterinary Studies, Faculty of Veterinary Medicine in the University of Edinburgh:

> Per pale; dexter, Argeant, on a saltire Azure between a thistle in chief proper and a castle on a rock in base Sable, a book expanded Or; sinister, Azure, a saltire between a horse's head couped in chief and in base a triple towered castle all Argent, masoned Sable, windows, flags and portcullis Gules situated on a rock proper. (Arms, 1977)

This was recorded and matriculated on 4 July 1978.

Keith Dyce, the Mary Dick Professor of Veterinary Anatomy, became Dean from 1980 until 1984 (Figure 11.6c). His time in office coincided with Britain embarking upon a period of national austerity. The reduction in Government expenditure had a direct impact on the availability of university funds for the next ten years. On 10 December 1981 the University introduced a moratorium on the filling of teaching, technical and other posts throughout the veterinary and other faculties. The target BVM&S

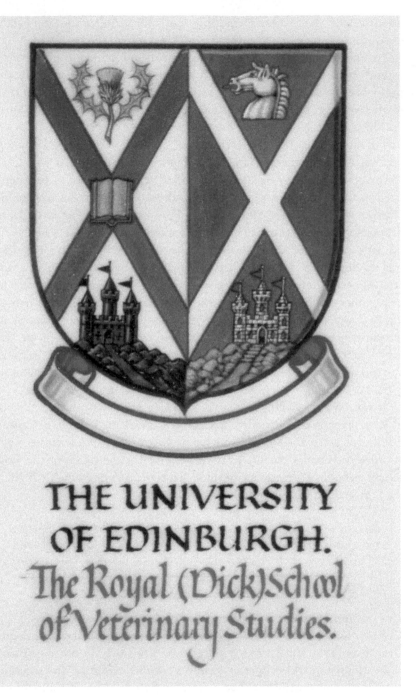

Plate 11.1   Second Coat of Arms awarded to the Dick Vet by the Lord Lyon King of Arms. Photographer: Colin M. Warwick.

student intake for 1981 and 1982 was sixty-two students. Session 1981–2 saw the introduction of a new first-year syllabus which incorporated much of the anatomy material formerly presented in second year. During the following Session a substantial portion of the Veterinary Biochemistry course was successfully transferred into the second year. The first diet of the new second-year Degree Examination in Veterinary Anatomy, Biochemistry and Physiology was operated successfully that Session.

James T. Baxter, the Professor of Veterinary Medicine, was made Dean from 1984 to 1985 (Figure 11.6d). During his short time in office, the structural remodelling of Hope Park Congregational Church (Figure 6.9) in 1985 provided an additional eight rooms for research offices and laboratories, a dark room, and a toilet on the top floor. On the floor below that, a large students' common room, three tutorial rooms and two toilets were built. The ground floor housed the long-awaited new refectory for staff and students.

Changes to the Biochemistry examination arrangements were agreed at the Board of Studies meeting in January 1985. Oral examinations would only be held for students who had failed the written examination or who were potential distinction candidates. In the June diet, nineteen candidates (out of a class of sixty-three) were given orals. Of these, eleven had failed the written papers (five subsequently passed) and eight were distinction candidates. The Examination Board was pleased with the operation of the new system. These arrangements eased the burden of the examination for the students, most of whom were now subjected to a single examination for this subject instead of three as previously. Timetabling arrangements were also eased, and the external examiner was only required to attend on one day instead of two. These new arrangements rapidly and sequentially spread with approval to other departments in the Veterinary Faculty.

Restructuring of Faculty departments from nine to four

The effect of the staff moratorium on the filling of the Chairs in the Departments of Veterinary Pharmacology, Animal Health and Veterinary Anatomy (with the early retirement of Professor Dyce in 1984), followed by the death of Professor James Reid Campbell, the William Dick Professor of Veterinary Surgery, on 9 March 1985, stripped the established professoriate of the Veterinary Faculty down to four. Discussions were therefore held within Faculty about the possible reformation of the nine old departments into four larger units. The death in post on 11 November 1985 of Professor James T. Baxter prompted urgent action to be taken. Ainsley Iggo was once again appointed Dean, from 1985 until 1990. On 1 April

1986 the Veterinary Faculty was restructured into the four Departments: Preclinical Veterinary Sciences, Tropical Animal Health (Centre for Tropical Veterinary Medicine), Veterinary Pathology and Veterinary Clinical Studies. The Department of Preclinical Veterinary Sciences was formed from the amalgamation of the former Departments of Veterinary Anatomy, Veterinary Physiology and Veterinary Pharmacology and the Biochemistry Unit. The Department of Veterinary Clinical Studies was formed from the Departments of Animal Health, Veterinary Medicine and Veterinary Surgery and the Veterinary Practice Teaching Unit. On 2 July 1986, as part of these changes, the titles of the Chairs in the Department of Veterinary Clinical Studies were changed and three William Dick Chairs of Veterinary Clinical Studies were created (Senatus 1986b).

Teaching innovations occurred at this time too. In Preclinical Veterinary Sciences, Dr Simon S. Carlyle introduced self-teaching facilities that he had developed and made available to students via a microcomputer. Teaching of the subject previously named Animal Management was reorganised to form the practical component of Animal Husbandry and now covered the first two years of the undergraduate course. For the first time, in June 1986, the Second Professional examination combined Animal Management and Animal Husbandry. The first-year lambing course was reorganised to incorporate both Animal Husbandry and Reproduction. In this way it prepared students to assist at on-farm lambing during the Easter vacation and acted as an introduction to Reproduction. For the benefit of new University staff, an introductory series of lectures and demonstrations was staged to indicate methods of best teaching practice. Every year, at the end of the summer term, a one-day programme of good teaching practice events was made available to lecturing academic staff. In addition, peer observation of teaching was sometimes arranged between colleagues to provide feedback on each other's teaching.

The old byre which had formed part of the Easter Bush Home Farm Stables was converted into a farriery and was established as the Scottish Farriery Training Centre. This was leased from the University by the Worshipful Company of Farriers and the Farriers' Registration Council, with a generous donation from the International League for the Protection of Horses. This Centre was opened by HRH The Princess Anne, Past Master of the Worshipful Company of Farriers, on Tuesday, 29 July 1986. The Centre was used to advance and improve the existing skills of Registered Farriers and to help those who shoe horses in the more remote parts of Scotland. Tuition was also made available for veterinary undergraduate students and veterinary surgeons.

During Session 1985–6 there were approximately equal numbers (160) of male and female BVM&S students studying at the Dick Vet. Of the five Directors of Studies, Dr Janet M. Nicholson, one of the seven female members of staff, was appointed Director of Studies for Final Year Studies. She also had some responsibilities for all the women students.

The following academic Session the Principal of the University drew Senate's attention to the prospect that the financial outlook for the University was going to be considerably worse than in 1981–4 (Senatus 1986a).

During 1987–8 three of the students taking the Tropical Veterinary Medicine course, Eric Feron, Nicholas Short and Graeme Thirlwell, set up Vets for the World (VETAID), specialising in worldwide primary animal healthcare. VETAID was based in Edinburgh and was actively supported by students at the Dick Vet. In 1988 those graduating BVM&S comprised twenty-seven men and twenty-six women (Plate 11.2).

The proposal to merge Glasgow and Edinburgh Veterinary Faculties

Several joint discussions were held by the Universities of Edinburgh and Glasgow in 1988 on the possibility that a single Scottish Veterinary School might be suggested by Government as a method for increasing the efficiency of veterinary education in Scotland. The maintenance of both veterinary teaching and research sites at Summerhall in Edinburgh and Garscube in Glasgow was central to these discussions. The Riley Committee, which had been set up to examine the subject of veterinary education for the future, reported in January 1989. It recommended that 'a single Scottish School of Veterinary Studies should be created by merging parts of the veterinary activities at the University of Edinburgh and Glasgow' and that this new school 'should be in the University of Edinburgh . . . [and] . . . should have the capacity to teach 85 students'.

The two Universities deplored the proposal that Edinburgh and Glasgow Veterinary Schools should be closed and that 30 per cent of their combined resources in relation to veterinary education be distributed elsewhere. The Edinburgh Veterinary School wanted expansion of its student numbers and the income to teach them. It was recruiting staff worldwide to further the cosmopolitan strengths of the Veterinary School and the University's teaching and research staff. There was already an emphasis in Edinburgh on collaboration between different disciplines in teaching and research. The general response to the report throughout the UK was widespread criticism, based, among other things, on the inappropriate estimate of a decrease in the need for veterinary graduates in the future and the failure to take into account the acclaimed research expertise in Glasgow. This

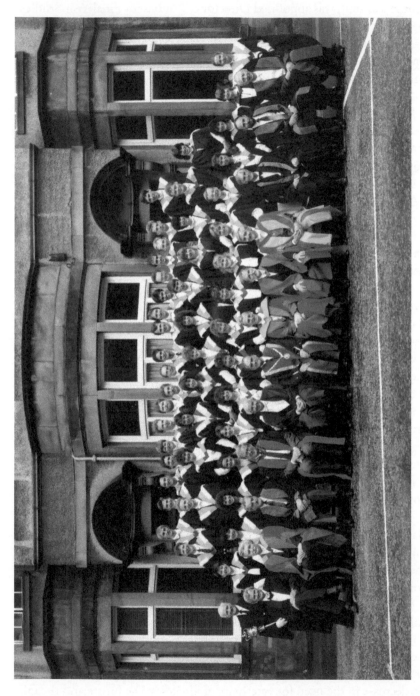

Plate 11.2 BVM&S Graduation, 1988, with Servitor George Costello holding the Dick Vet mace. Photographer: Fiona Manson.

was despite the fact that Sir Ralph Riley had himself stated that Glasgow was the 'only British veterinary school which contained a department of high international standing'.

Considerable political lobbing took place. The outcome was that the quinquennial Review of Veterinary Manpower was brought forward in the following terms:

> assess the need for veterinary manpower in the UK, both for the public service and the private sector and the demand for veterinary education from home and overseas students
>
> . . . make recommendations on how any increased manpower requirement might be met having regard to constraints on public funding and to potential funding from the UFC [Universities Funding Council] and other sources
>
> . . . [suggest] what future arrangements should be developed to assess the demand for veterinary manpower and determine the number of student places.

Chaired by Dr Ewan Page, the Vice Chancellor of Reading University, a preliminary report was expected before Christmas 1989. The UFC for its part had been expected to reach a decision in May that year but deferred a decision until it could take into account the findings of the Page Veterinary Manpower Review. This led to a further period of uncertainty for the Dick Vet. The University responded to invitations to present further evidence on the sizes of veterinary intake that the Dick Vet could handle in various circumstances and gave evidence to the Manpower Review. Although uncertainty continued, there were hopeful omens in the form of firstly, new appointments of junior staff to all departments in the Dick Vet, made despite the enforced economies largely met through early retirement of senior staff, and secondly, the research funds which continued to flow into all departments. By February 1990 the Government had accepted the Page recommendations that the restrictions on student intake should be lifted and that they should be determined in the future by student demand instead of fixed ceilings (Anonymous 1990a). Quinquennial reviews were abandoned. The consequence of these decisions on student intake at the Dick Vet can clearly be seen in Figures 11.1 and 11.5.

Dick Vet personalities and characters

Mrs Marion McIvor retired from the Faculty Library in 1988. She had seen the Summerhall library expanded into the basement and refurbished, supervised the computer automation of the book and journal collection, and had been delighted to see the Dick library as the first in the University's

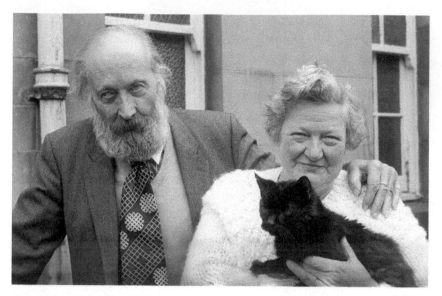

Figure 11.7 Mr and Mrs Cairns and Arthur, their cat. Photographer: Colin M. Warwick.

online system to 'go live'. The library had been termed 'the best in a UK Veterinary School'.

Gordon and Margaret Cairns (Figure 11.7), who owned the bookshop across the road from the front door of Summerhall, had been associated with the Dick Vet for fifty years (Anonymous 1989). Mrs Cairns recalled the long-gone days when the 'Dick Hops' were held in the Summerhall basement. She also remembered the strong associations with the girls from the 'Dough School', Edinburgh College of Domestic Science, in Atholl Crescent and how at the Dick Vet they met their match in more ways than one. Gordon Cairns sold veterinary books all over the world 'to the ambassadors from the Dick spreading the message'. Arthur, their cat, who had lived with them for twenty-eight years, had been a stray from the cat and dog home, and was now quite frail and 'beginning to feel his age'.

Mr Bill Dempsey, MM, mentor and father figure to hundreds of students, retired in April 1987 after twelve years a Servitor. Mr Arthur McKernan, another of the great 'characters' of the Dick, left in September 1989 after some ten years' service to the Faculty. The third man, Mr Freddie Simmonds, was rarely noticed. He remained for some more years our valued boilerman (Figure 11.8). The cleaning ladies were the 'angels in blue' (Figure 11.9). They were led by Mrs Josie Tully, eighteen years at Summerhall, and Mrs Jean Liddle, fifteen years at Easter Bush. Rarely seen by most folk in the Dick Vet, they started work at about 5.30 a.m. and were away before the 9 a.m. lectures began. It was due to the

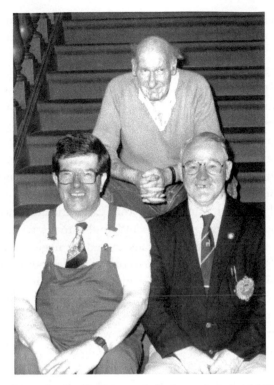

Figure 11.8 Left to right: Freddie Simmonds (boilerman), Arthur McKernan (yard maintenance) and Bill Dempsey (servitor) on the Summerhall stairway. Photographer: Colin M. Warwick.

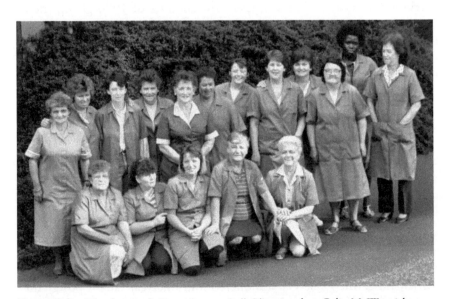

Figure 11.9 The cleaning ladies at Summerhall. Photographer: Colin M. Warwick.

crack-of-dawn best efforts of the twenty Summerhall and ten Easter Bush ladies that the staff had a clean and disinfected environment in which to work.

On 28 June 1989, at the Royal Mews in London, an international equine welfare project was launched, resulting from collaboration between the International League for the Protection of Horses (ILPH) and the World Farriers Association (WFA). The three-year programme was co-ordinated by Dr Tina MacGregor, lecturer in Farriery and Equine Orthopaedics at the Dick Vet. The project work in Morocco, Mexico, the Indian subcontinent and countries of the Middle East included training farriers, veterinarians, saddlers and other caregivers in the correct practices of animal husbandry and equine foot care. The aim was to increase the productivity of horses, donkeys and mules to better people's lives, and to reduce the suffering of animals caused by neglect and poor care (Anonymous 1989b). Educational material on farriery and good foot care was produced in English, French, German, Spanish and Arabic and was distributed throughout the world to farriers, vets, horse-related organisations and animal welfare bodies (Anonymous 1990b). Another educational contribution to the general public was *The Royal (Dick) School of Veterinary Studies Horse and Pony Feeding Guide*. It provided a central table of daily feed rates for ponies and horses from 11 to 17 hands, in activities ranging from complete rest to heavy work. It was distributed to stables, livery yards and major equestrian centres throughout the country.

On the other side of the world, Jim Methven, the superintendent in Preclinical Veterinary Sciences, spent the summer of 1990 giving training in the maintenance of medical equipment on the islands of Vanuatu (previously called New Hebrides) in the mid-Pacific. In 1991 he travelled to Kuala Lumpur, Malaysia to advise on legislation and equipment for hospital use (Anonymous 1990b).

Progress and optimism in the Veterinary Faculty

A new BVM&S curriculum was prepared for introduction in October 1990. In addition, undergraduate students now had the choice of seven Honours schools: Anatomy, Anatomy and Physiology, Biochemistry, Neuroscience, Pathological Sciences, Physiological Sciences (Biochemistry and Physiology) and Physiology. The BSc Honours Neuroscience course was unique among these in that it was an inter-faculty effort, with students and staff from the Faculties of Science, Medicine and Veterinary Medicine participating. The Dick Vet also offered four one-year taught postgraduate Diploma/MSc courses: Neuroscience, Tropical Veterinary Medicine,

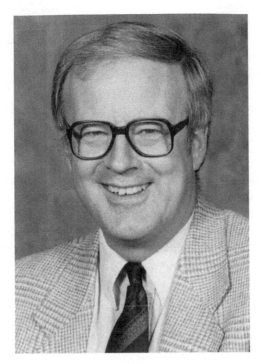

Figure 11.10   Richard Halliwell. Photographer: Bob Munro.

Tropical Veterinary Science and Tropical Animal Production and Health. In addition, all veterinary departments accepted registrations for MPhil and PhD research degrees. Moreover, graduates and members of staff of the Dick Vet could also register for the DVM&S, a research degree for which advice rather than supervision was provided. About fifty postgraduate degrees and diplomas were being awarded each year.

Richard Halliwell became Dean in 1990 (Figure 11.10). On 12 June 1990 a letter from Buckingham Palace to the University of Edinburgh said that HRH Princess Anne had accepted the invitation to become Patron of the Royal (Dick) School of Veterinary Studies (Patron 1990). The Dick Vet had survived the cuts of the 1980s, but its physical plant left much to be desired. In particular, the small-animal hospital was deemed not to be up to the standards to permit the satisfactory practice of modern-day veterinary medicine and surgery. Although many of the older staff had taken early retirement, some outstanding replacements had been recruited (Halliwell 1990). The energy and drive to make improvements were now in place.

Another statement of optimism that year was the International Symposium held at the University in July 1990 to mark Professor Ainsley Iggo's considerable contribution to sensory physiology through his own work and by inspiring and furthering the interests of many associates and students (Figure 11.11). The scientific programme covered the three major subject areas in which Ainsley had been active: 1. The saga of C fibres. 2. From Merkel cells to the Platypus bill. 3. The spinal cord . . . and beyond. Colleagues from many parts of the world – Europe, the Soviet Union, India, the Far East, North America and Australia – gathered together. This cosmopolitan veterinary outlook was also evident daily at Summerhall and Easter Bush. In Session 1990–1, of the total student population (under-graduate and postgraduate) in the School, 24 per cent were from overseas (Anonymous 1991a). Beginning from 1991, five Norwegian students per year were to be nominated for admission to the Dick Vet (Hackel 1996). The fees and living costs of these students were met by the Norwegian authorities as there was a shortage of undergraduate veterinary spaces in Norway at that time. Many more followed the initial five to Edinburgh. That Session twenty international and/or second-degree full fee-paying students were accepted, with thirteen of these from overseas (Finland, Iceland, Norway, USA). The new undergraduate BVM&S curriculum, introduced in October 1991, ensured that didactic teaching was reduced by about 12 per cent, and that the final year was to be made 'lecture-free'.

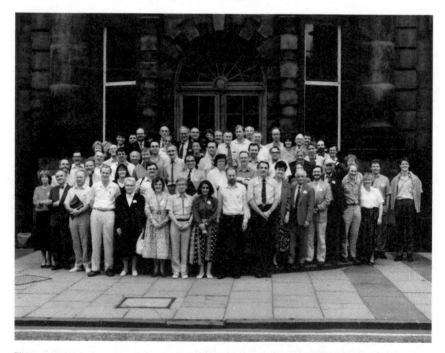

Figure 11.11 A symposium entitled 'The Edinburgh Connection', held to honour Ainsley Iggo on his retiral in 1990, was attended by his friends and colleagues from all over the world. Photographer: Colin M. Warwick.

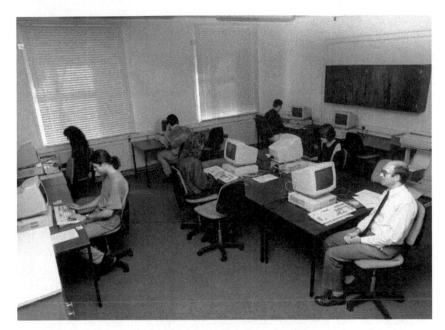

Figure 11.12 The Summerhall computing suite. Photographer: Colin M. Warwick.

There was to be increased horizontal and vertical integration between the classical disciplines, and the modularisation of the clinical teaching. Those aspects of parasitology previously taught in the Faculty of Science and Engineering at King's Buildings were also to be transferred to the Veterinary Faculty. A computing suite was established at Summerhall (Figure 11.12). Twelve research machine PC-386s and two Apple SE /30s were linked in a network, allowing communication with local and international academic networks. The laboratory was very popular with both staff and students and was a valuable addition to the Faculty's teaching facilities (Anonymous 1991b).

Sadly, Mr and Mrs Cairns died in 1991. In their memory the newly refurbished and extended North (Pharmacology) lecture theatre at Summerhall was renamed the Cairns Lecture Theatre (Anonymous 1991c).

At Easter Bush a new equine intensive care unit (ICU) was constructed. It consisted of a padded box for adult horses, a small, padded room for sick foals and an observation room so that staff could watch patients in the ICU without disturbing them. This allowed for easier and better twenty-four-hour care of horses and foals. The second part of the new equine development involved splitting the large existing operating theatre into two smaller theatres – one for clean operations, for example joint surgery, and the other for dirty operations, for example teeth and sinus problems. This reduced the incidence of post-operative infections and allowed more operations to be done. Two new induction/recovery boxes, one into each new theatre, enabled horses to be anaesthetised in a padded box next to the theatre and to be returned afterwards so that they could come round in safety (Anonymous 1991d).

In June 1991, following an invitation issued by the Principal and Vice Chancellor of the University, Sir David Smith, the Council of Friends of the Dick Vet was formed. Comprising alumni, representatives of commerce and Parliament and other friends, its role was to advise the Principal and the Dean on matters relating to the Dick Vet and to assist the School in obtaining resources to achieve its goals. The group, which met several times each year, was chaired by Brian Singleton (grad. 1945), former director of the Animal Health Fund (Anonymous 1993). During the following years the Council of Friends had many discussions about the possible rebuilding of the Summerhall stables area and central part of the Summerhall site to accommodate the expanding numbers of students (Figure 11.5). However, the student population at Summerhall was rapidly outgrowing the available space.

The Dick Vet was successfully training larger numbers of postgraduate research students. Its clinics were serving a greater number of clients, both first opinion and referred. The clinical staff were offering increasing numbers of highly successful postgraduate clinical courses which attracted veterinarians from all over the UK. The staff at the Dick Vet were also attracting higher levels of research funding than ever before and were publishing more (Halliwell 1993). The Dick Vet became the lead institution in a consortium involving all of the UK Veterinary Schools, developing computer-assisted learning. The integrated curriculum also encouraged the development of a great deal of inter-departmental collaboration and co-ordination of teaching. As a consequence, an additional new post of Associate Dean was created, charged specifically with streamlining the teaching within the School (Halliwell 1994).

In July 1993 the bicentenary of the birth of William Dick was celebrated, as was the fifty-year anniversary of the founding of the Polish Veterinary Faculty at the Dick Vet (Anonymous 1994a). On 8 July 1993 the Princess Royal received her first Honorary Degree, the DVM&S (Anonymous 1994b) (Plate 11.3). From Wednesday, 7 July to Saturday, 10 July 1993, a series of bicentenary symposia attracted speakers from nine countries and four continents (Anonymous 1994c). There was a two-morning farm animal symposium, one on equine neonatology and another on adult horse conditions, a small-animal symposium and a small-animal dermatology symposium, a wildlife symposium, and the final symposium centred on the future of veterinary education. A Gala Dinner was held in the Royal Museum of Scotland on 10 July.

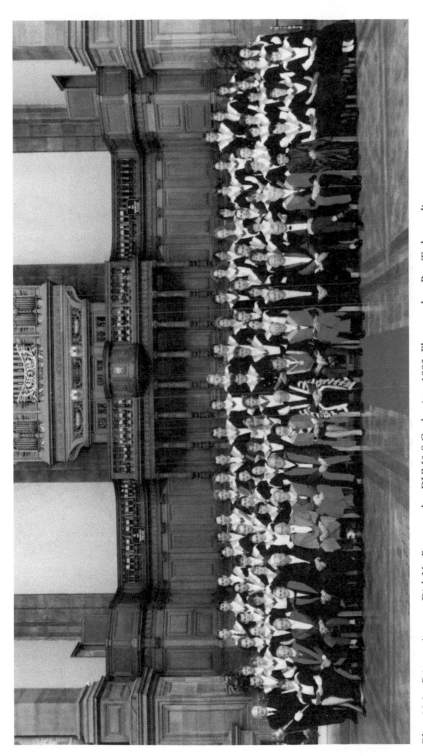

Plate 11.3 Princess Anne, as Dick Vet Patron, at her DVM&S Graduation, 1993. Photographer: Ron Taylor studio.

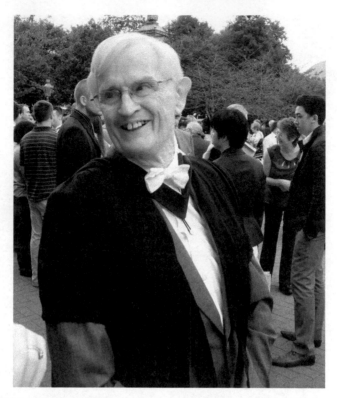

Figure 11.13   Morley Sewell. Photographer: Lois Saddler, née Packer.

Morley Sewell served as Dean from 1994 to 1997 (Figure 11.13). During his time, an Honorary Doctorate was given to Sir David Attenborough on 26 November 1994. A Centre of Excellence in Applied Respiratory Pathophysiology was established at Easter Bush. It was also discovered that student languages in one class at Summerhall included English, Norwegian, French, German, Welsh, Irish, Japanese, Russian and Italian. In 1995–6 there were approximately 1,300 applications to study at the Dick Vet submitted through the Universities and Colleges Admission Service (UCAS), with 250 candidates being interviewed at the Dick Vet and 135 offers being made for the sixty-five Scottish Higher Education Funding Council (SHEFC) funded places (Hackel 1996). Professor Sewell explained that the Veterinary Faculty had for some time been admitting full fee-paying students from overseas as well as UK graduates in other disciplines who wished to undertake veterinary medicine as a second 'first degree'. In 1995 the student intake into first year was forty-four men and forty-nine women giving a total of 93, of whom twenty-eight were from overseas or were second 'first degree' students.

The Dick Vet's Small Animal 'Continuing Professional Development' (CPD) in 1995–6 was centred around two programmes, the Evening Seminars and the Small Animal Medicine modular programme. Evening Seminars ran monthly or bi-monthly from October to May, and included Antibiotics, Gastroenterology, Ophthalmology, Endocrinology, Cardiology and Practical Oncology. The Small Animal Medicine modular programme was designed to be of assistance to those studying for the Royal College of Veterinary Surgeons Certificate in Small Animal Medicine, although it would also be of considerable interest to general practitioners wishing to update their knowledge and skills. Modules scheduled included Gastroenterology, Diagnostic Imaging, Haematological Disorders, Infectious Diseases of the Dog and Cat, and Ophthalmology. A new area of CPD that the Dick Vet was able to offer from 1995 was that of Exotic Species. Evening Seminars on reptiles and birds were scheduled, as was a weekend module in July 1996 as part of the annual Zoo Animal Behaviour and Welfare Summer School, which the University co-presented with Edinburgh Zoo. The third World Congress of Veterinary Dermatology was held in Edinburgh in September 1996; 1,175 delegates from thirty-eight countries attended.

The new Hospital for Small Animals

The high-priority Hospital for Small Animals began to take shape in 1996–7. The groundwork began in January 1997. The Provost of Medicine and Veterinary Medicine also decided to give first priority for building works in 1997–8 to the large-animal isolation facilities and the upgrading of a laboratory to extend the Dick Vet's computer-aided learning provision. The lecture-free final year was fully operative by 1997, which helped give the 1997 Teaching Quality Assessment (TQA) an 'excellent' result. A survey had been undertaken of Edinburgh graduates from 1988 to 1993. On the whole, Edinburgh graduates and their first employers appeared very happy with the education. Ninety-nine per cent of the graduates had a job within six months. Over 90 per cent of the employers would hire other Dick Vet graduates. Eighty-five per cent of the employers felt that the Edinburgh course had prepared the graduate properly for the veterinary profession. Ninety per cent of the graduates said that they would choose the Dick Vet again, if choosing to go to a veterinary school (Anonymous 1997). The Research Assessment Exercise (RAE) was performed in 1996 and in its report, early in 1997, the Veterinary Faculty maintained its rating of '4B'.

Hugh Miller became Dean from 1997 until 2001 (Figure 11.14). The Hospital for Small Animals opened for teaching and clinical services on

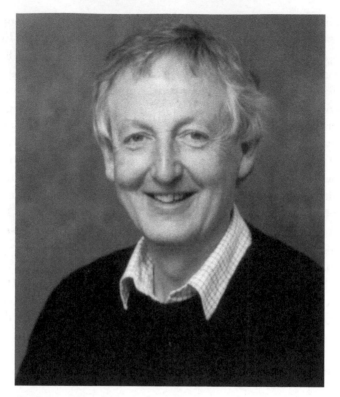

Figure 11.14 Hugh Miller. Photographer: Bob Monro.

11 January 1999 (Plate 11.4). The physical space of the Hospital was certainly a pleasure to work in. Important to achieving this was the fact that during the planning process, a senior member of the staff, together with the architect, had visited key new hospitals in the UK, continental Europe and North America to observe their strong and weak points.

The airy and spacious reception area provides a warm welcome for clients and their pets. At the entrance to the Hospital area there are eight large and well-appointed consulting rooms that can readily accommodate enlarged 'small groups' of final-year students. At the end of this corridor is the Quiet Room, in which discussions with clients regarding their pets can be held away from the bustle and general activity of the Hospital. Behind these is the main concourse and then Main Street', which runs the whole length of the Hospital. Both extend in height to the equivalent of four storeys, allowing an influx of natural light from all directions. There are three specialist rooms, one for cardiology and one each for ophthalmology and dermatology. The wards wing contains two isolation wards, a cytotoxic ward and three general wards. There is also a special ward for wildlife, with an external enclosed grassed area and a pond, and one for exotic animals.

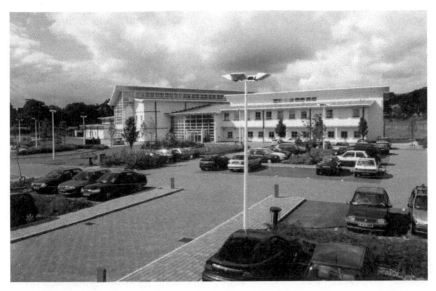

Plate 11.4   The Hospital for Small Animals at Easter Bush. Photographer: Bob Monro.

The surgery suite contains three main theatres, a minor procedures theatre, an anaesthetic suite and an intensive care unit. Situated next door is the diagnostic imaging suite with rooms for major and minor X-ray, for endoscopy and for ultrasound.

The first floor contains three seminar/tutorial rooms, a large quiet study and IT area and a laboratory suite. In the east wing are self-contained flats for four to five students, three nurses and three junior clinical scholars (interns). Forum Architects, Newmarket had designed different kinds of space for the work of staff and students. The Hospital for Small Animals was officially opened on 14 May 1999 by the Princess Royal.

Just before entering the new and flourishing Hospital, clients can pause before the bronze statue of a sprinting Afghan hound sculpted by Mathew Lane Sanderson. It commemorates the memory of a very special woman, Olive Smith, VN, MBE, who was Head Nurse at the Dick Vet from 1971 to 1996. Her concern for the animals in her care and her role in the training of veterinary nurses and veterinary undergraduates were well captured and commemorated in this lively sculpture.

The William Dick Large Animal Hospital

Across the road, a modern building was required to replace the old ruminant hospital. The new structure provided covered ventilated accommodation for two bull pens, divisible areas for cattle and areas for sheep. Linked to existing buildings, it comprised updated animal handling facilities and a refurbished operating theatre, wash area and pharmacy. The complex is serviced from a new yard created between the ruminant and equine buildings. The old equine accommodation was replaced to incorporate a new undercover outpatient clinic containing an examination room, holding boxes, ultrasound room, hard surface trot-up lanes and a lunging area, as well as areas suitable for students and clients. In the inpatient hospital there are three large teaching/diagnostic rooms, thirty-one large hospital boxes and ancillary rooms plus a diagnostic and treatment area. With student intake having risen from fifty-five to an average of over a hundred in First Year (Figure 11.1), the staff were confident that the new clinical facilities were spacious enough to educate these increased numbers.

The William Dick Large Animal Hospital was opened by the Principal, Professor Sir Stewart Sutherland, on 1 September 2000 (Anonymous 2000c). These purpose-built areas for the care of large animals provided state-of-the-art facilities for the training of veterinary undergraduates, and for the provision of continuing professional development of veterinary surgeons and nurses. Teaching was now conducted (safe from the weather) in an atmosphere that was conducive to learning, while at the same time providing for hands-on experience without risk of injury to either patient or student. The facilities had been designed to support a veterinary service devoted to the treatment, care and welfare of horses, ponies, donkeys and farm animal species such as cattle, sheep and goats, as well as more exotic species such as alpaca, llama, camels and water buffalo.

On Thursday, 15 July 2000 the statue of William Dick was moved to Easter Bush (Anonymous 2000a) and was repaired and restored by conservator Christa Gerdwilker of Croma working for David Lindsay of Stoneworks (Figure 11.15). When the statue was inspected it had a green surface appearance due to an abundant growth of algae (Anonymous 2000b). Many areas had suffered from surface fragmentation and loss due to internal stresses compounded by the action of water, frost and pollution over the eighty-three years it had been out in the open at Summerhall. Christa cleaned out and consolidated the cracks, pinning them where necessary, before filling them with special resins. Parts of the eroded left side of the face were built up without remodelling the whole side of the face, to resemble the original features (as discovered on an old photograph of the statue taken in the late nineteenth century). Christa was even able to reconstruct the badly eroded left whisker and left ear in this way. Other parts that required similar treatment included the right hip, left wrist and sleeve, as well as the feet and back of the chair. Christa's instructions were: 'Do not clean with water, chemicals or abrasives. Dust should be removed with nothing more than a feather duster.' The statue was temporarily

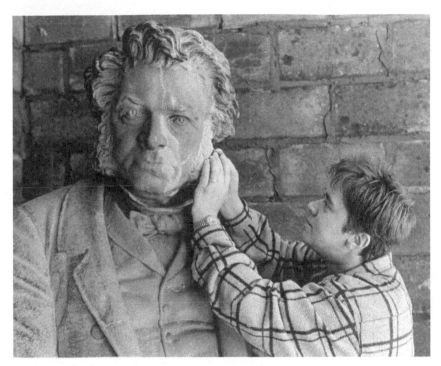

Figure 11.15 William Dick statue being cleaned and repaired by Christa Gerdwilker of Croma for David Lindsay of Stoneworks. Photographer: Bob Monro.

housed in a room at the front of the Field Station building (Anonymous 2002). It was later transferred to the New Teaching Building.

University restructuring into three Colleges

Research in the Faculty Group of Medicine and Veterinary Medicine had undergone a radical change in the past year, 1999–2000, with the creation of Interdisciplinary Research Groups (IDGs) and Interdisciplinary Research Centres. The objective had been to bring like-minded research groups together in order to give critical mass to important areas of medical and veterinary science. One such grouping had been centred at Summerhall. The Department of Veterinary Pathology hosted an IDG in basic and clinical virology. This brought virologists from the Department of Medical Microbiology to link with those in Veterinary Pathology. Thus, the Laboratory for Clinical and Molecular Virology (LCMV) began in October and had over seventy staff occupying six floors of the Tower.

A large amount of refurbishment of the Tower was necessary. The classroom on the ground floor was enlarged and re-equipped to serve both biochemistry and pathology practicals, thereby optimising the use of class-room space. A large open-plan research laboratory was created on Level 2, with additional rooms for tissue culture and molecular studies. New laboratories were created on Levels 3, 4 and 5, and office accommodation was centralised at Level 1.

Richard Halliwell became Dean again for 2001–2, and the teaching facilities at Summerhall were enhanced with the refurbishment of the dissection room, the Cairns Lecture Theatre and the Ainsley Iggo Undergraduate Laboratory.

During the summer of 2002 there was a further restructuring of the University into three Colleges, and an additional reduction in the number of departments within Veterinary Medicine. The three Colleges comprised twenty-one Schools. In the College of Medicine and Veterinary Medicine, there were three Schools of Medicine plus the Royal (Dick) School of Veterinary Studies. No longer were there any Faculties, Deans of Faculties or Faculty meetings. Instead, there were Schools, Heads of Schools (HoS) and School meetings. Much of the University estate at that time was scattered and housed in a wide variety of listed buildings. Many of these were no longer fit for purpose and were very costly to maintain. Summerhall fell into this 'high cost' category, with an estimated £8 million projected for roof repairs alone in the following few years. The Dick Vet was, therefore, actively planning for 'estate rationalization'. Two options for relocating the preclinical years were being evaluated. In line with the University estate strategy at that time, it had been proposed to move the preclinical division of the School into a central site, remote from the clinics at Easter Bush. The alternative was to move out of the city, perhaps close to the Medical School at Little France. It was recognised that changes were unlikely to occur before 2006, during which time several million pounds would have to be invested to accommodate the relocation. In preparation for these changes, £970,000 had been spent that summer on rebuilding the two lecture theatres at Easter Bush.

Hugh Miller became Dean again from 2002 to 2003. In 2002 the Dick Vet again achieved 'Excellent' in teaching and a '5' in the Research Assessment Exercise (RAE). Following careful inspection, accreditation for the maximal period of seven years came from the American Veterinary Medical Association (AVMA) in March 2002. The AVMA team found that the students were committed, articulate and pleased with the educational experience provided at the Dick Vet, and that the staff were enthusiastically devoted to student success. Further insight had been provided in 2000 by George Costello, who had been Servitor at the Dick Vet from 23 March 1987 until his retirement that year:

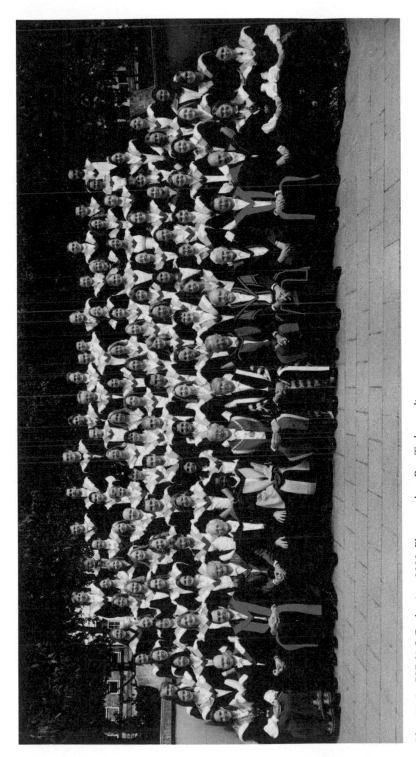

Plate 11.5 BVM&S Graduation, 2003. Photographer: Ron Taylor studio.

> The college, to my way of thinking in those early days, was very much a family concern. It had its own identity separate from the University. Everyone enjoyed the climate they worked in, and the traditions of the College were held in very high esteem. (Costello 2000)

As Janet Hackel, the Veterinary Faculty Officer, also said in 2000: 'The staff and students of the Dick Vet are without a doubt the friendliest at the University.'

Administrative and technical staff such as Janet, and before her, others such as Jim Nisbett, Betty Nash, Chris Bell, Gordon Goodall and the long-serving Summerhall and Clyde Street characters before them, such as Richard C. W. S. Hood, Hubert (Joe) Peapell, Willie Brewser, Willie Angus and Charlie Craig, and of course 'Bean' Phillips, Vince Molony, Padraic (Paddy) Dixon, Alan Rowland and Eileen Burdekin, were and are each 'repositories' of the institutional memory of the Dick Vet.

The results of the third survey since 1996 of student views conducted by the Association of Veterinary Students were published in February 2003. Almost one-third of all veterinary students were experiencing severe financial problems, and over 70 per cent indicated that their debts would have some effect on their choice of job. Edinburgh students rated the relevance of their course the highest, with over 88 per cent classifying it as 'good' or 'very good'. Edinburgh students gave the highest score (80.7 per cent) for their interest in the course. Dick Vet students also rated most highly (79.6 per cent) their satisfaction with the coverage of the subjects in the course. The quality of practical teaching at Edinburgh scored most highly, with 70.7 per cent of students rating it in the 'good' or 'very good' range, and the balance of lectures and practicals at Edinburgh was also rated highest, at 77.9 per cent.

The first undergraduates from North America came in 1835, those from Ireland first enrolled in 1840, one from Russia came in 1844, and students from Norway started to come in 1845 (Pringle 1869). In 2002–3 there were undergraduate students from fifteen countries, and postgraduate students from twenty-three countries, contributing to a total of 106 students from overseas. The total number graduating in 2003 was eighty-one, of whom fifty-eight were women and twenty-three were men (Plate 11.5).

References

Anonymous, 1971. New buildings for veterinary school. *The Scotsman*, 25 November 1971.

Anonymous, 1978. Universities 'hold back' veterinary school cash. *Times Higher Education Supplement*, 12 May 1978, p. 4, col. 2.

Anonymous, 1989a. Mr and Mrs Cairns who have been associated with the Dick Vet for 50 years. *Dick Vet News*, 1, 10–11.

Anonymous, 1989b. Working together for equines. *Dick Vet News*, 2, 1.

Anonymous, 1990a. Closure threat to Glasgow vet school is lifted. *The Herald*, 15 February 1990. <heraldscotland.com/news/11974235.closure-threat-to-glasgow-vet-school-is -lifted/> (accessed 16 July 2022).

Anonymous, 1990b. Farriery and Vanuatu work. *Dick Vet News*, 3, 6.

Anonymous, 1991a. Tomorrow's world today. *Dick Vet News*, 4, 11.

Anonymous, 1991b. Computing suite. *Dick Vet News*, 4, 6.

Anonymous, 1991c. Gordon and Margaret Cairns. *Dick Vet News*, 4, 9.

Anonymous, 1991d. Equine Intensive Care Unit. *Dick Vet News*, 4, 7.

Anonymous, 1993. The Council of Friends. *Dick Vet News*, 5, 10.

Anonymous, 1994a. 50th anniversary of the establishment of the Polish Veterinary School. *Dick Vet News*, 6, 5.

Anonymous, 1994b. HRH the Princess Royal awarded honorary degree. *Dick Vet News*, 6, 8–9.

Anonymous, 1994c. Bicentenary symposia. *Dick Vet News*, 6, 5–7.

Anonymous, 1997. Listening to our graduates. *Dick Vet News*, 10, 3–4.

Anonymous, 2000a. Oor Wullie's made the move. *Dick Vet News*, 12, 1.

Anonymous, 2000b. The reconstruction of William. *Dick Vet News*, 12, 6.

Anonymous, 2000c. All smiles as hospital opens. *Dick Vet News*, 13, 1 and 6.

Anonymous, 2002. Visit of the AVMA team. *Dick Vet News*, 14, 4.

Arms, 1977. *Public Register of All Arms and Bearings in Scotland*, Vol. 59, 70; The 'Ensigns Armorial' of the University of Edinburgh were registered on 22 October 1789 and recorded in Vol. I, folio 485.

Costello, G. 2000. George retires. *Dick Vet News*, 13, 5.

Faculty, 1973. *Veterinary Faculty Minutes*. 20 November 1973.

Faculty, 1980. *Veterinary Faculty Minutes*. 5 January 1980. 1337. Fees.

[Hackel, J., ed.] 1996. Self-assessment for Teaching Quality Assessment. Edinburgh: Royal (Dick) School of Veterinary Studies.

Gardiner, A. 2014. The 'Dangerous' Women of Animal Welfare: How British Veterinary Medicine Went to the Dogs. *Social History of Medicine*, 27 (3), 466–87.

Halliwell, 1993. Our path to the future. *Dick Vet News*, 5, 3.

Halliwell, 1994. We must take stock of the present and look to the future. *Dick Vet News*, 6, 3.

Letter, 1974. Manuscript dated 13th May to University Principal from Veterinary Faculty. CRC, University of Edinburgh.

MAFF, 1964. *Report of the Departmental Committee of Inquiry into Recruitment for the Veterinary Profession*. HMSO, cmnd 2430.

Patron, 1990. *Letter*. Archives of the Royal (Dick) School of Veterinary Studies, CRC, University of Edinburgh.

Pringle, R. O. 1869. *Memoir. In W. Dick, Occasional papers on veterinary subjects; with a Memoir by R. O. Pringle*. Edinburgh: William Blackwood and Sons, i–xci.

Senatus, 1970. *Senatus Academicus Signed Minutes*, Degree of BVM&S, Appendix XVIIB. Page 733, 13 May 1970.

Senatus, 1986a. *Senatus Academicus Signed Minutes*, 38, p. 160.

Senatus, 1986b. *Senatus Academicus Signed Minutes*, 37, p. 199.

Swabe, J. 1998. *Animal disease and human society; Human-animal relations and the rise of veterinary medicine*. London: Routledge.

Chapter 12

From Summerhall to the Easter Bush Campus (2003–11)

Elaine Watson: The first woman Head of the Dick Vet

On 1 August 2003 Elaine Watson was appointed Head of the Royal (Dick) School of Veterinary Studies. She was the first woman to become Head of the Dick Vet since it was founded in 1823 (Figure 12.1). She took up office in the year that eighty-one students – fifty-eight women and twenty-three men – had graduated with BVM&S (Plate 12.1A). Those numbers would continue to increase to a peak of 123 graduates in 2010, of 104 women and nineteen men (Plate 12.2). The ongoing international distribution of the Dick Vet's 2,650 graduates in 2005 was depicted (Plate 12.1B). The student intake numbers had risen to about 110 by Session 2002–3 and remained fairly steady for the next three years (Figure 12.2). One consequence of these numbers was that many of the lectures to first- and second-year students had to be presented in the larger University lecture theatres around George Square. As was indicated earlier, two lecture theatres at Easter Bush had been rebuilt to provide accommodation for the large veterinary class sizes during the clinical years. There was now more general discussion about whether the Summerhall site could ever be structurally modified to support the preclinical years of veterinary teaching and research.

Selection of a new site for the Dick Vet

The Erskine Medical Library on George Square closed in June 2004. This event prompted a group of Dick Vet senior staff to be assigned to look at the possibility of the preclinical part of the school moving to this vacated,

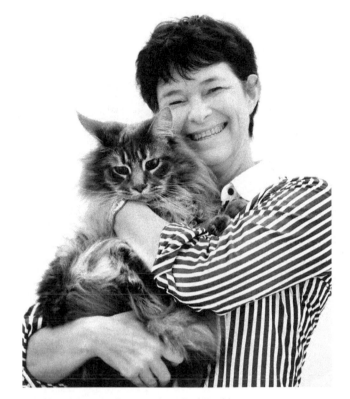

Figure 12.1 Elaine Watson. Photographer: Paul Dodds.

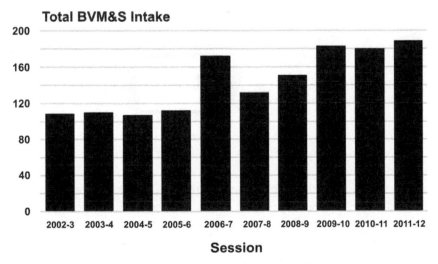

Figure 12.2 Graph of undergraduate (BVM&S) student intake, 2002–11.

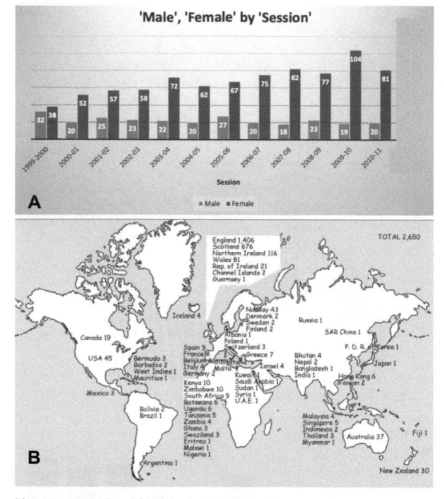

Plate 12.1 A. Male and female student BVM&S graduating numbers, 2000–11; B. The 2005 distribution of Dick Vet graduates.

more modern but much more restricted accommodation. Another alternative was to in some way join the Medical School at Little France. However, the danger of animal disease transmission to the Royal Infirmary on that site did not support that suggestion. Following consultation with senior staff and other interested parties, a consultant-led options appraisal was performed. The compelling case was for consolidation of the Veterinary School adjacent to the veterinary clinics at Easter Bush. This option would allow expansion of the Dick Vet's teaching, clinical and research activities and was perceived to provide the best possible educational experience for the undergraduates. Unprecedented opportunities would arise from this choice; the move would be into a modern, purpose-built facility, which

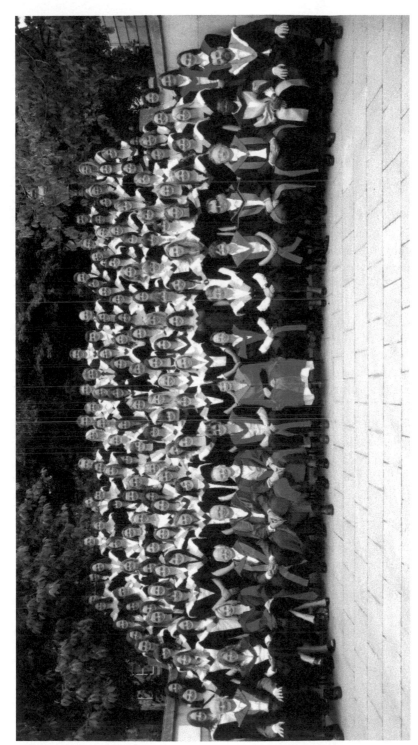

Plate 12.2 Graduation photo, 2010. Photographer: Ron Taylor studio.

would enable the development of a vertically integrated veterinary curriculum. It would also facilitate close collaborative research with neighbouring veterinary research institutes, grow and strengthen the Dick Vet's own research base, and expand the breadth and depth of the Dick Vet's clinical services. There was a feeling of optimism within the Dick Vet that renewal was under way.

Detailed studies had been carried out to identify the scale and association of the spaces needed for the consequential teaching and staff accommodation requirements of the Dick Vet. There needed to be a logical flow through the new building. Much of this early design work was thanks to Tom Bostock, the Managing Director of Reiach and Hall, who worked tirelessly with the Dick Vet staff through many iterations in the early stages of planning the proposed new teaching facilities. After performing rigorous studies on the feasibility of the move, in May 2005 the University Court enthusiastically approved this vision for the future of the Veterinary School (Watson 2005). Planning began immediately, led by the Head of School and the School Facilities Coordinator, Dr Tudor Jones. The architects (BDG Architecture + Design) produced outline plans for the new school based on the preparative work done earlier. These were subjected to extensive scrutiny and substantial revision following a series of consultation exercises with teaching staff and students.

In the autumn of the preceding year, preparation work had begun for the 2005 RCVS visitation (Anonymous 2005a). A 'Self-evaluation' report, in which the School reviewed itself against UK and European criteria, was compiled; senior staff wrote the content of the areas for which they had responsibility. The document, which comprised 120 pages plus fourteen appendices, was finalised by the Head of School and sent to the RCVS. Several weeks later, in March 2005, the RCVS team, consisting of seven specialists covering different interests, visited the School (Anonymous 2005b). During the course of the week, they had meetings with over fifty staff and seventy students, both in formal sessions and over refreshments. In addition, there were tours of Summerhall and the Easter Bush Veterinary Centre, together with a trip to the Veterinary School's dairy herd at Langhill Farm. At the end of the week, the RCVS team met with the Head of School and the Principal of the University to deliver their findings – a very positive outcome for the School, with much praise for the Dick Vet staff, the facilities at Easter Bush and the BVM&S course. The final report gave full accreditation from the Royal College of Veterinary Surgeons (Anonymous 2005b). The visitors were unanimous in their view of the high international standing of the Dick Vet. This reinforced the earlier full accreditation from the American Veterinary Medical Association, with special commendation for the plans to move to Easter Bush, for the new research institute and for the Dick Vet's outcomes-based approach to curriculum revision (Anonymous 2005b).

One year later, on Monday, 12 June 2006, in the grandeur of the University's Playfair Library at Old College, the Dick Vet's Patron, the Princess Royal, unveiled the plans of the brand-new teaching facility. The overall design was to bring the teaching, research and veterinary practice of the Dick Vet onto one site at Easter Bush. Guests also learned of the new 500-person Research Institute to be built next to the Dick Vet at Easter Bush. This was to house a hundred of the Dick Vet's own researchers, as well as researchers from The Roslin Institute, the Institute for Animal Health's Neuropathogenesis Unit and the Scottish Agricultural College.

The research to be undertaken there would benefit the health and welfare of animals, as well as shed light on zoonotic threats to the human population. This development was in close association with the Moredun Research Institute and together represented one of the largest concentrations of animal bioscience research in the world. When placed in the context of other major projects within the University, these included capital development at King's Buildings to house the Dick Vet's prestigious Centre for Infectious Diseases, the refurbishment at Teviot Place to house the Dick Vet's world-class Centre of Neuroscience Research, and the investment at the Medical School at Little France, including a Centre for Regenerative Medicine, led by Professor Ian Wilmut. It had been planned that the veterinary educational programme would benefit greatly from this proximity to world-class biomedical researchers. Some aspects of the global shortage of trained veterinary researchers could be addressed by closely involving the Dick Vet's undergraduate students with the staff of these centres of research expertise.

Teaching expertise recognised

In February 2006 the Veterinary Teaching Organisation (VTO), led by Dr Susan Rhind, learned that the Dick Vet's Virtual Learning Environment, together with that in the Medical School, had won a prestigious Queen's Anniversary Prize for Higher Education (Anonymous 2006a). These awards were given, every two years or so, to reward and recognise innovation, excellence and impact on the wider community. The Dick Vet award was for the development of the Virtual Hospital Online as an integral part of the adaptable, home-grown Virtual Learning Environments, EEVeC and EEMeC for the veterinary and medical curricula. One veterinary example in the project was 'The Virtual Farm'. This was designed to increase student involvement in the every-day activities of the University's farms. Students were assigned an 'adopted' cow and calf and received data feeds on progress such as milk yields from their cow. Additionally, there were newsletters, a farm tour, a discussion board and a webcam, which were used to show selected events on the farm. The Dick Vet has had a long-established record of excellence in the use of educational technology. The Veterinary Learning Environment was supported by a dedicated team from the College of Medicine and Veterinary Medicine Learning Technology section and was key to the development of the Dick Vet's new curriculum, due to be rolled out in 2007–8 (Anonymous 2006a).

Graduate Entry Programme (GEP)

Also in February 2006, two senior staff visited the USA as part of a recruitment search for international students (Anonymous 2006b). In Portland, Oregon they were hosted by the Banfield Pet Hospital Group Headquarters. On the east coast, they held a reception at the American University in Washington, DC (a University of Edinburgh partner). In both places potential veterinary candidates and their families were invited to presentations given on Scotland, Edinburgh, the R(D)SVS and the veterinary curriculum. These generated a lot of good will, and the detailed question-and-answer sessions focused particular interest in the new Graduate Entry Programme (GEP) to be introduced for the 2006–7 Session. This bespoke four-year programme was tailored for students who already had an appropriate first degree. Featuring a case-based approach to learning, the course was designed to fully prepare graduate entry students to enter the same third year as students pursuing the traditional five-year course (Watson 2006). Seventy-two graduate entry students (sixty-three women and nine men) were admitted to a specially designed 'second year' programme of studies. These well-educated and socially experienced individuals had a very positive and long-lasting impact on the tone of student education at the Dick Vet. The declining prevalence of the earlier school-leaver cohort as the main undergraduate intake was replaced by the intake of a largely postgraduate group of older students; these students shared knowledge from many different academic coursework backgrounds, commercial experience and international lifestyles. The total BVM&S student intake for the 2006–7 Session was 172 (Figure 12.2). The student intake peaked at 189 in Session 2011–12 (Figure 12.2). In line with this commitment to undergraduate education, the School now employed an Educational Development Manager, two Teaching Fellows dealing with projects including curriculum mapping and e-assessment, and an e-learning Development Officer (Watson 2006).

In 2006, with the heightened awareness worldwide of the risks to poultry and humans of the Highly Pathogenic Avian Influenza A (HPAI) virus, called bird flu, the School worked on the relevant contingency plans. The focus was on negating the risk to students, staff, clients and patients while maintaining full diagnostic and treatment capabilities (Soutar 2006).

In 2007 Susan Rhind was appointed to the first Chair of Veterinary Education in the UK, a clear demonstration of the high value that the Dick Vet placed upon excellence and innovation in teaching and learning. On 9 August she received the Chancellor's Award for Teaching from the Duke of Edinburgh in recognition of her innovation and developments in teaching and learning at the Dick Vet (Anonymous 2007). In her response to the award, Susan emphasised the need to acknowledge the changing requirements of the profession and expectations of students by designing a more flexible programme and making appropriate use of information technology. As Director of Veterinary Teaching since 2003, she had led a major curriculum review which increased clinical integration in the early years of the course, as well as developing a 'Virtual Veterinary Practice'. During Session 2006–7 a new clinical skills and study facility was developed at Summerhall to provide students with enhanced opportunities to practise core clinical techniques on surrogate mannequins from the earliest stages of the curriculum. Development of the Virtual Veterinary Practice continued apace, encompassing the Virtual Farm, Virtual Clinic and Post-mortem Room.

In November 2007 a weekend training course was organised for vets to brush up on their emergency techniques. The Dick Vet's canine mannequins were used to simulate a whole range of emergency situations and the delegates worked in teams against the clock putting what they had learned into practice (Anonymous 2008a). The School also began developing a range of e-learning programmes aimed at students who wanted to continue their education but who were not able to study full-time in Edinburgh. In 2006 an e-learning Masters Programme in International Animal Health (IAH) had been launched and attracted students from around the globe (Anonymous 2008b). The new online Masters programmes in Equine Science and Emerging and Neglected Infectious Diseases (ENID) were designed to be available from autumn 2008. These new courses attracted considerable interest from prospective students. The IAH and ENID programmes were supported by the Commonwealth Scholarships Commission and enabled many more students from developing countries to gain higher degrees (Anonymous 2008b). Similarly, specialised online courses for vets in practice and the first course in small animal internal medicine were started in 2008. The idea was that small groups of vets could enrol on a course at the same time, allowing for the formation of an online community where participants would be able to share experiences and knowledge online, allowing group learning. Online courses permitted distance learning that was available to everyone, regardless of their location or their ability to be away from their practice. They also provided the support and motivation gained from discussion with other vets with similar interests, together with direct access to experts' opinions at the Dick Vet (Anonymous 2008c).

New research and teaching buildings at Easter Bush

The construction of the new Dick Vet teaching block by Balfour Beattie Construction Ltd, beginning in the autumn of 2008, was routinely photographed from a high vantage point. Other photographs were taken at ground level (Plate 12.3). The traditions of building were upheld; a topping-out ceremony was carried out on Thursday, 24 September 2009, when a fir branch was hung from the tallest point in the building to symbolise good luck. Persistent snowy weather between December 2009 and the following January delayed the outer cladding (Jones 2010). Nevertheless, the building was completed on 5 December 2010, followed by an approximately twelve-week fit-out period (Anonymous 2010c)

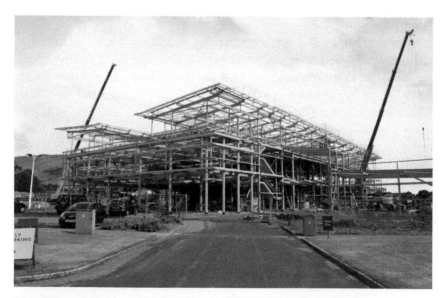

Plate 12.3 The Dick Vet Teaching Building under construction, June 2009. Photographer: Colin M. Warwick.

During roughly the same period of time, after its official launch on 7 April 2008, The Roslin Institute was administratively incorporated within the Dick Vet and joined the University of Edinburgh; it thereby became the research arm of the Veterinary School (Watson 2008; Anonymous 2008d). The integration of The Roslin Institute with the Dick Vet created an organisation with around fifty research groups in the fields of genetics and genomics, infection and immunity, neurodegeneration and developmental biology. Bench researchers at The Roslin Institute and clinicians from the Hospitals at the Dick Vet were now encouraged to work together thanks to a new programme. A group of fourteen Dick Vet clinicians became the first Clinical Research Associates (CRAs). The CRAs brought to the bench-based researchers in The Roslin Institute a wealth of experience in veterinary science and expertise in a number of companion and production animal diseases that could be compared to similar diseases in humans. Also, discoveries made in the research labs could now be translated much faster into cures in the clinics for life-threatening diseases in pets such as cancer. This was seen as a great opportunity to advance CRAs' research by introducing many of the genetic and molecular aspects of animal bioscience that had been refined at The Roslin Institute (Hart 2010). It also offered increased opportunities for undergraduate research studies. The Easter Bush Research Consortium, which was also launched on 7 April 2008, focused 'on animal and human health, identifying new and emerging diseases that can pass from livestock and wild animals to humans and understanding the ways in which these diseases work' (Anonymous 2008d). The threat of the deployment of biological weapons, and the role veterinary surgeons would have in dealing with these, was highlighted by Bruce Vivash Jones in the William Dick Memorial lecture presented in London on 3 July 2008 (Bonner 2008).

Extra-mural studies

'Seeing Practice' for twenty-six weeks had been an extra-mural studies (EMS) requirement for all veterinary students in the UK since 1932 (Anonymous 2015). Modern EMS consists of two distinct phases. The preclinical or animal husbandry phase comprises a total of twelve weeks carried out during the first two years of the BVM&S course. The Clinical EMS comprises twenty-six weeks towards the latter part of the degree course. Clinical EMS should include time in abattoirs, research laboratories and with the Government veterinary services, as well as in clinical practices. Students could spend time working on research projects or attending research summer schools as part of EMS.

Veterinary practices provided a vital contribution to this part of the veterinary student's training. The Dick Vet encouraged students to follow their interests with their EMS, offering advice on placement planning and distributing information about new opportunities that arose. While this was an important part of learning the core skills required of all vets, it was also an opportunity to travel and see the wide range of careers open to Dick Vet graduates. For example, in 2008, thirty-six Dick Vet students and staff visited Beijing to learn about veterinary medicine as practised in China. Over the two weeks they were there they learned about Chinese herbal medicines and the application of massage from veterinary staff at Beijing's Agricultural University. Information previously learned in the Dick Vet's topographic anatomy classes was recalled and brought into sharp focus during practical classes on acupuncture when applied to dogs, a horse and a donkey (Plate 12.4A). Each student received a detailed handout, prepared in English, to assist their practical learning of this technique. The students also visited private veterinary clinics in the city. Important components of the trip included working and learning with Chinese veterinary students, discovering daily life in Beijing, visiting historical and cultural sites nearby such as the Ming Tombs and the Great Wall, and explaining to the many Chinese people they met who they were and why they were there (Metcalf 2008). In effect, they were Dick Vet and University of Edinburgh ambassadors. Dick Vet students were also involved in research projects in Kenya (Bronsvoort 2008) and others worked with wildlife conservation in South Africa and in Indonesia. Visits to these and other countries gave Dick Vet students the opportunity to see how their profession was taught and practised in different cultures. It also gave them a deeper understanding of what they had learned at the Dick Vet and how they might apply it in a range of different and often quite new (to them) settings. They each discovered that veterinary medicine is truly global. Experiences such as these have long helped prepare Dick Vet graduates to practise their profession wherever in the world they end up (Plate 12.1B). Chinese postgraduate and undergraduate students were attracted to come to Edinburgh to study in subsequent years.

In 2009, over a two-week period, another group of Dick Vet students visited two of Japan's top veterinary schools, Tokyo University and the beautiful Sapporo campus of Hokkaido University (Bradshaw 2010). They also took a behind-the-scenes look at Asahiyama Zoo and spent two days observing deer and tracking bears with the rangers at Shiretoko World Heritage Site. Visits to beef and dairy farms enabled the students to see and discuss local animal husbandry with the farmers. They also learned from the veterinarians at the Japanese Racing Association and saw the elaborate facilities that were available there. Some of the differences

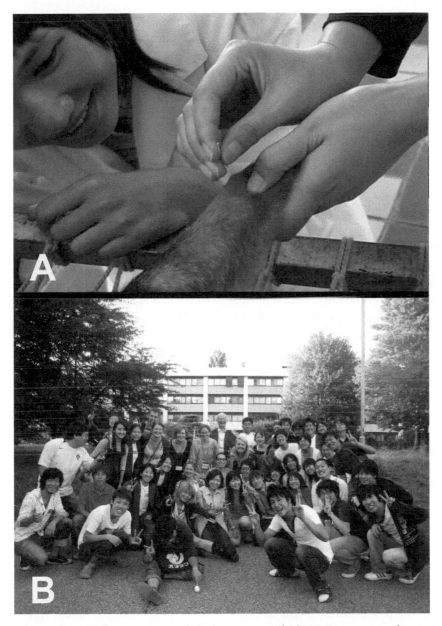

Plate 12.4 A. Tiffany Tsz Ting Ho happily attentive at the Beijing acupuncture class. Photographer: Cynthia Metcalf. B. Sapporo University student welcome. Photographer: unknown.

in social Japanese etiquette were learned at mealtimes while enjoying the wonderful presentation and varied tastes of the food. Other etiquette differences were learned during clothing for and while enjoying onsen, the natural hot-water bath, first thing in the morning and last thing at night. Calm courtesy was everywhere very apparent. The staff and students at both universities made the students very welcome (Plate 12.4B). The level of hospitality shown by the hosts was enormous and very much appreciated (Bradshaw 2010). Naturally, arrangements were made for a return visit of Japanese students and staff to Scotland the following year.

From August 2009, graduate entrants to the Dick Vet were able to enrol on a new combined BVM&S/PhD degree programme. This allowed them to carry out research towards a PhD alongside their BVM&S veterinary training, thereby producing veterinary clinicians who had a unique insight into veterinary research. The programme was the first of its kind in a UK Veterinary School and entrance to the programme was highly competitive, with only a few top students enrolled each year.

In 2009 the Dick Vet again passed the AVMA accreditation inspection with flying colours and came first in the RAE that year (Watson 2009).

Presentations to the general public

Engagement with the general public, other than through client visits with their animals to the clinics, took on a new form in 2009. The School featured in a new five-part documentary television series on Scottish Television (STV) called *Vet School*. The cameras went behind the scenes, focusing on the Small and Large Animal Hospitals, to follow the stories of our staff and students, along with our patients and their owners. This was a wonderful opportunity for the Dick Vet to showcase to the public the work its clinicians were doing (Watson 2010; Anonymous 2010a). In 2010 the Dick Vet shared a meet-the-public showcase stand with The Roslin Institute at the Royal Highland Show at Ingliston. Also in 2010, for the first time, Veterinary Services presented lectures for the general public on preventative healthcare for animals. The four lectures, funded by money donated to the University, were held throughout the spring and focused on some of the most popular pets and animals. The events were free to the public and were held on the central area campus of the University of Edinburgh. Some 350 people attended. The following year, a second Scottish Television fly-on-the-wall *Vet School* documentary series in six parts followed the work of the vets and students in the Hospital for Small Animals as well as the work of the Equine and Farm Animal teams (Soutar 2011). The second series built on and outstripped the success of the first series. It included more advanced work, imaging and oncology and a wider range of interesting cases. In addition to pets with major problems, there were also cases concerning herd health and farm issues.

An in-house self-training event in 2010 was the Veterinary School's first Agricultural Day. It was designed to help second-year and GEP students further their knowledge and practical skills in certain aspects of livestock husbandry. The day was made up of a series of lectures given by senior students with an agricultural background, followed by competitions and demonstrations. With the help of staff and local farmers, there was breed identification, estimation of age, weight and height, lameness scoring, stock-judging, sheepdog training and conformation scoring (Johnson 2010). The same year the Veterinary Teaching Organisation (VTO) created a new online learning tool to prepare vet students for EMS placements (Bell 2010). It resembled a driving theory test. The 'EMS Driving Licence' was full of tips and checklists. It also had a handy FAQ section with advice on issues such as confidentiality and other aspects of professional behaviour. The importance of modifying personal body language was explained, and students were shown how they could make a huge difference by being interested and enthusiastic. It was explained that improved body language often influenced how much additional experience the student would gain during a placement (Bell 2010).

In 2010 the Hospital for Small Animals opened an exotic animal teaching facility, where students could learn the best ways to care for exotic animals (Anonymous 2010b). It was the UK's first specialist training facility for veterinary students. The unit housed a range of animals, including rabbits, guinea pigs, hamsters, chinchillas, rats, lizards, snakes and tortoises. Students learned about the correct environment in which to keep these exotic pets and their dietary requirements. Animal-handling classes were held to complement the taught course. One-to-one sessions were made available for students who had phobias about snakes or rats to help them overcome their fears. Students were also able to carry out supervised placements at the new unit. It was estimated that in 2010 there were 1.4 million pet rabbits in the UK, making them the third most popular pet after cats and dogs. About 100,000 households had snakes and 80,000 homes had pet rats (Anonymous 2010b).

The new buildings begin work

Staff and postgraduate students of The Roslin Institute moved from their old buildings beside Roslin village into their new Institute building at Easter Bush in March 2011 (Plate 12.5A). The £60 million building, the design of which was inspired by the shape of a pair of chromosomes, has coloured-glass panels representing the DNA 'fins' which link the office and research laboratory blocks together. The building provides office and laboratory accommodation for over five hundred scientists, not only from The Roslin Institute, but also the Dick Vet, the Neuropathogenesis Unit and the Scottish Agricultural College (Anonymous 2011a). Together they incorporate expertise in areas such as genetics, developmental biology, immunology and infectious disease, neuroscience and behaviour and animal sciences (Anonymous 2011b). The ground floor and basement provide office space, a cafeteria, a three-hundred-seat auditorium, seminar rooms, cell-sorting and imaging facilities and laboratory support services. The two upper floors house laboratory space, office accommodation, meeting rooms and breakout areas.

Shortly thereafter the New Teaching Building was completed and fitted out (Plate 12.5B). The William Dick statue had been temporarily located in the William Dick Room of the Easter Bush Veterinary Centre (EBVC) main building for careful restoration (Figure 11.15). On 24 March 2010 (Figure 12.6) it was transferred with great care to its new indoor home in the atrium of the New Teaching Building (Jones 2010). This was the fourth time that the statue (Figure 6.4) had been moved. The first move was from the original Clyde Street courtyard (Plate 6.1) into safe keeping while the north end of the new 1887 building on Clyde Street was being constructed, and then back again onto its new plinth (Figure 6.5 and Plate 6.2B). It was then removed in 1916 from its indoor Clyde Street site to an outdoor setting in the Summerhall courtyard (Figure 8.5). The third move was indoors to the William Dick Room at Easter Bush in 2000 for repairs (Anonymous 2002; Jones 2010). Finally, it was transferred to its present location (Plate 12.6).

The focus of the new building started with the students themselves. They had been involved with planning it from its early stages. The various learning spaces were designed to be at the cutting edge of educational development. This was due to Tudor Jones's untiring quest for excellence with input from various members of the VTO. Each cohort of specialist staff planned their own area, such as the Study Landscape where the expertise of clinicians and librarians overlapped (Plate 12.7A).

Following the completion of The Roslin Institute building and the new Veterinary Teaching building, all activities previously carried out at the old Roslin Institute building in Roslin and at the Summerhall Campus in Edinburgh were transferred to the single site of the Easter Bush Campus. The Princess Royal opened the Vet School's new £42 million Veterinary Teaching building on 27 September 2011 (Plate 12.7B). The Princess, Patron of the Royal (Dick) School of Veterinary Studies and now also

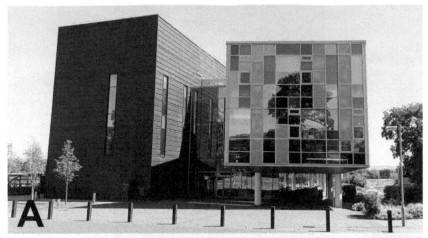

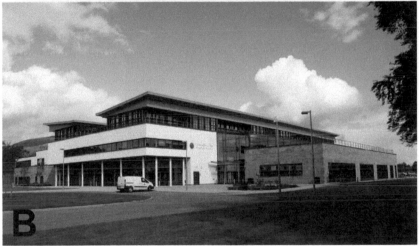

Plate 12.5   A. Façade of The Roslin Institute, Easter Bush. Photographer: Alastair A. Macdonald; B. Façade of the Dick Vet Teaching Building, Easter Bush. Photographer: Colin M. Warwick.

Chancellor of the University of Edinburgh, toured the facilities which can accommodate more than a thousand staff and students, one of the world's largest veterinary school campuses. To enable future generations of students and staff to enjoy and be inspired by the stained-glass windows from Summerhall, the position of the large windows in the new building's atrium was specially designed, like a flying kite (Plates 12.8A and B), by Douglas Hogg, an architectural glass artist from Berwickshire. The windows were carefully restored by Jim Jordan, a specialist stained-glass restorer based in Fife, and installed at the heart of the new building overlooking the statue of William Dick in the atrium (Anonymous 2011d).

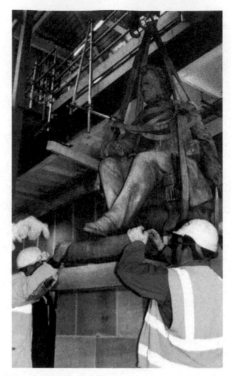

Plate 12.6 The William Dick statue arriving in the New Teaching Building. Photographer: unknown.

The Veterinary Teaching building provided most of the formal teaching facilities, student support facilities and administration offices capable of accommodating the needs of all five years of undergraduates (Anonymous 2011c). Students from all years were now able to meet socially, eat together and learn from one another in the same environment. The ground floor has a large atrium and reception area (Plate 12.8B). Two large lecture theatres were centrally placed in the building. Each one has the capacity for 202 and thereby fulfils the current requirements for formal lectures (Anonymous 2015). Each seat has power and internet connections. Both theatres have video links to a larger external audience via the internet. To the east of these theatres, across the atrium, are two formal group-study teaching rooms, each with a capacity for forty-eight students (Plate 12.8B). These can be subdivided when smaller class sizes are required; they have access to computers. Alongside these to the south is a hundred-seat seminar room.

On the west side of the building there is a 120-seat anatomy dissection room (Plate 12.9B). The general layout of the tables in the room has little changed since Summerhall (Plate 12.9A) or indeed since Clyde

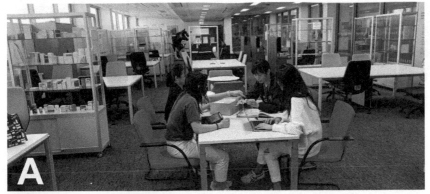

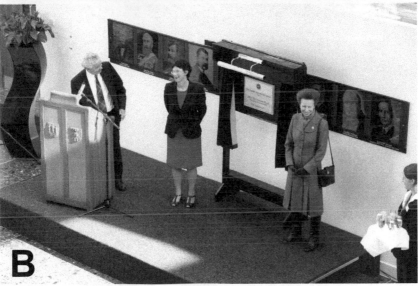

Plate 12.7   A. The students' Study Landscape. Photographer: Alastair A. Macdonald;
B. The Princess Royal opening the Teaching Building with Elaine Watson and the
University Principal Timothy O'Shea. Photographer: Colin M. Warwick.

Street (Figure 14.5) a century earlier; an observation and study balcony
was constructed in all three. Next door, to the north of the dissection
room, is a large chill room and a walk-in freezer. The large necropsy suite
is situated further to the north. The latter can accommodate most species and like the anatomy dissection room is fully serviced with hoists. It
has a hydraulic table to allow safe handling and examination of carcases.
A smaller necropsy room contains a Class I safety cabinet, which is suitable for higher-risk necropsies (for example, psittacines). There are dedicated changing facilities to allow safe access to the anatomy and necropsy
facilities. There is also a forty-seat bio-secure viewing area, permitting

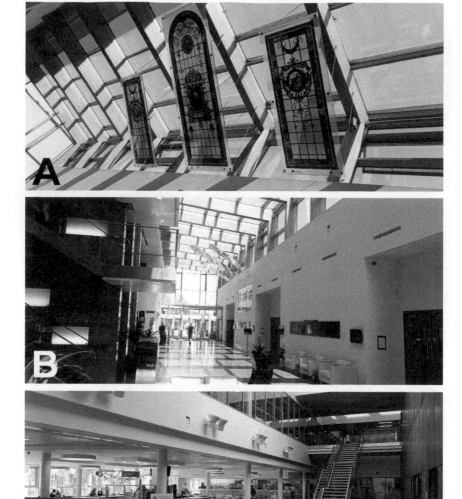

Plate 12.8 A. 'Kite formation' of the three large stained-glass windows in the atrium of the Dick Vet Teaching Building; B. The atrium looking east from the front door, with the entrances to the two study rooms on the right, the stair and lift to the upper floors on the left, the 'kite formation' of the stained-glass windows hanging from the ceiling and beyond them the back door; C. Entrance to View cafeteria with stair up to the Study Landscape and Lady Smith of Kelvin Veterinary Library. Photographer: Alastair A. Macdonald.

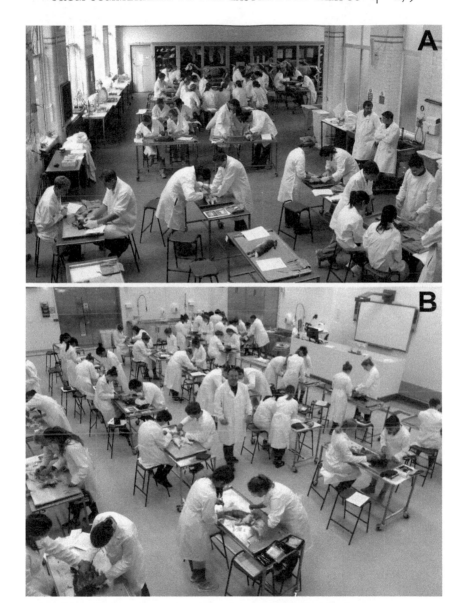

Plate 12.9 Anatomy dissection of the rabbit. A. Summerhall. Alasdair Cannon and Craig Johnstone attending; B. Easter Bush. Alasdair Cannon smiling to camera. Photographer: Colin M. Warwick.

the demonstration of necropsy material to students without the need for them to enter the necropsy suite (Anonymous 2015). This viewing gallery is serviced with intercom and cameras to allow close viewing of such material and discussion with the pathologist. Next door is a multi-head microscope teaching room. Nearby, to the north inside the building, are

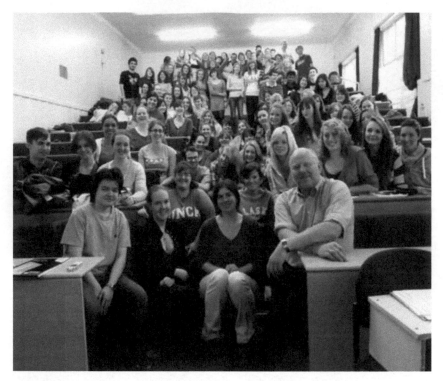

Plate 12.10 The end of the last lecture at Summerhall. Photographer: Heather Thomson.

two large teaching laboratories (ninety-seat and sixty-seat) for histology, biochemistry, physiology and microbiology. A student locker room with showers is situated close to the rear entrance to the building. The gymnasium, which is managed and run by the student body, was positioned to the north of the group-study teaching rooms (Anonymous 2015). The cafeteria is close to the front entrance and offers a range of catering (Plate 12.9C). Nearby, the undergraduate veterinary students have a dedicated common room with table games and soft seating, and the stair to the first floor. Students can bring their own food to eat in these areas and microwave ovens are provided. Between the teaching building and the Hospital for Small Animals is the sizeable Dick Vet Garden, designed for relaxation and contemplation.

On the first floor is the large Lady Smith of Kelvin Veterinary Library, with journals, textbooks, and ninety-five study places. There are six open-access computers. Five ten-seat tutorial/meeting rooms and a quiet-study room lead directly off the library. There are five twenty-seat tutorial/meeting rooms on the same floor. All these tutorial rooms are used for private study when not in timetabled use (Anonymous 2015). For more practical-based study there is the long Study Landscape, with teaching aids, specimens and group-study areas with computer access (Plate 12.7A). Nearby is an animal clinical skills laboratory, which houses further specimens, clinical equipment and surrogate mannequins of different animal species. On this floor there is also the BVM&S student hub, which houses student support services, teaching administration and the admissions team (Anonymous 2015). The top floor consists of academic and administration staff offices, meeting rooms, a second multi-head microscope room for teaching and a staff breakout area.

Dr Robert Dalziel gave the last-ever Dick Vet lecture at Summerhall on 17 May 2011 (Dalziel 2011). The lecture, on viruses and cancer, was attended by 110 first-year students (Plate 12.10).

References

Anonymous, 2002. Visit of the AVMA team. *Dick Vet News*, 14, 4.

Anonymous, 2005a. RCVS visitation – 'very positive'. *Dick Vet News*, 16, 5.

Anonymous, 2005b. Visitation to the Royal (Dick) School of Veterinary Studies University of Edinburgh 14–18 March 2005. London: Royal College of Veterinary Surgeons.

Anonymous, 2006a. Queen's prize: Queen's anniversary award for further and higher education. *Dick Vet News*, 17, 5.

Anonymous, 2006b. Student recruitment. *Dick Vet News*, 17, 6.

Anonymous, 2007. Novel posts for Edinburgh. *Dick Vet News*, 18, 2.

Anonymous, 2008a. New course in emergency surgery and medicine. *Dick Vet News*, 19, 5.

Anonymous, 2008b. E-learning opportunities. *Dick Vet News*, 19, 4.

Anonymous, 2008c. E-learning specialists join CPD team. *Dick Vet News*, 19, 4.

Anonymous, 2008d. Double boost for Dick Vet research: Official launch of the Roslin Institute and the Easter Bush Research Consortium. *Dick Vet News*, 20, 4–5.

Anonymous, 2010a. Vet school on TV. *Dick Vet News*, 23, 3.

Anonymous, 2010b. A first for exotics. The Dick Vet has created the UK's first specialist training facility for veterinary students. *Dick Vet News*, 23, 12.

Anonymous, 2010c. New building news. *Dick Vet News*, 24, 6.

Anonymous, 2011a. Embracing the future. *Dick Vet News*, 25, 3.

Anonymous, 2011b. Roslin Institute moves to new buildings. £60 million building for research institute. *Dick Vet News*, 25, 9.

Anonymous, 2011c. The new veterinary teaching building, Easter Bush. *Dick Vet News*, 25, 4–5.

Anonymous, 2011d. Something old, something new. Summerhall windows provide a permanent link to the past. *Dick Vet News*, 25, 28.

Anonymous, 2015. *Self evaluation report*. Edinburgh: The University of Edinburgh, Royal (Dick) School of Veterinary Studies.

Bell, C. 2010. 'Driving licence' for student vets. A new online learning tool is set to help students prepare for 'the real world'. *Dick Vet News*, 23, 11.

Bonner, J. 2008. Vets and biological warfare. *Dick Vet News*, 20, 8.

Bradshaw, J. 2010. Japan experience. *Dick Vet News*, 23, 22.

Bronsvoort, M. 2008. University of Edinburgh's Kenyan lab. *Dick Vet News*, 20, 20.

Dalziel, R. 2011. Last of the Summerhall. *Dick Vet News*, 26, 7.

Hart, P. 2010. Clinical research connections. *Dick Vet News*, 23, 19.

Johnson, H. 2010. Students learn to crawl to raise funds. *Dick Vet News*, 23, 23.

Jones, T. 2010. New buildings for the Bush. *Dick Vet News*, 23, 6.

Metcalf, T. 2008. Dick Vets in Beijing, Summer, 2008. Video. Edinburgh: Royal (Dick) School of Veterinary Studies.

Soutar, R. 2006. Avian Influenza: contingency plans in place. *Dick Vet News*, 17, 5.

Soutar, R. 2011. Vet school on TV. Second series of the popular documentary broadcast. *Dick Vet News*, 25, 6.

Watson, E. 2005. Head of School news. *Dick Vet News*, 16, 2.

Watson, E. 2006. Head of School news. *Dick Vet News*, 17, 2.

Watson, E. 2008. Message from Head of School. *Dick Vet News*, 19, 2.

Watson, E. 2009. Message from Head of School. *Dick Vet News*, 21, 2.

Watson, E. 2010. Message from Head of School. *Dick Vet News*, 23, 2.

Chapter 13

The Easter Bush Dick Vet (2011–22)

Complexities of the local and international environment

The teaching infrastructure of the Royal (Dick) School of Veterinary Studies was now once again in one geographical place (Anonymous 2019a). Over the next dozen or so years, improvements would continue to be made to the older existing structures at Easter Bush. The replacement of and additions to some veterinary clinical facilities also took place, with the opening of the Equine Diagnostic Surgical and Critical Care Unit and the Large Animal Research and Imaging Facility, and the expansion of the Hospital for Small Animals (Anonymous 2015, 2019a, 2022a). Underlying these physical adjustments, the rolling impact of the administrative restructuring of the University from Faculties into Schools within three Colleges generated changes at many levels of Dick Vet management. As these continue, now is not the time to attempt to analyse them. Indeed, the current data-protection laws obscure and thereby prevent any competent overview.

The wider environmental background to the next decade contained a number of very relevant uncertainties. There was a growing consciousness of world climate change (IPCC 2007) and accelerating scientific understanding of the need for urgency in dealing with rising world temperatures (Pörtner et al. 2022; IPCC 2022). The University's positive reaction to this information was internationally recognised (Anonymous 2013a, 2022b). The architecture of the New Teaching Building included several appropriate elements, such as the green roof and the harvesting of rainwater for toilet flushing (Anonymous 2010a). A low-carbon Energy Centre was later built on the Easter Bush Campus (Gorman 2016). In December 2019 the sudden and unexpected appearance in China of the 'severe acute respiratory syndrome coronavirus 2 (SARS-CoV-2)', and the very rapid worldwide spread of the COVID-19 disease through the human population, directly impacted veterinary education in Edinburgh from March 2020. Brexit, on 31 January 2020, resulted in the dismantling of trouble-free links with the rest of Europe and placed barriers on what had been highly productive teaching and research contacts. The 2022 escalation of the Russo-Ukrainian War, started in 2014 (Ukraine 2022), and the ongoing threat of a wider European conflict, added to the external uncertainties surrounding the Dick Vet as the 2023 bicentenary approached. The world's human population was estimated by the United Nations to have reached eight thousand million on Tuesday, 15 November 2022 (<https://www.un.org/en/dayof8billion>), double that in 1974.

David Argyle appointed Head of the Dick Vet

Most of these circumstances were not apparent on 1 November 2011 when David Argyle became the twenty-second Head of the Royal (Dick) School of Veterinary Studies (Figure 13.1). That Session and those that

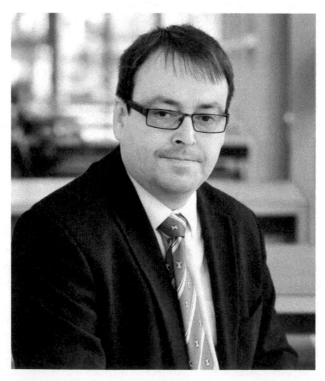

Figure 13.1   David Argyle. Photographer: Paul Dodds.

immediately followed it may justifiably be characterised as a 'settling in' period for all those students and staff who were 'newcomers' to studying and working on the Easter Bush Campus. Everything was very new (Day 2016). In addition to the arrival of the previously Summerhall-based staff and students, The Roslin Institute staff had also moved from their former premises near Roslin village to the new three-storey building across the road from the Dick Vet Teaching Building (Plate 12.5A). The human population now working and studying on the Easter Bush Campus had increased by more than 1,200 staff and students. Their arrival brought together onto the one academic site a plethora of very different institutional cultures and ways of thinking and working.

Preceding these moves, considerable efforts had been made by highly motivated library and other academic staff to safely transfer books and partially catalogued historical and archival materials from Roslin, Easter Bush and Summerhall into the appropriate University of Edinburgh library and the Centre for Research Collections (CRC) storage facilities at the Gyle. Retiring staff members also passed into these archives various teaching and other relevant materials that they had held 'in trust' or as part of their own personal collections. The detailed cataloguing of most of this material had to await the arrival of funding support ten years later. Sadly, as can happen with any sort of 'flitting', precious historical materials appear to have been overlooked and lost. However, where very careful attention was paid, much of the traditional Dick Vet memorabilia, in the form of sculptures, paintings, plaques, sports trophies and stained-glass windows, did get gathered up and brought from Summerhall to Easter Bush (Figures 13.2a, b, c and d). These were variously placed outside the equine reception office, in lecture theatre 2 and along corridors of the teaching building. Other paintings from Summerhall, together with additional works of art from the University's collections, were placed in seminar rooms, teaching laboratories, offices and along corridors on all three floors of the New Teaching Building as well as in the Dick Vet's clinical buildings. Further artworks were sought from the University and elsewhere to assist with the firm establishment of the Dick Vet in the integrated countryside setting of Easter Bush (Figure 13.3). Representative of the latter were the shadow-carved portraits of former Deans and Heads of School which were placed in a long row on the east wall of the atrium (Plates 12.7B and 12.8B).

On the human side, however, many of the familiar faces of the older teaching, technical, research and administrative staff had chosen to retire around the time of the move out to Easter Bush. Summerhall's 'institutional memory' was thereby summarily dismantled and has also been partially lost. Events over the next few years would add to this 'forgetting'. By way of compensation there were many examples of fresh human 'newness'

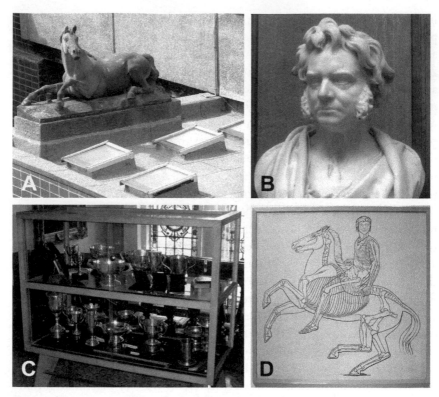

Figure 13.2 A. The rising horse sculpted by A. Wallace of Wallace and White, 6 Shrub Place, Edinburgh; B. The marble bust of William Dick by George Clark Stanton; C. The cabinet of silver trophies and other memorabilia; D. The anatomical horse and rider by James T. Murray. Photographer: Colin M. Warwick.

to be seen on the Easter Bush site. Young growth and the gradual exploration of different Dick Vet 'traditions' became evident in the New Teaching Building (Anonymous 2012a, 2013b, 2014a, 2014b). Relaxed celebrations saw expression in the new teaching setting (Anonymous 2014c).

The BVM&S student population of the Dick Vet was 754 in 2011, comprising 602 women and 152 men. The intake in 2011 was 189, of whom 123 were first year students and 66 were GEP entrants; of the total, 153 were women and 34 were men. There were some fluctuations in both first-year and GEP student intake numbers over the next eleven years, with the total BVM&S student intake averaging 175±7 (Figure 13.4). The total numbers of students graduating increased from 139 in 2011–12 to 155 in 2013–14 (Figure 13.5 and Plate 13.1A) and subsequently rose to 162 in both 2015–16 and 2016–17 and topped at 181 in 2022. During the first half of the decade the number of women graduates increased (Figure 13.5a), while the numbers of men decreased (Figure 13.5b). The total

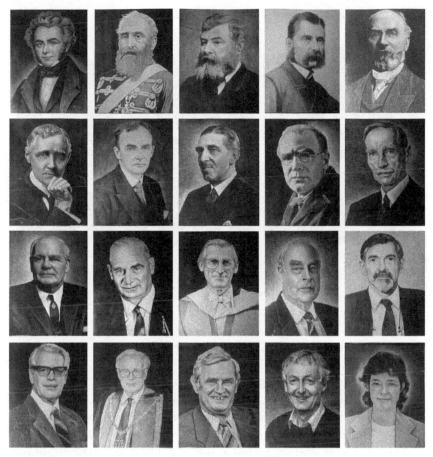

Figure 13.3 The initial unique set of twenty stone portraits, representing previous Principals, Directors, Deans and Heads of the Veterinary School, from the founder, William Dick, to Elaine Watson, on the east wall of the Teaching Building atrium. The set, a gift from an anonymous donor, was 'shadow-carved' by hand at the ancient walled city of Chong Wu by the craftsmen Lv Ting Yan and Wang Shi Peng in Lin Ting Fan's workshop. Photographer: Colin M. Warwick.

number of overseas graduates in 2011–12 was sixty-five, by 2013–14 it was sixty-nine and by 2020–1 it had reached seventy-eight.

The Student Welfare Committee, made up of both staff members and students, was formed in 2011. It organised the Dick Vet's first-ever Student Welfare Awareness Week in February 2012 (Anonymous 2012b), which included lunchtime talks, daily relaxation and meditation workshops and an afternoon of fun activities. The workshops were well attended during the week, reflecting the popularity of the School's regular twice-weekly relaxation sessions that took place throughout the term. A new, perhaps more countryside-aware social atmosphere had begun to develop.

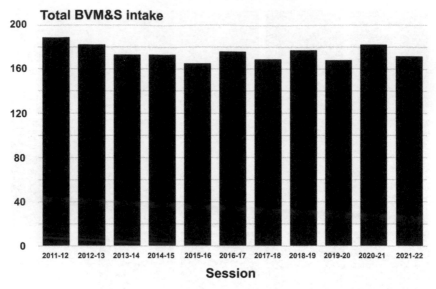

Figure 13.4 Graph of total BVM&S intake from Session 2011–12 to 2021–2.

Massive Open Online Courses (MOOCs)

The Royal Highland and Agricultural Show in June 2012 provided the first opportunity to showcase the now Easter Bush-based Dick Vet's teaching, clinical practices and research. Over the four days of the Show, staff and students met around six hundred people, including youngsters/budding vets who tried their hand at milking 'Daisy' the mannequin cow (Anonymous 2012c.). An additional kind of 'outreach' occurred in July 2012, when the University of Edinburgh joined the Coursera consortium, the organisation set up by senior academics at Stanford University to provide free online undergraduate-level courses to anyone who wishes to access them (Coursera 2016). Coursera offered short online courses, called Massive Open Online Courses or MOOCs, entirely free of charge. In January 2013 the Dick Vet was one of the first Schools within the University and the first Veterinary School to launch a course as part of this programme. A five-week course of Equine Nutrition, covering the anatomy and physiology of the equine digestive tract, was presented together with discussion of dietary management for different kinds of horses and ponies, particularly those with nutrition-related disorders (Murray 2014). Over the years since then, 53,000 individuals have taken the course. By the summer of 2014, 10,000 students from 146 countries had signed up to the MOOC entitled 'Do you have what it takes to be a veterinarian?' (Argyle 2014).

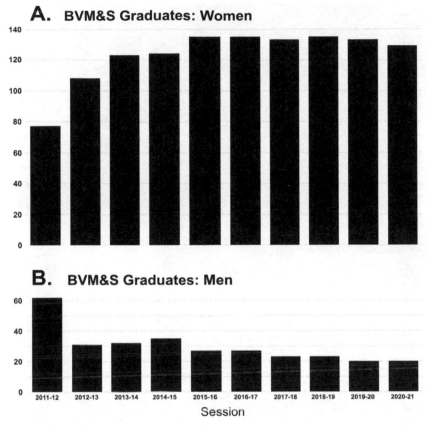

Figure 13.5 Graphs of women (A) and men (B) graduates from Session 2011–12 to 2020–1.

By 2022 the Dick Vet was offering the following MOOCs:

Virtual work experience and exploring the veterinary profession. This course has been developed by the UK Vet Schools to mitigate the impact of Covid-19 on applicants' work experience. The course is two weeks long and aimed at prospective undergraduate veterinary medicine applicants.

EDIVET: 'Do you have what it takes to be a veterinarian?' This course is for anyone interested in learning more about veterinary medicine, giving a 'taster' of courses covered in the first year of a veterinary degree and an idea of what it is like to study veterinary medicine.

Animal Behaviour and Welfare. This course allows learners to develop an understanding of some of the main welfare issues that animals have to cope with, as well as gain an insight into the behavioural needs and emotions of dogs, cats, farmed animals and captive wildlife.

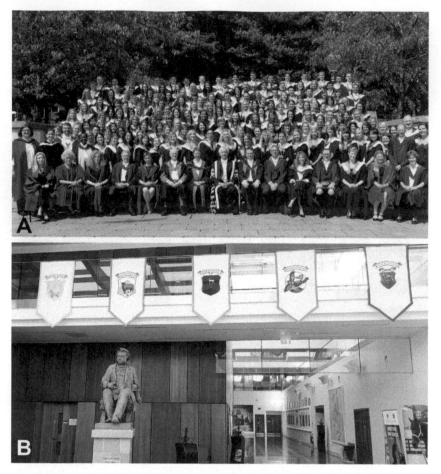

Plate 13.1   A. Summer Graduation photograph taken on 5 July 2014. Photographer: Ron Taylor studio. B. Statue of William Dick in the atrium with the two lecture theatres behind him and examples of the student house banners displayed from the first-floor balcony railing above him. Photographer: Alastair A. Macdonald.

The Truth about Cats and Dogs. What is your cat revealing to you when she purrs? What is your dog expressing when he yawns or wags his tail? Understanding cats' and dogs' behaviour and the way they communicate with you will enable you to better understand their needs and strengthen your relationship with them.

Chicken Behaviour and Welfare. The course looks at the behavioural and physiological indicators that can be used to assess welfare in chickens kept in hobby flocks through to commercial farms. The focus is primarily on laying hens and meat chickens (broilers), although many of the principles are relevant to other types of poultry. The course is likely to be of interest to people who own chickens as pets or keep a small hobby flock, commercial egg and chicken meat producers, veterinarians and vet nurses.

Sustainable Global Food Systems. How do we feed 11 billion people? Discover the importance of sustainable food systems globally with our new online course on @edXOnline.

The number of participants from around the world who had engaged with the Dick Vet MOOCs by June 2022 totalled over a third of a million.

Further contact with the general public occurred in 2012 with the summer filming of ten thirty-minute television episodes of *Junior Vets* by True North Productions for CBBC. The programmes presented a group of six young animal enthusiasts undertaking a range of veterinary challenges to find out who had what it takes to become a 'Junior Vet' at the Dick Vet. By their nature, these programmes gave another insightful and entertaining series of public viewings of clinical and preclinical life in the Dick Vet (Anonymous 2013c).

Enhancing the student experience

The key strategic theme for the School that largely characterised the decade was defined in 2013/14 as 'enhancing the student experience' (Argyle 2013; Paterson 2015; Dhinoja et al. 2020). To this end the School made new appointments in teaching and student support, including a new Student Experience Officer. Student support was revamped by the creation of a new organisation of personal tutors. A student 'house-system' was also created to enhance the interaction between students in different years, now that all five BVM&S years were studying on the Easter Bush Campus site (Anonymous 2013d). Between seventy and eighty students became members of each house. These houses were named after the ten local hills; Capelaw, Castlelaw, Turnhouse, Carnethy, Scald Law, West Kip, East Cairn, Spittal, Allermuir and Caerketton. Banners were displayed on the balcony overlooking the atrium to signify these houses (Plate 13.1B). Academic and pastoral support was provided through personal tutors, who were each assigned to a specific house. Students were allocated a personal tutor in each house, but also had access to three other house tutors as well as the senior house tutor. To encourage social interaction between students from different years, each house had its own committee in charge of organising events. These could include walks on the hill after which the house was named, inter-house sports days and inter-house quiz nights.

Widening student access had for some decades been routinely undertaken at the Dick Vet (Murdoch, Bergkvist and Kristruck 2021).

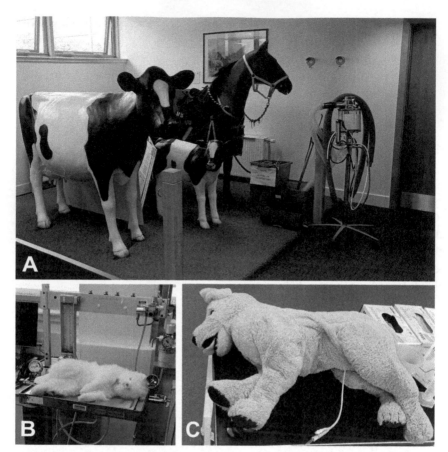

Figure 13.6 Veterinary training mannequins: A. Cattle and horse. B and C. Canine mannequins for catheter and intubation practice. Photographer: Alastair A. Macdonald.

Continued enhancement of the general student experience occurred on both the academic and pastoral fronts. This included providing direct study development advice to students, for instance through one-to-one or group sessions or through workshops. There was also an additional focus in providing support to the international student body and developing the Dick Vet's peer-support system. Help was given to improve student learning strategies, and these included support for students with specific learning difficulties. The teaching of clinical skills was enhanced with the provision of a range of simulators, which included bovine, canine and equine training models and mannequins (Anonymous 2022a; Figure 13.6a, b and c). These mannequins provided students with a flexible means of learning basic clinical skills in the welfare-friendly environment of the School's Clinical Skills Lab (Anonymous 2013e). The models enabled students to hone practical skills, such as rectal palpation to detect the different stages of pregnancy in cows. Different canine simulators allowed students to practise endotracheal intubation and intravenous injections, as well as a simulator to help them identify irregular heart sounds. The realistic attributes of these models allowed students to initially learn and then refine their basic clinical skills before undertaking the procedures on live animals. By way of an extension of this teaching approach, in 2014 staff at the Dick Vet and the Edinburgh Dental Institute (EDI) came together to offer an intensive two-day course in dental prophylaxis for fourth-year veterinary students. The students spent time in the EDI's clinical skills laboratory, where they practised dental techniques on phantom human heads. The teaching prompted a lot of discussion about the similarities between veterinary and human dentistry and the necessity for optimum client communication and education (Gardiner 2014).

Veterinary outreach

For many years the Dick Vet has offered a broad range of Clinical Training Scholarships to vets who want to specialise in a particular discipline (Anonymous 2013f). Residents undertake three- and four-year Residency Programmes, also known as Senior Clinical Training Scholarships. These cover areas of veterinary anaesthesia, dermatology, diagnostic imaging, small animal surgery, small animal internal medicine (canine and feline), cardiology, oncology, equine medicine and surgery (soft tissue and orthopaedics) and exotic animal medicine and surgery. In 2012–13 the School announced additional scholarships in farm animal practice and residencies in anatomical and clinical pathology. The Dick Vet also offered a number of one-year Junior Clinical Training Scholarships (Internships) within the Hospital for Small Animals.

Outreach veterinary training stretched as far as China. The Dick Vet's Jeanne Marchig Animal Welfare Education Centre, which opened in 2011 (Anonymous 2010b), was invited to host a forum on animal welfare at the third annual conference of the Chinese Veterinary Medicine Association (CMVA) in Suzhou, Jiangsu Province (Anonymous 2013g). It was attended by veterinarians and Government officials and provided an overview of animal welfare from an international perspective, the role of veterinarians and the challenges as well as opportunities for China in the animal welfare arena.

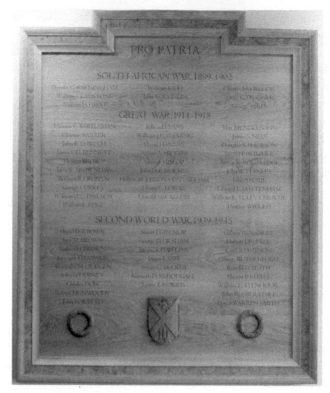

Figure 13.7 New War Memorial placed in the Quiet Study Room on 7 November 2014. Photographer: Colin M. Warwick.

The new War Memorial

Following detailed research (Matthews et al. 2016a), a new War Memorial (Figure 13.7) was made to commemorate the students, graduates and staff of the Royal (Dick) Veterinary College who died during or following active service in the South African (2nd Boer) War (1899–1902), Great War (1914–18) and Second World War (1939–45). The plaque was created by Dovetailors, designed by David Wilson and made in European Oak by Craig Dalziel, with individual carving of the coat of arms and the wreaths by Graham Gamble. It was placed in a decorative frame featuring oak burr detailing (Matthews et al. 2016b). On 7 November 2014 it was placed in the Teaching Building on the east wall of the first-floor quiet-study room beside the marble plaque donated in 1944 by the staff and students of the Polish Faculty (Figure 8.4).

One Health – One Medicine

The Edinburgh students' One Health Society hosted the inaugural National Students' One Health Conference in November 2016 (Herrington, Stirling, Cassie and Ford, 2017). The Conference's main aim was to inspire a new generation of professionals from across these areas to engage in One Health research, and open communication between disciplines, breaking down traditional barriers. The hundred delegates came from across many institutions, including London, Dublin, Vienna and Nottingham.

The Edinburgh Clinical Academic Track for Veterinarians (ECAT-V) programme enhances the School's One Health – One Medicine philosophy, where traditional boundaries between veterinary and human medicine no longer exist (ECAT-V 2013). It is intended to develop a new generation of veterinary researchers, able to conduct internationally competitive research while still being grounded in clinical practice. Veterinary clinical lectureship posts are designed to be flexible to the requirements of individual trainees. They combine parallel specialist clinical training with the opportunity to undertake a fully funded PhD and postdoctoral research in a supportive and scientifically stimulating environment. During the first twelve months their time is divided between 30 per cent clinical training (in their chosen discipline within the Veterinary School) and 70 per cent research time (to identify ideal PhD supervisors and develop a tailor-made PhD project). Successful candidates are encouraged to undertake three mini-projects with the aim of developing a tailor-made PhD project in one of the labs that have hosted a project. Years 2 to 4 are dedicated to 100 per cent research towards a PhD in one of the University's major research centres.

Postgraduate research and teaching at the Easter Bush Campus had gone from strength to strength (Anonymous 2014d). The number of postgraduate research students doubled between 2009 and 2014. There were five online distance-learning Masters programmes in 2014. The National Postgraduate Research and Taught Student Surveys found 96 per cent of taught postgraduate students and 93 per cent of research postgraduate students expressed overall satisfaction with their programmes. In 2014 there were more than 170 postgraduate research students. The Dick Vet's online postgraduate community – with courses including Equine Science; International Animal Welfare, Ethics and Law; Conservation Medicine; Bioimaging; and One Health – incorporated 159 students from across the world (Anonymous 2014d). Its Masters courses in Animal Biosciences and Applied Animal Behaviour and Animal Welfare, run on-site, had a student cohort of thirty-six. In addition, the Dick Vet played an active role in the postgraduate training of veterinary clinicians, with seven interns and twenty-nine residents, some of whom were also undertaking Masters by Research.

Accreditation visitation

In November 2015 the Dick Vet received its seven-yearly accreditation visitation from the major international veterinary accrediting bodies (Argyle 2016). The visitation teams included representatives from the Royal College of Veterinary Surgeons (RCVS), American Veterinary Medical Association (AVMA), Australasian Veterinary Boards Council (AVBC) and European Association of Establishments for Veterinary Education (EAEVE). Once again, full accreditation was received from all bodies for a further seven years. This came with a comprehensive endorsement of the Dick Vet's strong teaching, research and clinical programmes and its commitment to delivering an outstanding student experience. The joint submission with Scotland's Rural College (SRUC) to the recent Research Excellence Framework (REF) exercise was ranked as the most powerful in the UK (Anonymous 2016a). The most recent accreditation visit took place in November 2022. The results will be made known during 2023, the bicentenary of the establishment of the Dick Vet. Currently Dick Vet graduates are qualified and accredited to practise veterinary medicine in the UK, Europe, North America, Australasia and South Africa.

In 2016 the Easter Bush Campus won the Community Engagement Award at the Scottish Enterprise Life Sciences Awards held in Edinburgh (Anonymous 2016b). This highlighted wide-ranging Dick Vet engagement with the local community. It reflected Dick Vet involvement in the Midlothian Science Festival, the Campus Open Day (Anonymous 2016c) and contributions to the schools programme. It also included the outreach visits, and such activities on the Easter Bush Campus as 'Science Insights', the innovative work-experience programme, and the 'Hands-On Pathology – Understanding Disease' event. In addition, it profiled the work carried out by clinical staff and students who provide advice and a basic veterinary service across a number of Edinburgh Housing Associations, including the student-led veterinary care provided to the homeless in the area (Anonymous 2016b).

In 2016 Professor Susan Rhind, the Dick Vet Chair of Veterinary Education and Deputy Head of School, was made Assistant Principal with responsibility for Assessment and Feedback (Anonymous 2016d). In her new role, she led on developing strategies to improve the timeliness and quality of feedback across the University in addition to her responsibilities at the Veterinary School.

Progressively from 2014 to 2016, the education of equine clients has taken on a variety of new forms, with a move away from the traditional evening talk towards discussion, audience participation and practical sessions (Anonymous 2016e). For example, the 'Colic Evening' drew 150 horse owners from across Edinburgh, the Lothians and further afield to the New Teaching Building. They saw the gastrointestinal tract of a horse from the new post-mortem room viewing suite, got their hands on 'Rodney' the plastic horse in order to rehearse post-surgery intensive care, and saw innovative 3D modelling demonstrating how the guts can move around during a bout of colic. This very practical approach was well received. The Equine Practice's education programme created another first by organising a four-week evening course for horse owners (Anonymous 2016e). The sessions covered preventative healthcare, first aid, biosecurity, yard policies, infection control and behaviour and finished with a live 'ask the expert' session.

Peer-assisted learning

Dick Vet students had long wanted more contact with students from other years. Studying on the same geographical site and having the house system enabled those from earlier years to benefit from the experience of students who were further through their course. Peer-assisted learning had happened informally at Summerhall and Easter Bush for a number of years. In recent years it has been brought into the curriculum (Hudson 2017). Dick Vet students are now helping their first-year counterparts to study more effectively through the use of VetPals. There are two schemes: one for GEP students joining the four-year programme and one for those on the five-year programme. These are student-to-student support systems where more senior students facilitate discussion on specific topics with junior students. Feedback has shown that this has been highly beneficial to all taking part. This project recently received an Impact Award for Best Peer Assisted Learning Scheme (PALSs) at a student-led event on campus. The VetPals initiative encourages students to pass on study tips to first years. They cover topics such as how to take notes in lectures, write essays and lab book reports, revision techniques and how to prepare for exams. Ten one-hour sessions are held throughout the academic year, led by a team of trained VetPal leaders selected from senior students.

Since 2016 Dick Vet students have had the opportunity to gain an undergraduate Certificate in Veterinary Medical Education (Anonymous

2016f). The modular programme – believed to be the first of its kind in the veterinary sector – is open to students in the third year of their degree. It incorporates core and elective components and is completed over the final three years of a veterinary degree. It also includes visiting local secondary schools and holding veterinary science workshops for pupils there to both boost teaching skills and to inspire pupils to consider scientific careers. By 2017 some 107 students had enrolled in the programme (Anonymous 2017). Four of them, with exceptional teaching potential, were honoured by a leading higher education body; they were thought to be the first undergraduate veterinary students in the UK to receive an Associate Fellowship from the Higher Education Academy (AFHEA). The Associate Fellowship is normally awarded to academics further on in their careers in recognition of their contributions to education and learning.

The new Equine Diagnostic, Surgical and Critical Care Unit was completed in 2017. It comprised four integral and connected parts (Anonymous 2018): a diagnostics and triage area for evaluating and triaging emergency cases; two state-of-the-art theatres with adjacent induction and recovery boxes, plus a new standing surgery suite to reduce the risk of complications associated with general anaesthesia, leading to faster recovery rates; a dedicated unit of six boxes for adult horses and neonatal foals which require intensive and/or perioperative care, with twenty-four-hour video monitoring and an on-site laboratory; and a support hub to deliver on-site teaching in surgery, critical care and anaesthesia, incorporating surgery viewing and an education area for students, to counsel and support clients, to provide facilities for clinicians and nurses to plan treatments, and to encompass office and teaching facilities.

The Charnock Bradley Building

The Charnock Bradley Building, designed by Atkins (Plate 13.2A), was officially opened by the Princess Royal on 1 May 2017 (Anonymous 2019). She also unveiled the 4.6 metre steel sculpture representing a working horse's head, *Canter* by Andy Scott, which forms the centrepiece of the landscaped entrance plaza (Plate 13.2B). This building houses the Roslin Innovation Centre and new facilities for students, including a shop, gymnasium, multi-faith contemplation space and teaching and exhibition space. Spread over the two upper floors, the Innovation Centre has provided flexible, open-plan, cellular office and laboratory space for a broad range of companies undertaking research in the animal and veterinary sciences, agri-tech and One Health industries. There is also space for science outreach. The theme of commercialising research and growing companies

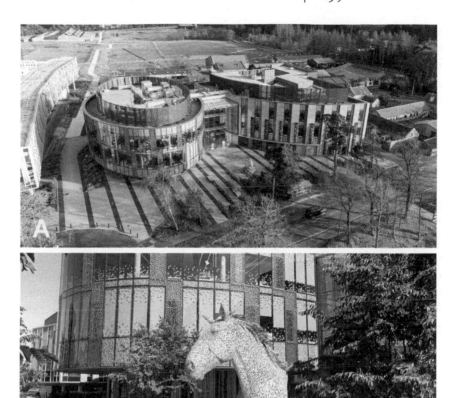

Plate 13.2   A. Aerial view looking south of the Charnock Bradley Building, with the west wing of The Roslin Institute on the left. Photographer: Lee Live; B. 'Canter' the workhorse statue by Andy Scott at the entrance to the Charnock Bradley Building. Photographer: Alastair A. Macdonald.

formed a central point of the Centre's strategy. The aim was to attract up to thirty tenant companies, and at January 2023 there were twenty-four resident tenants, four organisations 'hot desking' and two 'Academia in residence' (Roslininnovationcentre 2023).

Somewhat ironically, in 2016 a European collaboration of veterinarians, scientists and technical specialists began work to identify at a very early stage any new emerging diseases in livestock and companion animals. The collaboration involved the Easter Bush Research Consortium, The Roslin Institute, the Dick Vet, Scotland's Rural College (SRUC) and the Moredun Research Institute, together with the health company Zoetis. Expertise was co-ordinated through a hub in Edinburgh incorporating genetic sequencing, molecular biology, laboratory diagnostics and infectious disease surveillance, along with Zoetis's research and development and specialist infectious disease capabilities. The collaborative initiative involved a multi-disciplinary team with knowledge relating to emerging infectious disease surveillance and rapid response. This also included detecting new pathogens through genomic sequencing and identifying routes to diagnostics and therapeutics (DVN 30 2016).

The impact of SARS-CoV-2 virus on teaching

Four years later, the identification in March 2020 of the severe acute respiratory syndrome coronavirus 2 (SARS-CoV-2) causing the (Covid-19) human infection in Britain prompted the Veterinary School to set up a Covid-19 task force (Argyle 2020). It was created to deal with the potential impact of the pandemic on teaching, student support, research, clinical care and staff wellbeing. Key people from across the campus were called upon to help co-ordinate the School's response, including moving teaching and assessment online, repatriation of staff and students from across the globe, moving clinics to emergency only, and setting up the infrastructure for home working. A large proportion of the staff began working from home from March. Many have continued to do so. There was considerable innovation from everyone involved. The teaching and support staff, Digital Education Unit and student support teams co-ordinated to ensure that the students had an immersive student experience despite the challenges (Ferguson 2022). A system of hybrid learning saw all possible lectures and tutorials move online. The School's long-established expertise in, and the technology for, online postgraduate education meant that the Dick Vet was in an excellent position to quickly ensure that the online experience would facilitate effective learning outcomes. The clinical teaching teams faced challenges as practical training is a key part of the BVM&S programme. This was not only important for the development of clinical skills but essential to meet the RCVS requirements for accreditation. Close working with the accrediting bodies ensured that all of the standards required of the School's programmes were met.

However, the repeated – approximately bi-monthly – appearance of a wave of one or more new Omicron variants of the Covid-19 virus extended the need for caution (Figure 13.8). The arrival of the Omicron variant BA.2 in March and April 2022, with its replacement by BA.5 and BA.5.1 through the summer of 2022, the presence of the Omicron BQ.1.1 variant (a sub-lineage of BA.5) in November and December, with the cluster of BA.2.75 and its sub-lineages XBB.1.5 and CH.1.1 in late January 2023 have together played important roles in the University preparations being made for the teaching sessions 2022–3 and 2023–4. In the background,

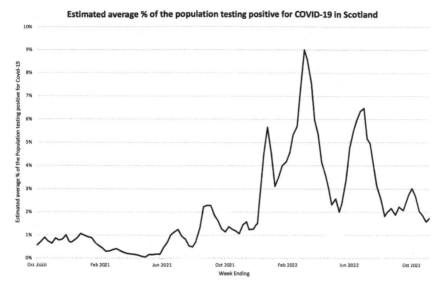

Figure 13.8 Timeline of peaks and troughs of the percentage of people in Scotland infected with the variants of Covid-19 since October 2020. Data from the Office of National Statistics (ONS 2022). Image: John Frace.

the accumulating economic effects of Brexit, increasing austerity and the Russian threats of war spilling out of Ukraine have had a negative impact on the previous normality of everyday life, travel and the supply of consumables for living and laboratory work.

In 2020 the annual National Student Survey (NSS) results reported an overall satisfaction of more than 95 per cent for the School's undergraduate veterinary programme, and *The Times and Sunday Times Good University Guide* named the Royal (Dick) School of Veterinary Studies as the top UK Veterinary School for the sixth year in a row (Anonymous 2020).

Global Academy of Agriculture and Food Systems

The Global Academy of Agriculture and Food Systems has evolved from University approval in 2016 and formal establishment on 26 January 2019, and is now based in the Charnock Bradley Building (Plate 13.2A). Geoff Simm has been appointed as its head. The Academy sits within the Royal (Dick) School of Veterinary Studies, and its remit is to catalyse interactions University-wide, and with partners globally, to drive progress towards regenerative and ethical food systems and land use for healthy people and a healthy planet. Recognising that the global population is expected to approach 11 billion by the end of this century and that the world is in the midst of climate, biodiversity, malnutrition and inequity crises, the Academy will seek new approaches to transform agri-food systems, exploring decision making at a range of scales from policy through to farm and consumer and how these decisions might be altered for better, more equitable outcomes (Simm 2022). It will also seek to understand the determinants of and risks to health and wellbeing at local, national and international levels, spanning infectious, non-communicable and emerging neglected diseases associated with food and land use systems. A third cluster of themes will use training and education in good practice, including data-driven innovation, governance and ethics, and the science policy–industry interface. The current key areas of activity include food and nutritional security north and south of the equator, and the interconnections between human, animal and environmental health. The Academy, in partnership with Scotland's Rural College (SRUC), offers a suite of three BSc (Hons) Agricultural Science programmes: Global Agriculture and Food Security; Animal Science; and Crop and Soil Science, as well as a BSc (Hons) Agricultural Economics programme (Jarvis 2019). The early student intake of fourteen nationalities reflected the Academy's ambition to be a centre for international study. To this end, recruitment visits have been made to India, China and countries of South-east Asia.

In 2022, from 25 July to 5 August, fifty-two undergraduates with mentors and researchers from leading European research universities were hosted by the Academy at the first Una Europa One Health Summer School. The focus was on the inter-related health of people, animals, plants and the environment.

Science Insights

Science Insights is a flagship work-experience programme initiated in 2014 by The Roslin Institute and the Institute of Genetics and Cancer (previously the Institute of Genetics and Molecular Medicine) that runs across the College of Medicine and Veterinary Medicine (CMVM) and is organised by the School's Roslin Institute and Easter Bush Science Outreach Centre (EBSOC), along with the Institute of Genetics and Cancer, Centre for Regenerative Medicine and Centre for Inflammation Research.

Annually groups of up to forty fifth-year high school pupils spend five days visiting the Central, Easter Bush, Edinburgh BioQuarter and Western General campuses and engage with researchers and technicians in laboratories, explore the science behind the scenes, discuss a variety of ethical issues around science, investigate the relationship between science and the media, and receive advice on studying and applying to university. Due to the Covid-19 pandemic, an online programme was delivered to sixty S5 pupils across Scotland in 2020 and 2021, and these pupils heard from researchers involved in tackling Covid-19. Using the overarching theme 'Science is for Everyone', this annual programme provides an incredible opportunity for young people to learn more about studying and working at the University.

In 2022 Science Insights returned to an on-campus programme, attracting pupils from Scottish high schools who were just about to start their final year at school and had a strong interest in biological, biomedical and/or animal sciences. Raising young people's aspirations around studying and making a career in science-related areas is at the heart of Science Insights, so the Science Insights Team works closely with the University's Widening Participation team to ensure that the forty pupils taking part include at least twenty who are likely to have lower Science Capital and whose personal circumstances entitle them to extra consideration in the University of Edinburgh admissions process. The 2022 programme took place Monday 25 – Friday 28 July and was once again based at all four CMVM campuses – Central, Western General, Easter Bush and BioQuarter. All pupils spent Wednesday 27 July at Easter Bush.

Online taught MVet.Sci. and MSc programmes

Since 2005 the Dick Vet has offered a range of online taught Master of Veterinary Science (MVet.Sci.) and Master of Science (MSc) programmes for candidates with a first degree in veterinary medicine, or in a relevant biological or animal science subject. Many of the programmes are also available as a Postgraduate Diploma (PgDip) or Certificate (PgCert), or as Postgraduate Professional Development (PgProf.Dev. or PPD). The Postgraduate Taught (PGT) community has continued to grow and flourish despite the pandemic (Anonymous 2021). Its 2021–2 distribution in the UK and the rest of Europe has been depicted (Plate 13.3). The numbers and breadth of the 2021–2 distribution across the world has likewise been illustrated (Plate 13.4). In 2021–2 over eight hundred students were studying for postgraduate taught qualifications (Certificate, Diploma and MSc/MVet.Sci.) across fourteen different programmes. Twelve of these were online: Advanced Veterinary Practice; Applied Conservation Genetics with Wildlife Forensics; Applied Poultry Science; Clinical Animal Behaviour; Conservation Medicine; Equine Science; Food Safety; Global Food Security and Nutrition; International Animal Welfare; Ethics and Law; One Health; and Veterinary Anaesthesia and Analgesia. With more than 550 students, the delivery of teaching online is treated as seriously as

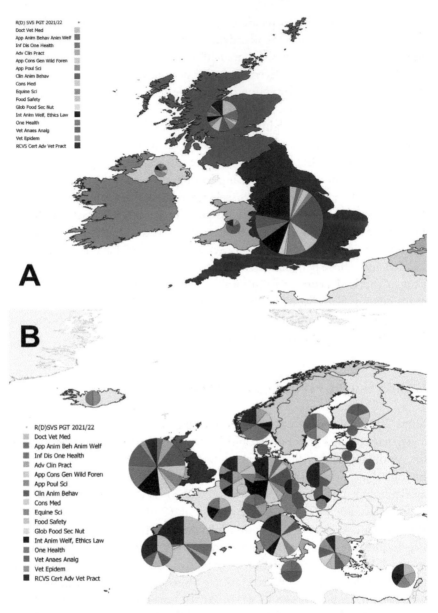

Plate 13.3 A. The 2021–2 distribution of Taught Postgraduate courses in Britain; B. The 2021–2 distribution of Taught Postgraduate courses in Europe excluding Britain. Figure produced by D. J. Shaw and K. Ainsworth.

it is on campus. Every programme has an experienced team of programme director, co-ordinator and administrator, and each student is provided with a personal tutor, to give full support in all aspects of the student's experience. The vast majority of the PGT students were online intermit-

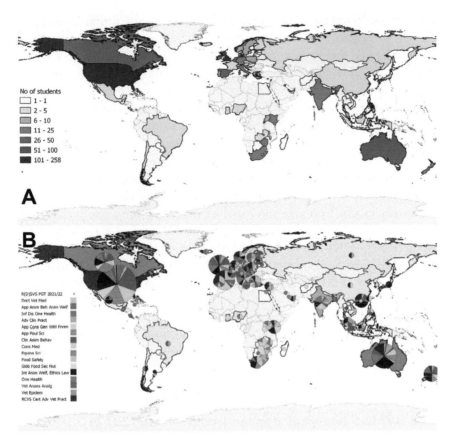

Plate 13.4 A. The numbers and worldwide distribution of students matriculated in 2021–2 to take Taught Postgraduate courses; B. The worldwide distribution of students taking Taught Postgraduate courses in 2021–2. Figure produced by D. J. Shaw and K. Ainsworth.

tent students, carrying out their studies in over seventy countries across the world, from Fiji, Rwanda and Argentina to North America, continental Europe and the UK. The Dick Vet was delighted to be the top-rated School in the University of Edinburgh in the 2021 Postgraduate Taught Experience Survey, achieving more than 95 per cent Overall Satisfaction. In 2021, despite the Covid-19 pandemic, the Postgraduate Research (PGR) students numbered over 170.

International veterinary outreach

As part of its international programme of veterinary outreach, the Dick Vet has established partnerships with a number of international universities. Veterinary students from the China Agricultural University (CAU) in Beijing who have successfully completed the first two years of their degree there can enter onto the accelerated four-year BVM&S Programme. This agreement allows the students to graduate with an internationally accredited veterinary degree in a combined total of six years and receive a qualification from both CAU and the University of Edinburgh. A similar programme pathway is offered to students from the Northwest Agriculture & Forestry University in Xianyang. Students from the University of Alberta, Edmonton, Canada, McGill University, Montreal, Canada and California Polytechnic State University, San Luis Obispo, USA who have successfully completed three years of study on an eligible BSc programme can likewise enter onto the accelerated four-year BVM&S Programme. In partnership with the University of Hong Kong (HKU), the Royal (Dick) School of Veterinary Studies offers B.Biomed.Sc. students from HKU the opportunity to undertake a year of study at the Dick Vet following the second year of their degree. Students can subsequently elect to return to Edinburgh after completing their HKU degree and enrol for the remaining three years of the veterinary degree to gain a BVM&S By the autumn of 2022, eight of the students from these universities had graduated and about thirty were on programme.

The BVM&S five-year degree programme (2022)

The change in the BVM&S admissions process, with the incorporation of multiple 'mini interviews', was highly appreciated by prospective students and enhanced the admissions process and the positive impression made by the School (Anonymous 2022a). The curriculum was reviewed in 2013 by a curriculum development group reporting to the Learning and Teaching Committee (LTC). All recommendations of the group were approved (Anonymous 2015). Curriculum content, design and review is the overall responsibility of the LTC.

The current BVM&S five-year degree programme (Degree, 2020–1) comprises:

Year 1, starting in September

The Animal Body (1)	50 credits
The Animal Body (2)	40 credits
Professional and Clinical Skills (1)	10 credits
Animal Life and Food Safety (1)	40 credits

Year 2, starting in August

The Animal Body (3) 60 credits

The Animal Body (4)	20 credits
Professional and Clinical Skills (2)	10 credits
Animal Life and Food Safety (1)	40 credits
Student Research Component (Foundation Skills)	10 credits

Year 3, starting in August

Professional and Clinical Skills (3)	10 credits
Clinical Foundation Course (Yr 3) 40 credits	
Veterinary Pathology	0 credits
Integrated Clinical Course: Cat and Dog	40 credits

Year 4, starting in August

Integrated Clinical Course: Farm Animal	40 credits
Integrated Clinical Course: Equine	30 credits
Integrated Clinical Course: Exotic	10 credits
Veterinary Public Health	20 credits
Professional and Clinical Skills (4) 60 credits	

Year 5, starting in August

Student Research Component 20 credits	
Final Year Core	100 credits
Final Year Selected Rotations	60 credits

The BVM&S four-year degree Graduate Entry Programme currently comprises:

Year 2, starting in August

The Animal Body (1)	30 credits
The Animal Body (2)	40 credits
The Animal Body Systems & Cases	60 credits
Animal Life and Food Safety	60 credits
Professional and Clinical Skillss	10 credits

Years 2–4 of the Graduate Entry Programme are the same as Years 3–5 of the BVM&S five-year degree programme (Degree, 2020–1). A student

Research Component course runs from the third to the final year and gives each student the opportunity to develop their own research project (Anonymous 2022a).

The BVM&S student population of the Dick Vet was 776 in 2022–3, comprising 671 women, 103 men and two who 'preferred not to say'. The intake in 2022 was 198, of whom 132 were first-year students and 66 were GEP entrants; of the total, 175 were women and 23 were men. The number of students graduating in 2022 was 181, comprising 159 women and 22 men.

References

Anonymous, 2010a. New building news. Teaching building close to completion. *Dick Vet News*, 24, 6.

Anonymous, 2010b. Improving animals' lives. School to open Marchig Centre for Animal Welfare Education. *Dick Vet News*, 24, 4.

Anonymous, 2012a. Students and staff celebrate together. Inaugural Burns Night in new Teaching Building. *Dick Vet News*, 27, 25.

Anonymous, 2012b. The feel-good factor. Great reception for student welfare week. *Dick Vet News*, 27, 21.

Anonymous, 2012c. Applause for the milking . . . *Dick Vet News*, 27, 7.

Anonymous, 2013a. Our Changing World celebrates success. <ed.ac.uk/about/annual-re view/1213/news-in-brief/ourchangingworld-221112> (accessed 11 September 2022).

Anonymous, 2013b. Hallowe'en event. *Dick Vet News*, 28, 21.

Anonymous, 2013c. 'Junior Vets' star on-screen. *Dick Vet News*, 28, 5.

Anonymous, 2013d. Student experience. The names of the Pentland Hills that surround the Dick Vet have taken on a new meaning for the veterinary students. *Dick Vet News*, 28, 24.

Anonymous, 2013e. Practice makes perfect. Major investment in state-of-the-art equip-ment. *Dick Vet News*, 28, 9.

Anonymous, 2013f. Senior clinical training scholarships. Broad spectrum of specialisms offered. *Dick Vet News*, 28, 8.

Anonymous, 2013g. Improving animal welfare in China. Edinburgh vets are contributing to efforts to improve animal care in China's zoos. *Dick Vet News*, 28, 7.

Anonymous, 2014a. Burns night. *Dick Vet News*, 29, 19.

Anonymous, 2014b. Hallowe'en. *Dick Vet News*, 29, 19.

Anonymous, 2014c. Animal-tastic. *Dick Vet News*, 29, 18.

Anonymous, 2014d. Postgraduate success. *Dick Vet News*, 29, 17.

Anonymous, 2015. *Self evaluation report*. Edinburgh: The University of Edinburgh, Royal (Dick) School of Veterinary Studies.

Anonymous, 2016a. Campus leads UK in Research Excellence Framework. *Dick Vet News*, 30, 6.

Anonymous, 2016b. Easter Bush campus recognised for Community Engagement. *Dick Vet News*, 30, 12.

Anonymous, 2016c. Easter Bush Open Day – Midlothian Science Festival. *Dick Vet News*, 30, 17.

Anonymous, 2016d. Professor Susan Rhind appointed Assistant Principal. *Dick Vet News*, 30, 18.

Anonymous, 2016e. The Dick Vet equine practice's education programme continues to expand! *Dick Vet News*, 30, 22.

Anonymous, 2016f. New undergraduate education certificate students visit Liberton High School. *Dick Vet News*, 30, 16.

Anonymous, 2017. Vet students make their mark in teaching. *Dick Vet News*, 31, 28.

Anonymous, [2018]. Easterbush Campus Virtual tour. R(D)SVS Equine Hospital. <https://www.csl.vet.ed.ac.uk/resources/tours/Equine_VR/index.htm> (accessed 11 September 2022).

Anonymous, 2019a. Veterinary Medicine at Easter Bush Campus. <https://www.youtube.com/watch?v=13orDPFlx-o> (accessed 11 September 2022).

Anonymous, 2019b. Princess Royal opens Charnock Bradley Building. <https://www.ed.ac.uk/estates/news/news-archive/princess-royal-opens-charnock-bradley-building> (accessed 11 September 2022).

Anonymous, 2020. Continued league table success for the Dick Vet. *Dick Vet News*, 32, 21.

Anonymous, 2021. Teaching update. *Dick Vet News*, 31, 6–8.

Anonymous, 2022a. *Self evaluation report November 2022: AVMA, avbc, RCVS, SAVC.* Edinburgh: The University of Edinburgh, Royal (Dick) School of Veterinary Studies.

Anonymous, 2022b. Our Changing World. <https://www.ed.ac.uk/biomedical-sciences/news/our-changing-world> (accessed 11 September 2022).

Argyle, D. 2013. Message from Head of School. *Dick Vet News*, 28, 2

Argyle, D. 2014. Message from Head of School. *Dick Vet News*, 29, 2.

Argyle, D. 2016. Message from Head of School. *Dick Vet News*, 30, 2.

Argyle, D. 2020. Welcome. *Dick Vet News*, 32, 2.

Bergkvist, G., Bradley, K., See , J., Wilhelm, A. and Ma, C. 2019. Veterinary medicine experience – study abroad science pathway. <youtube.com/watch?v-dRkUw-zNHMI> (accessed 11 September 2022).

Coursera, 2016. Dick Vet joins US online partnership. <https://www.ed.ac.uk/vet/news-events/archive/2012/mooc> (accessed 11 September 2022).

Day, 2016. Day in the life of a first year vet student. <youtube.com/watch?v=D7dI5QaVXeE> (accessed 11 September 2022).

Degree, 2020/21. Degree Programme Table: Veterinary Medicine. (Preclinical) (BVMS) <http://www.drps.ed.ac.uk/20-21/dpt/utclivms.htm> (accessed 30 November 2022).

Degree Programme Table: Veterinary Medicine. (Preclinical) (Graduate Entry) (BVMS). <http://www.drps.ed.ac.uk/20-21/dpt/utcliv2.htm> (accessed 30 November 2022).

Dhinoja, S., Towell, I., Raborn, E., Poll, D. and Podgurski, A. 2020. The student experience – Edinburgh Veterinary School. <youtube.com/watch?v=NNpX_DV7l4c&list=PLCB1_5xg9L8boRYN-9x7PuoSR290Xd6gL&index=18> (accessed 11 September 2022).

ECAT-V, 2013. Edinburgh Clinical Academic Track for Veterinarians programme. <https://www.ed.ac.uk/medicine-vet-medicine/research-support-development-commercialisation/edinburgh-clinical-academic-track/wellcome-trust-training-fellowships/ecat-veterinary-clinical-lectureships> (accessed 11 September 2022).

Ferguson, C. 2022. Dick Vet undergraduate vlog. <youtube.com/watch?v=Roo1SJj6m4sA> (accessed 11 September 2022).

Gardiner, A. 2014. 'One Health' approach to teaching core skills in dentistry. *Dick Vet News*, 29, 8.

Gorman, D. 2016. £11m Energy Centre for Easter Bush Campus. *Dick Vet News*, 30, 27.

Herrington, R., Stirling, H., Cassie, G. and Ford, S. 2017. Inaugural One Health Student conference in Edinburgh. *Dick Vet News*, 31, 24.

Hudson, N. 2017. Teaching Matters Undergraduate Certificate in Veterinary Medical Education. <youtube.com/watch?v=j7lGIubiRac> (accessed 11 September 2022).

IPCC, 2007. Climate Change 2007: Synthesis Report. Contribution of Working Groups I, II and III to the Fourth Assessment Report of the Intergovernmental Panel on Climate Change [Core Writing Team, Pachauri, R. K and Reisinger, A. (eds)]. Geneva, Switzerland: IPCC.

IPCC, 2022. *Climate Change 2022: Impacts, Adaptation and Vulnerability. Contribution of Working Group II to the Sixth Assessment Report of the Intergovernmental Panel on Climate Change* [H.-O. Pörtner, D. C. Roberts, M. Tignor, E. S. Poloczanska, K. Mintenbeck, A. Alegría, M. Craig, S. Langsdorf, S. Löschke, V. Möller, A. Okem, B. Rama (eds)]. Cambridge and New York: Cambridge University Press, 3,056 pages. < doi:10.1017/9781009325844> (accessed 6 December 2022).

Jarvis, S. 2019. Global Academy undergraduate programmes. *Global Academy of Agriculture and Food Security Newsletter*, 1, 2.

Matthews, P. K., Macdonald, A. A. and Warwick C. M. 2016a. The War Memorial and Roll-of-Honour of the Royal (Dick) School of Veterinary Studies. *Veterinary History*, 18, 117–64.

Matthews, P. K., Warwick C. M., McTier, B. and Macdonald, A. A. 2016b. Royal (Dick) School of Veterinary Studies War Memorial – Update. *Veterinary History*, 18, 242–3.

Murdoch, F., Bergkvist, G. and Kristruck, H. 2021. Widening access at the Royal (Dick) School of Veterinary Studies. <youtube.com/watch?v=z0Uva1efxEg> (accessed 11 September 2022).

Murray, J.-A. 2014. Participants' perceptions of a MOOC. Insights. *The UKSG Journal*, 27 (2), 154–9. <doi: 10.1629/2048-7754.154> (accessed 11 September 2022).

ONS, 2022. Office for National Statistics (ONS), released 2 December 2022, ONS website, statistical bulletin, Coronavirus (COVID-19) Infection Survey, UK: 2 December 2022.

Paterson, J. 2015. The student experience. <youtube.com/watch?v=uj-mZjwh9jA&list=PLCB1_5xg9L8boRYN-9x7PuoSR290Xd6gL&index=11> (accessed 11 September 2022).

Pörtner, H.-O., D. C. Roberts, H. Adams, I. Adelekan, C. Adler, R. Adrian, P. Aldunce, E. Ali, R. Ara Begum, B. Bednar-Friedl, R. Bezner Kerr, R. Biesbroek, J. Birkmann, K. Bowen, M. A. Caretta, J. Carnicer, E. Castellanos, T. S. Cheong, W. Chow, G. Cissé, S. Clayton, A. Constable, S. R. Cooley, M. J. Costello, M. Craig, W. Cramer, R. Dawson, D. Dodman, J. Efitre, M. Garschagen, E. A. Gilmore, B. C. Glavovic, D. Gutzler, M. Haasnoot, S. Harper, T. Hasegawa, B. Hayward, J. A. Hicke, Y. Hirabayashi, C. Huang, K. Kalaba, W. Kiessling, A. Kitoh, R. Lasco, J. Lawrence, M. F. Lemos, R. Lempert, C. Lennard, D. Ley, T. Lissner, Q. Liu, E. Liwenga, S. Lluch-Cota, S. Löschke, S. Lucatello, Y. Luo, B. Mackey, K. Mintenbeck, A. Mirzabaev, V. Möller, M. Moncassim Vale, M. D. Morecroft, L. Mortsch, A. Mukherji, T. Mustonen, M. Mycoo, J. Nalau, M. New, A. Okem, J. P. Ometto, B. O'Neill, R. Pandey, C. Parmesan, M. Pelling, P. F. Pinho, J. Pinnegar, E. S. Poloczanska, A. Prakash, B. Preston, M.-F. Racault, D. Reckien, A. Revi, S. K. Rose, E. L. F. Schipper, D. N. Schmidt, D. Schoeman, R. Shaw, N. P. Simpson, C. Singh, W. Solecki, L. Stringer, E. Totin, C. H. Trisos, Y. Trisurat, M. van Aalst, D. Viner, M. Wairiu, R. Warren, P. Wester, D. Wrathall, and Z. Zaiton Ibrahim, 2022: Technical Summary. [H.-O. Pörtner, D. C. Roberts, E. S. Poloczanska, K. Mintenbeck, M. Tignor, A. Alegría, M. Craig, S. Langsdorf, S. Löschke, V. Möller and A. Okem (eds)]. In: *Climate Change 2022: Impacts, Adaptation and Vulnerability. Contribution of Working Group II to the Sixth Assessment Report of the Intergovernmental Panel on Climate Change* [H.-O. Pörtner, D. C. Roberts, M. Tignor, E. S. Poloczanska, K. Mintenbeck, A. Alegría, M. Craig, S. Langsdorf, S. Löschke, V. Möller, A. Okem and B. Rama (eds)]. Cambridge and New York: Cambridge University Press, 37–118. <doi:10.1017/9781009325844.002> (accessed 6 December 2022).

Roslininnovationcentre, 2023. A growing community of collaborators. <https://www.roslininnovationcentre.com/assets/contentfiles/pdf/Tenant_Directory_Jan23_AZ.pdf> (accessed 14 February 2023).

Simm, G. 2022a. Why study Agricultural Science? Launching a new Global Academy of Agriculture and Food Security. <https://www.ed.ac.uk/global-agriculture-food-sy

stems/gaafs-news/news/launching-new-global-academy-of-agriculture> (accessed 11 September 2022).

Simm, G. 2022b. Personal communication.

Ukraine, 2022. Timeline of the 2022 Russian invasion of Ukraine. <https://en.wikip edia.org/wiki/Timeline_of_the_2022_Russian_invasion_of_Ukraine> (accessed 11 September 2022).

Chapter 14

Student Activities at the Dick Vet (1823–2022)

Dick Vet student experience

This chapter seeks to capture some measure of the enormous variety and richness of the student experience at the Dick Vet over the last two centuries. It recognises that all ages of human life, from the unborn to the most aged, contributed significantly, at an individual level, to the social milieu within which veterinary education in Edinburgh was carried out. We shall attempt to give some indications of those personal reflections while placing most focus on the 'organised' aspects of student social life – the sports, clubs, societies, dances, expeditions and other activities. Most of the available information of necessity refers to the last 120 years. However, some indications of student life in nineteenth-century Edinburgh can be gathered from these detailed, lively, and varied accounts (Mansfield 1854; Fraser 1884; Worthington 1897). Undoubtedly climate played a significant role. Edinburgh in November and December was described as 'airy, and perfectly free from damp'. Edinburgh's winters were often described as 'not cold enough. It is desirable that they were more keen.' The winter days were short too.

Outdoor games in the mid-nineteenth century tended to be physical and competitive (Tranter 1987). Quoiting was a popular sport in Scotland, in which heavy metal rings, usually weighing 3.5 to 5.5 kg, were thrown at a pin in the ground (Tranter 1992; 1998). The distance was 20 m, often on rough ground (Figure 14.1). Strength and stamina were required, attributes acquired daily by iron-hammering farriers. Golf was popular in Scotland, and the game flourished in Edinburgh (Tranter 1987; Burnett 2000). In winter, curling was the more popular sport, all over Scotland; it was highly likely that some of the lads studying in the

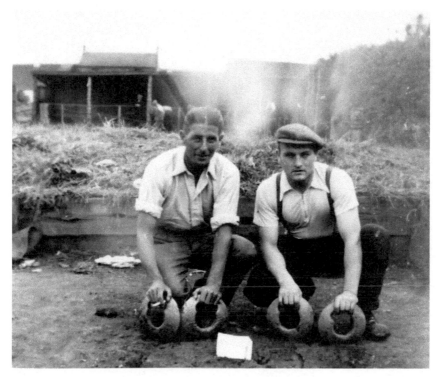

Figure 14.1 Mauchline quoiters J. Cartner and J. Kirkpatrick at the quoiting green. Photographer: J. Kirkpatrick. Permission granted by James Taylor, Ayrshirehistory.com.

Veterinary School would have participated (Burnett 2000). Duddingston Loch, to the south-east side of Arthur's Seat, was the local centre of attraction (Figure 14.2). In 1833 two to three thousand folk were reported on the 'thick-ribbed ice', with skaters and curling teams playing. Curling was, and is, a game of passion. Games in that period could be hoped for, but not planned, as it was cold weather-dependent.

Outdoor exercise was encouraged as recreation. Edinburgh is fortunate to have within its boundaries to the south the large free open spaces at the Bruntsfield Links, the avenue walks in the Meadows and the large Holyrood Park with Salisbury Crags and Arthur's Seat, in addition to Princes Street Gardens and Calton Hill (Figure 14.3). All of these will have been used by individual or groups of veterinary students. The indoor riding facility provided by John Gamgee's west Edinburgh college, in the former Royal Riding Academy, was most probably used by his students (Figure 3.3). The gymnasium built into the remodelled Clyde Street College building (Figure 6.8) indicated both a student and staff appreciation of the intrinsic values of regular exercise and physical fitness during the late nineteenth century.

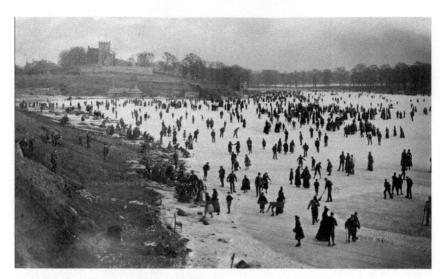

Figure 14.2 Skating on Duddingston Loch. Photographer: J. Patrick.

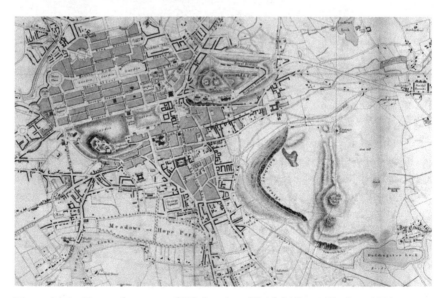

Figure 14.3 Extract from map of Edinburgh and Leith by James Gardner, 1832. Reproduced with the permission of the National Library of Scotland.

Indoors, several circuses and theatres provided a wide range of public entertainment from 1820 (Baird 1964). Examples include the Adelphi Theatre (1830–53), situated on the corner of Broughton Street and King Street at the top of Leith Walk, and the Theatre Royal (1830–59), situated in Shakespeare Square on Princes Street. The names and proprietors of these sites changed through the century. The Gaiety (or Moss's) Theatre of Varieties was on Chambers Street. Renamed the Operetta House, it remained in business until 1939. During the last quarter of the nineteenth century, the range of productions included operas, ballet, plays, musical events and, at the end of the year, pantomimes. For example, a *Cinderella* pantomime benefit night at the Theatre Royal on Wednesday, 24 February 1904; the Baron of the pantomime, 'Mr Sheridan, introduced several special items of his own, which never failed to find the mark, especially those directed to a gathering of some 200 veterinary students [from both veterinary colleges] whose behaviour, by the way, was altogether above reproach' (Anonymous 1904). The Edinburgh Choral Society drew large audiences for their annual concerts in the large Assembly Room on George Street. At a more local level, ceilidh music-making, ballad-singing, billiard-playing and dancing occurred. The published reports of celebratory meals held during the nineteenth century at the end of the veterinary teaching session provide some insight into student singing, speech-making and other elements of their relaxing activities, a commonplace at that time. Other aspects of Dick Vet student life between 1833 and 1841 have been described elsewhere (Macdonald 2020).

Who are the students?

The students who have studied veterinary medicine in Edinburgh cover a wide range of ages and circumstances. Both married and unmarried men were students during the nineteenth century. In the early years of the nineteenth century, they were young farriers recruited to William Dick's School by the advertisements of the Highland Society of Scotland (Macdonald and Warwick 2012). Later in the century, following the entry requirement to attain more advanced secondary school qualifications, more educated cohorts of students attended. Generally, these students tended to be nineteen to twenty-five years old. However, in 1837 Robert Olden, aged fifty-two, and his fifteen-year-old son, Robert Jun., came from Cork in southern Ireland and studied at the Dick Vet together. About a hundred years later, the retired Major General Philip Thomas, who was not allowed to serve in the Second World War, came to study for and obtained, aged sixty-five, his veterinary qualification at the Dick Vet instead. With the solitary exception of Aleen Cust's admission to Williams's New Veterinary College in 1895, the veterinary students in Edinburgh were exclusively male until 1943, when women were first admitted to the Dick Vet. Later in the twentieth and twenty-first centuries, some women graduate-entry students brought their children and grandchildren on organised teaching visits to Edinburgh Zoo.

Student 'dress code'

Not surprisingly, the outward physical appearance of veterinary students has changed over the past two centuries. Drawings by George Clark Stanton (1832–94) (Figure 14.4) give some indication of the working clothing worn during the first half of the nineteenth century (Gamgee 1858). Likewise, the drawing by William Gordon Burn Murdoch (1862–1939) (Figure 14.5) illustrates the clothing worn during dissection classes at Clyde Street towards the end of that century (Dollar 1894). Mid-century photographs of students in the courtyard of the old Clyde Street College (Figure 2.13) and outside the New Veterinary College at Gayfield House (Figure 5.4) give further indication of the 'dress code' of that period; staff wore top hats, while bowlers and bow ties were de rigeur for students. This appearance changed somewhat towards the end of the nineteenth century (Figures 5.11; 6.3; 14.6). The new College tie, maroon with silver bands, and the College crest in miniature on the silver ground, were approved in 1933 by students and alumni (Mitchell 1933).

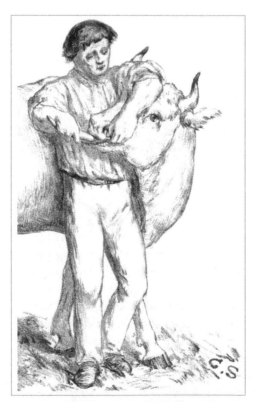

Figure 14.4 Medicine given orally to an ox – detail. Illustration: George Clark Stanton.

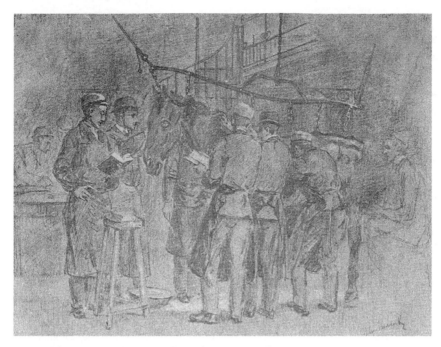

Figure 14.5 Equine dissection class, Clyde Street college, early 1890s. Illustration: William Gordon Burn Murdoch.

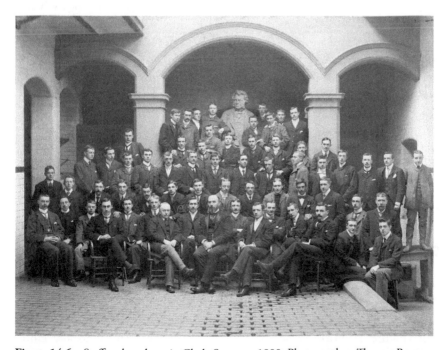

Figure 14.6 Staff and students in Clyde Street, c. 1900. Photographer: Thomas Burns.

White laboratory coats were worn by students for dissection, laboratory and clinical classes at Summerhall during the twentieth century and at Easter Bush thereafter (Figures 12.11a and b, Plate 14.1B; Nivan et al. 2016). During the last thirty years there has been considerable variation in normal appropriate clothing for attending lecture classes (Plate 14.1A). Students working with farm animals wore boiler suits and protective tunic tops (Figure 14.1c) (Nivan et al. 2016), whereas those working clinically in the Hospital for Small Animals wore red scrub tops. When the Covid virus appeared, face masks and other personal protective equipment (PPE) were required to be worn (Plate 14.1D and E). The most obvious sign of being in final year was the much-sought-after final year jacket (Figure 14.7).

Although accounts of student social life in the veterinary colleges during the nineteenth century were often fragmentary, during the following century many aspects of the veterinary students' experience were more clearly documented. Three magazines give a helpful and often detailed insight into student life: *The Royal Dick College Magazine*, which ran from 1906 to 1909; *The Representative*, which ran from 1909 to 1911; and *The Centaur*, which was published from 1930 until 1967 with a gap during the war years (Figure 14.8). A fourth, the *Dick Vet News*, was begun in 1981 and was briefly published (VSC 1980, 1981). Added to these were the Final Year magazines which were published from 1952 until 2014 (Figure 14.9) and the ongoing student internet blogs and vlogs which began in the 2010s (Claire, Patrick and Phillip 2013; Dhinoja, Towell, Raborn, Poll, Belanger and Podgurski 2020). The archived minutes of the Student Representative Council (Lexmond 2022), from 1908 until the present, give further detailed insights. In addition, there are the numerous books by graduates and the compilations of alumni recollections (for example, Auchterlonie 1968), many of which have been archived in the Lady Smith of Kelvin Veterinary Library at Easter Bush and the Centre for Research Collections in the University of Edinburgh Main Library in George Square. A detailed examination of this huge amount of readily accessible material awaits another time. However, a sampling of it here gives a series of meaningful glimpses.

Student team sports and social events

Student team sports, begun as football in 1895 and rugby in 1897 (Figures 14.10 a, b, c and d), were greatly expanded thereafter. By 1930 the Dick Vet had active participation in soccer, rugby, cricket, tennis and golf (Figure 14.11a). These sports and the newly formed hockey club were brought under the oversight of the original Athletics Committee

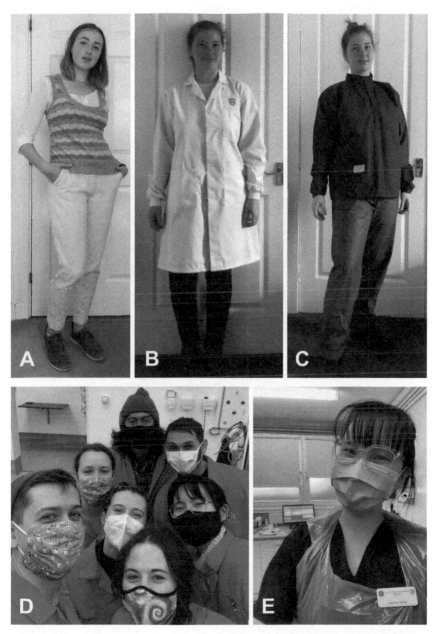

Plate 14.1 A. Joey Luxmoore, fourth year (2022–3), wearing a summertime lecture-going outfit. Photographer: Holly Smith; B. Sian Lexmond, fourth year (2022–3, wearing laboratory practical PPE. Photographer: Sian Lexmond; C. Sian Lexmond wearing farm practical PPE. Photographer: Sian Lexmond; D. Students wearing anti-Covid masks, with no dampening of enthusiasm; E. Covid-masked and clinical veterinary PPE protection, with a smile. Photographer: Vivian Yu.

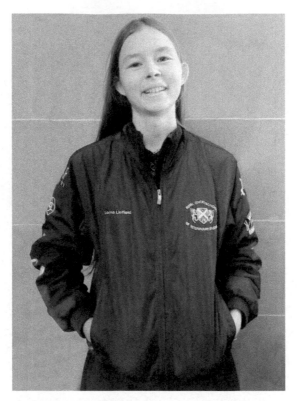

Figure 14.7 Lorna Linfield, final year (2021–2), wearing the 'fiercely coveted' Final Year jacket. Photographer: Ilona Linfield.

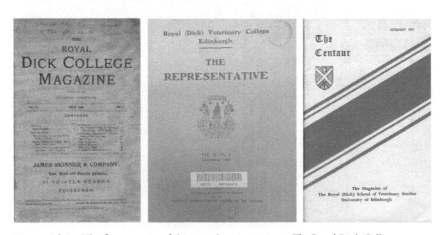

Figure 14.8 The front covers of three student magazines: *The Royal Dick College Magazine*, *The Representative* and *The Centaur*.

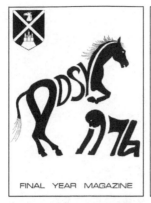
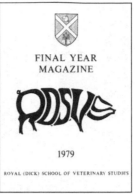
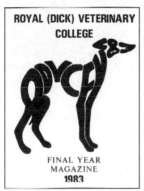
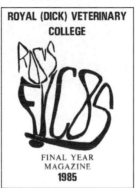

Figure 14.9 The front covers of the final-year magazines for 1976, 1979, 1983 and 1985.

that year. A swimming club was enthusiastically started in 1933 and field sports/athletics were organised into a separate club in 1940. In 1951 the badminton club appeared (Figure 14.11c), with basketball in 1962, pony trekking in 1963 and the squash club in 1966 (Figure 14.11b). Each of the Dick Vet sports clubs strived to maintain the College esprit de corps, and to retain a discrete 'independent' distance from Edinburgh University sports activities. However, the greater range of sports and clubs offered by the University gradually attracted the involvement of Dick Vet students. Nowadays there is a comprehensive mix of sporting opportunities, including mixed hockey (Figure 14.11d), ladies' rugby (Figure 14.12), polo, snow sports, netball, ladies' football, indoor climbing and many others. Early in the twentieth century, participation in a variety of non-sporting College-based activities such as the Officers Training Corps (Figure 14.13; Matthews et al. 2015), established in 1912, the Dialectic Society (inaugurated 1920), the Drama Society (1950s and early 1960s), and student magazine writing, contributed to the diversity of college life. In the 1990s the Veterinary Student Council (VSC) ran a shop selling 'the cheapest

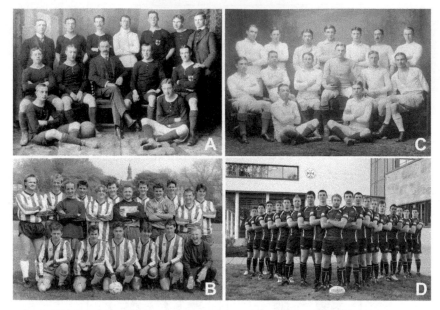

Figure 14.10 A. Football team 1904–5. Photographer: unknown; B. Football team, 1995. Photographer: Fiona Manson; C. Rugby team 1909–10. Photographer: unknown; D. Rugby team 2012. Photographer: 'Female team photographer'.

stationery equipment etc. in Edinburgh as well as second hand books, lab coats and so on'. Nowadays, visit the Dick Vet Promotions shop at https://dickvet.imagescotland.com/ for all R(D)SVS branded clothing and accessories. All profits from Dick Vet Promotions go directly to the Dick Vet Student Union to help improve the student experience.

Music-making and other events

Music-making has long been a Dick Vet student tradition, personified in the illustrations of two orchestras (Figure 14.14). The 1935–6 first-year students' orchestra played Haydn's Toy Symphony and was conducted by Henry Dryerre, the Professor of Physiology, on the Main Hall stage at Summerhall (Figure 14.14a). The annual winter music concerts in the University's Reid Concert Hall were begun on Saturday, 21 November 2009 (Figure 14.14b) after the formation of the Dick Vet Orchestra that year (Macdonald 2010). The Dick Vet pipers were established by Bob Beck (Animal Health) and Ramsay Borthwick (Surgery) and have been a core musical element of the Dick Vet since 1978 (Figure 14.15); they were an attraction at College balls and ceilidhs. The Summerhall students of the 1980s also had ceilidh bands in several incarnations, for example

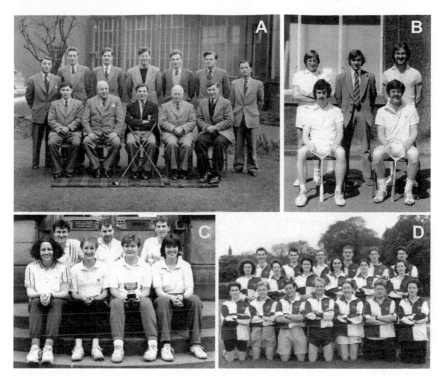

Figure 14.11 A. Golf 1st team 1953–4. Photographer: Yerbury & Sons; B. Squash team 1976–7. Photographer: Fiona Manson; C. Mixed badminton. Photographer: Fiona Manson; D. Mixed hockey team 1996. Photographer: Colin M. Warwick.

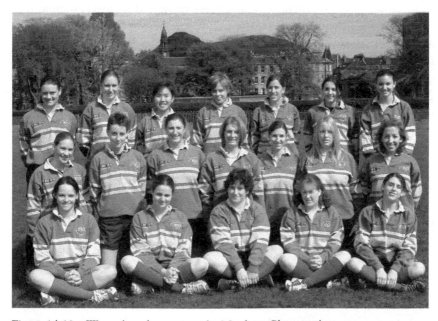

Figure 14.12 Women's rugby team on the Meadows. Photographer: Colin M. Warwick.

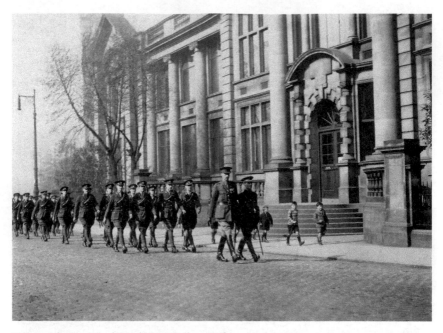

Figure 14.13 Royal (Dick) Vet College Officers Training Corps parading past the front of the College in 1927. Photographer: Charles B. Davidson.

Borborygmi and the Tricky Dicky Band, which featured many talented musicians. Nowadays there are many more clubs and societies, such as the pathology club, wildlife conservation club, art society and musical society, as was recently articulated in a student vlog (Grace 2021). An up-to-date listing can be found on the Dick Vet Student Union website (DVSU 2023).

Weekly student dances in the Main Hall became a prominent feature between and after the World Wars; they were held in the basement throughout the Second World War (Olver 1943). Annual College dinners originated almost two centuries ago and were held after student examination (Anonymous 1840). Final-year dinners have been held ever since. In relatively recent decades the idea of a half-way celebration came into being (Plate 14.2A):

> The **Halfway ball** – is an annual tradition for third years to celebrate being more or less exactly halfway through the course. [It is held] either towards the end of their first semester or at the start of their second semester in third year. This year [2022], it was held at the beginning of February. Everyone enjoys dressing up in formal wear to attend the ball and celebrating making it this far in the course! (Lexmond 2022)

Annual College dinner dances began in the early 1930s and have been maintained. Over the years they have visited many venues (once

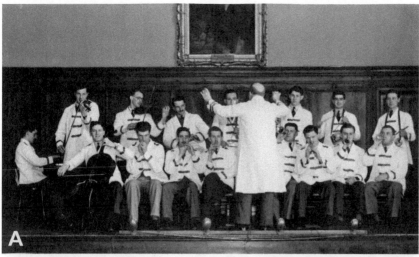

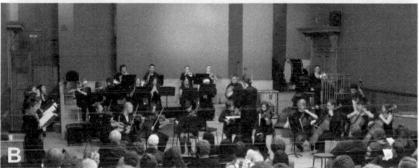

Figure 14.14 A. First-year orchestra, conducted by Henry Dryerre, Session 1936–7. Photographer: unknown; B. Dick Vet Orchestra and Choir, conducted by Chris Hutchings, 21 November 2009. Photographer: Alastair A. Macdonald.

only sometimes!) and been welcomed at the next venue. These have now morphed into the

> **College ball** – is similar to halfway ball in its vet school prestige, college ball is open to the entire vet school (instead of just third years) and has become a good mixing ground between staff and students. Again, it is usually well attended as we all love a good night of fun and celebration. Everyone also knows to bring a good, solid pair of comfortable shoes along too as there is always a ceilidh to close out the night. (Lexmond 2022)

Winter student concerts of music, comedy and variety acts were held annually in the Hall at Summerhall during the later years of the twentieth century and into the twenty-first century. With the move to Easter Bush these became referred to as '**Talent nights** – an event that . . . before covid,

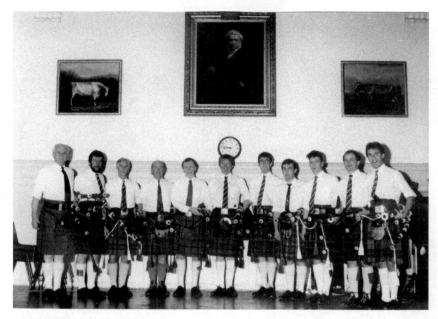

Figure 14.15 Dick Vet pipers, left to right: Bob Beck, Robin Beck, Ramsay Borthwick, Ian McAdam, Colin Warwick, Andy Cant, Alastair Ferguson, John Henderson, Stuart Gough, Matt Coulson and Stuart Ashworth. Photographer: unknown.

was a stage for staff and students to showcase their various talents and just have fun. It has not taken place recently, but lecturers have been heard talking about it with fond memories' (Lexmond 2022).

Burns Suppers were also held regularly. With the move to Easter Bush these became

> **Pre-Burns suppers** – usually held on the Tuesday evening before Burns night and is quite a traditional Burns night celebration with haggis, neeps and tatties followed by sticky toffee pudding and prosecco, all provided by the vet school. There is usually a pub quiz during the event and this year [2022] we organised a treasure hunt through the vet school campus as well. (Lexmond 2022)

These have been very well supported by students and staff (Anonymous 2014). In recent years, during the late spring/early summer before their final exams, the final year have presented the:

> **Final year review** – while mostly aimed at final years, this event is open to the entire vet school, and lecturers and clinicians often attend as well. It usually takes place on an evening towards the end of the second semester and is a platform for final year students to pay homage to their years in the vet school. Some students sing or dance, others tell vet school-based jokes or

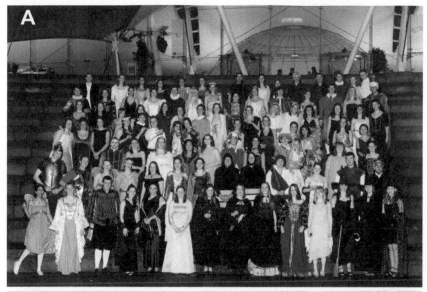

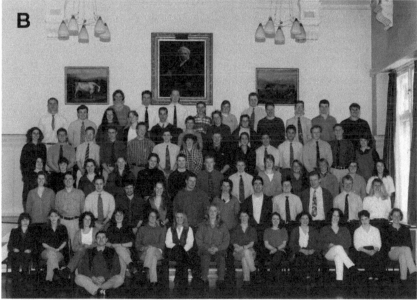

Plate 14.2 A. Half-way to Completion Party at Dynamic Earth, Edinburgh; B. Final Year, 1996. Photographers: unknown.

give photo presentations of all their memories. One year, one student also did impressions of some of the clinicians. (Lexmond 2022)

In the past the Final Year students also produced the Final Year magazines full of insight and mischief; these were written and published from

1952 until 2014 (Figures 14.9a, b, c and d). The Final Year group photo-graph (Plate 14.2B) and annual Graduation Ball in July rounded off the Session.

The emergence of new traditions is best illustrated by the

> **Last fourth year lecture** – the trend to wear onesies was started in 2014 and has become a beloved annual tradition for fourth years to wear a onesie for their last lecture before final year [Plate 14.3]. With lectures being online during covid, [the live gathering] was suspended in 2020–21 but there was a strong showing of onesies this year! (Lexmond 2022)

> Here are a few [additional veterinary] student traditions that we all look forward to each year!
> **Dick Day** – this is our annual sports meeting with Glasgow veterinary students. It takes place on a Wednesday in the middle of November (so not really a fixed date) and it alternates between us and Glasgow hosting the event. Glasgow hosted it last year (2021) so we will be hosting it this year (2022) and so on. The sports that are included are men's football, women's football, men's rugby, women's rugby, hockey and equestrian (dressage & show jumping). After the sports events conclude, there is always a well-attended pub crawl through whichever city is hosting.
> **Welcome week** – The week before the first semester starts in September is a big week for the first years that are new to the vet school. The final years will plan events for the first years to help them bond within and amongst the years. There is usually a vet pub crawl on the Monday, to show new students where all the best pubs/bars/hangout spots are. Safari Supper usually takes place on the Tuesday, where everyone dresses up as an animal and have supper together. Toga Night takes place on the Wednesday, and it is a time for clubs/societies to attract new students. Individual sports clubs will start the night by each hosting flat parties so first years can come and meet the other members of that club, before everyone meets together in a pre-booked club. This is also a chance for some first-year students to be adopted by second-year students as part of the mummies & daddies support structure we have amongst students in the vet school. The week then rounds out with a traditional ceilidh held on the Sunday. (Lexmond 2022)

On Wednesday, 11 February 1998, at a Veterinary Student Council meeting, the idea of a First Year **Mummies and Daddies** scheme was first proposed:

> this is something of an initiation for first years where groups of first years with the same second year 'parents' will get together for flat parties hosted by their 'parents'. Every year, Mummies & Daddies night has a specific theme which students have to dress up in. For example, in 2019 it was Aliens (first years as green aliens and second years as the army) and in 2021 the theme was Farms (first years dressed as pigs and second years as farmers). It is always a hotly anticipated event as it is a chance for students to mix among years and make new friends. The Mummies & Daddies support structure

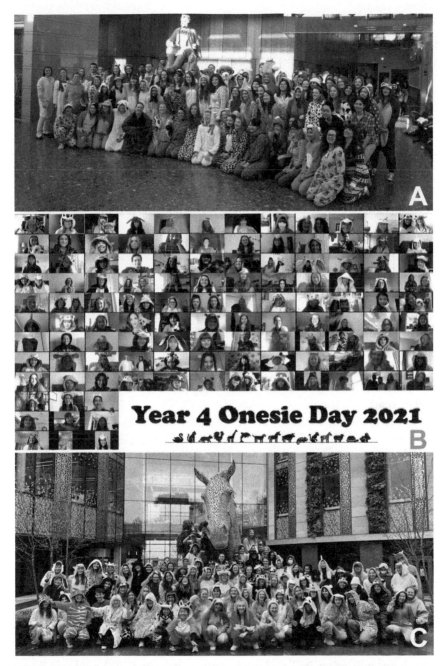

Plate 14.3 Expressions of the new onesies tradition: A. For the first time, in 2014. Photographer: Alastair A. Macdonald; B. 2021. Individual photos compiled and put onto Zoom. Photographer: Ali Humphreys; C. The Fourth Year can gather in person again, 2022. Photographer: Ali Humphreys.

is also helpful in passing knowledge, skills, resources and comfort between years. (Lexmond, 2022)

The launch in 2014 of the VetPals initiative has helped students transition into Vet School life; senior-year students mentor those from earlier years (Anonymous 2017). The expansion of internet connections and social media in recent years has also enabled insight into normal student life to be gained through the guided YouTube tours provided by the students themselves (Nivan, Mary, Rebecca and Ally 2016; Kirsten 2020; Bhagwan 2022).

> **Traditional holiday celebrations** – various holidays are celebrated throughout the year. The big one is Christmas with the statue of William Dick being dressed up in Christmas colours and a big tree being put up in the atrium of the vet school. There is also a Christmas market that is usually held on campus, with all the proceeds going to a chosen charity, and a Christmas bag appeal where items from staff and students are donated to those in need. Other celebrations like Halloween and Chinese/Lunar New Year are usually acknowledged with decorations going up and some small events (quizzes/ food and candy giveaways) during the day but we have not really organised any big events for these lately. In previous years, there has been a big Halloween party on campus where almost everybody dressed up. (Lexmond 2022)

Covid has unfortunately removed the enthusiasm to organise this event in recent years.

Other traditional student events include bake sales for the clubs and societies, second-hand book sales, Dick Vet Christmas card sales (in the past), Dick Vet art exhibitions (in the 1970s and 2010s), plus all the 'non-campus' entertainments and festivities, the various Edinburgh Festivals, rugby tours, international student exchanges (incoming and outgoing), skiing weekends, trekking with the Exmoor ponies, pub crawls, charity collections, film nights, the Dick Vet Car Club, birthday parties, bowling nights, dinners with friends, walking on Calton Hill and up Arthur's Seat and in the Pentland Hills . . . and many more.

How many students?

It is important to keep in mind that during the last two centuries of veterinary education in Edinburgh, approximately 8,700 students from approximately ninety countries became qualified as veterinary surgeons (Highland Society Certificate and/or MRCVS) from the Dick Vet, about sixty became MRCVS qualified from Gamgee's New Veterinary College and almost 650 graduated MRCVS from Williams's New Veterinary

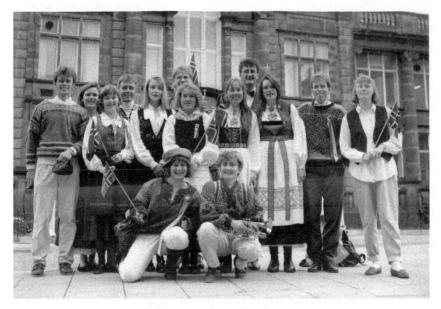

Figure 14.16 Norwegian students, 17th May. Photographer: Colin M. Warwick.

College. Each nationality, such as these Norwegians, brought with them their own traditions, in their case 'Constitution Day on 17th May' (Figure 14.16). Clearly there were and are many others which were/are being incorporated into the lives of the Dick Vet students and staff. The estimated total of veterinary graduates from Edinburgh is therefore about 9,410. Their undergraduate veterinary qualifications were obtained after studies lasting increasingly longer periods of time; one session (1823–8), two sessions (1829–75), three sessions (1876–94), four sessions (1895–1932) and five sessions (1933–), with Graduate Entry Programme (GEP) students taking four sessions (2006–23) before graduating. In addition, there have been several students from other universities' Veterinary Faculties who have spent part of their degree course study time in the Dick Vet's clinics. When taken together with an estimate of the number of students who took classes but did not qualify or seek to qualify (15 per cent), the total student body of about 12,000 men and women experienced the equivalent of approximately 45,000 'sessions' of veterinary undergraduate life in Edinburgh. And this doesn't take into account all the postgraduate students who took short courses, Diploma courses, Masters courses and Doctorates of Philosophy, Science and Veterinary Medicine.

The Dick Vet independent ethos

The independent ethos within the Dick Vet has gradually been formed and reinforced by the accumulated collective mindset of the students who have lived, worked and studied in the Clyde Street College, the Summerhall College and on the Easter Bush Campus. In 1840 the students proposed to the Highland Society that their Veterinary School should become a Veterinary College, and that William Dick should have the title of Professor (HASS 1840). The students recommended and, through their Edinburgh Veterinary Medical Association, collectively paid for books to be purchased for the library (Macdonald et al. 2022). The traditions, culture and pride in the Dick Vet were also transmitted through two centuries with the assistance of students who became staff members. The competitive success of the sport clubs, particularly the rugby clubs, regularly provided events for student expression of pleasure, self-esteem and independence. Membership of the Royal (Dick) Veterinary College Officers Training Corps (OTC) was also an important 'melding' factor from September 1912 until September 1939, as was the College membership of a Home Guard unit during the Second World War (Matthews et al. 2015). Pre-war and post-war international input from fellow students and alumni added to the quality of the mix (Bradley 1928).

Dick Vet students have always travelled abroad, and after qualifying the graduates of Edinburgh veterinary colleges have undertaken veterinary jobs overseas (Williams 1875). As one published series of examples of that tradition, from 1966 to 1986 teams of new graduates organised veterinary expeditions to Uganda (1966), Kenya (1969), Botswana (1971–2), Colombia (1973), the Seychelles (1974), Belize (1981), Botswana (1984–5) and Swaziland (1985) (Hunter and Hammond 1988). Since then, expeditions of one sort or another have become a regular feature of the School's graduate and undergraduate activities. Teams of students have been to many places, including the Gambia (1989), Indonesia (1991, 1993), China (2008), Ulaanbaatar in Mongolia (2010), Tokyo and Hokkaido Island in Japan (2009), the High Atlas of Morocco (2007), Kenya (2008) and many other countries more recently.

Coping with Covid

Finally, a series of student comments on the impact of Covid from 2020 and their advice to fellow students on how to deal with it:

All of our lectures have transitioned online; most of them are being delivered live by our professors, while a handful are pre-recorded ones from the previous year. Every week, we go onto campus, on a designated day, for our practical classes. Each year of study goes in on a different day, to minimize students mixing on campus. It feels quite bizarre to see the normally bustling Easter Bush campus so very quiet and empty. Although I do miss being able to attend lectures in person, with my friends, I'm very grateful for all the safety measures the school has in place to ensure everyone is healthy and minimize spread of disease. It's also times like these that I appreciate more than ever, topics that we learn in classes like Veterinary Public Health. (Yu 2020)

I try to follow a schedule I've written out for myself, and also make a list of some work and recreational activities that I would like to do that day . . . like quick 30 min YouTube workouts, sewing, walking outside, looking after my plants, calling my friends, chores around the house, etc. (Yu 2020)

Alaimo (2020) reported that 'with hybrid learning, the number of hours spent in front of a computer screen has significantly increased. I found it necessary to step away from the screen in between classes to give myself a break and give my eyes a rest. Going for a walk in between classes or calling friends to chat acted as a nice change of pace to look forward to.' She advised:

Plan virtual study groups. Studying in a group has always helped me reinforce the concepts that are taught in lecture. With physical distancing guidelines, it is not always possible to meet up with others in person. But coordinating virtual study groups with friends is helpful, fun, and a nice way to stay in touch! Studying with company also helped to keep me motivated and engaged. On the weekends, I turned to reading, cooking, baking, and going on walks. I also used my printed notes as a study aid instead of using online notes. Find hobbies/join clubs virtually. The university offers a wide range of clubs that have now transitioned to an online format. This makes it easy to learn new skills and interact with others, so definitely take advantage of this!

Alaimo (2020) also advised other students to

Take a day of the week off (this is so important). This semester, Thursdays were my practical day. When I came home from practical, I would take the day off from school. This helped me to recharge and make time for myself [and to] schedule things to look forward to. The way I spent my free time this semester drastically changed. As a result, I found new things to look forward to, including finding new recipes to try, taking baths, discovering new music, and watching new television shows.

Jessica (2020) reported:

we now have new online material to aid our learning such as postmortem images, online histology slide boxes (that you can navigate across and zoom into much like a real microscope) and my favourite of all is a suture kit that we have at home to practise what we have learnt in class. We have already learnt quite a few clinical skills such as bandaging techniques and hand ties for surgery so practising these in the comfort of your home makes you feel quite vet-like! . . . There are more interactive sessions than I anticipated with the opportunity to engage via discussion boards, writing answers live on screen and writing comments in the chat box during a lecture or seminar. The online layout also allows you to be more flexible with your day – studying more when you feel more productive and then taking breaks when you want, such as going for a walk when the sun is shining.

In 2021, Wulfsohn (2021) wrote:

Firstly, right now we have a blended learning model. This semester we have had an average of two days on campus with our Graduate Entry Programme (GEP) class. This includes a combination of labs, animal handling practicals and lectures delivered in person. The rest are delivered online through Blackboard Collaborate, which is an easy-to-use platform that allows for text chatting and microphone use for class participation. Sports teams and other societies are mostly meeting in person as well.

Dick Vet students are bright and very adaptable. Dick Vet students live life fully, just like they have done for the last two centuries.

References

Alaimo, M. R. 2020. *Tricks of the trade.* <https://blogs.ed.ac.uk/vetstudentlife/2020/12/20/tricks-of-the-trade> (accessed 11 September 2022).

Anonymous, 1840. Dinner of the friends and students of the Veterinary College, Edinburgh. *The Veterinarian*, 13, 364–72.

Anonymous, 1904. Benefit night at the Theatre Royal. *The Scotsman*, 25 February 1904, p. 4, col. 7.

Anonymous, 2014. Burns night. Hallowe'en. *Dick Vet News*, 29, 19.

Anonymous, 2017. Chancellor's Award recognises teaching excellence. *Dick Vet News*, 31, 14.

Auchterlonie, L. 1968. *Sixty Years Back: some light-hearted reminiscences of a Royal 'Dick' Veterinary College graduate.* Edinburgh: T. and A. Constable.

Baird, G. 1964. *Edinburgh theatres, cinemas and circuses 1820–1963.* Edinburgh. <scottishcinemas.org.uk/etcc/ETCC.0.Complete.pdf> (accessed 11 September 2022).

Bhagwan, P. 2022. *Unwinding in Edinburgh. Stories from the Vet School.* <https://blogs.ed.ac.uk/vetstudentlife/2022/05/30/unwinding-in-edinburgh/> (accessed 11 September 2022).

Bradley, O. C. 1928. *Royal (Dick) Veterinary College. Principal's report for session 1927–1928.* CRC, The University of Edinburgh.

Burnett, J. 2000. *Riot, revelry and rout: Sport in Lowland Scotland before 1860.* East Linton: Tuckwell Press.

Claire, Patrick and Phillip. 2013. *UK and Irish Dick Vet student vox pops.* <youtube.com/watch?v=BP6C7cCgocA> (accessed 11 September 2022).

Dhinoja, S., Towell, I., Raborn, E., Poll, D. Belanger, A. and Podgurski, A. 2020. *The student experience – Edinburgh Veterinary School.* <youtube.com/watch?v=NNpX_DV7l4c> (accessed 11 September 2022).

Dollar, T. A. 1894. *Inaugural address delivered by Thomas A. Dollar, M.R.C.V.S. at the opening of the 72nd session of Royal (Dick) Veterinary College Edinburgh, 3rd October 1894. Presentation to the trustees of Miss Dick's Portrait and report of the banquet given to the Lord Provost, Magistrates, and Town Council, and leading members of the medical and veterinary professions.* Edinburgh: Turnbull and Spears.

DVSU, 2023. *Dick Vet Student Union.* <dvsu.vet.ed.ac.uk> (accessed 11 September 2022).

Fraser, N. 1884. *Student life at Edinburgh University.* Paisley: J. & R. Parlane.

Gamgee, J. 1858. *The veterinarian's vade mecum.* London: T. C. Jack.

Grace, 2021. *Dick Vet undergraduate vlog.* <youtube.com/watch?v=TY7Pkfp_vpw> (accessed 11 September 2022).

HASS, 1840. Meeting of Directors, 24 April 1840, *Records of the Highland and Agricultural Society of Scotland,* 16, 514–17.

Hunter, A. G. and Hammond, J. A. 1988. University of Edinburgh veterinary expeditions: 1966–1986. *Veterinary Record,* 122, 532–5.

Jessica, 2020. *The semester so far . . .* <https://blogs.ed.ac.uk/vetstudentlife/2020/11/20/the-semester-so-far/> (accessed 11 September 2022).

Kirsten, 2020. *Day in the life of an Online Student. Stories from the Vet School.* <youtube.com/watch?v=UEgC3V4IQGg> (accessed 11 September 2022).

Lexmond, Sian. 2022. Personal communication to Alastair A. Macdonald.

Macdonald, A. A. 2010. Dick Vet musicians take to the stage. *Dick Vet News,* 23, 26.

Macdonald, A. A. 2020. Clyde Street 1833–1841: The veterinary teaching and learning environment. *Veterinary History,* 20 (3), 272–306.

Macdonald, A. A. and Warwick, C. M. 2012. Early teaching of the 'veterinary art and science' in Edinburgh. *Veterinary History,* 16 (3), 227–73. <era.ed.ac.uk/handle/1842/6277> (accessed 11 September 2022).

Macdonald, A. A., Johnston, W. T. and Warwick, C. 2022. The Edinburgh Veterinary Medical Society's library. *Veterinary History,* 21 (2), 168–93.

Mansfield, H. (ed.). 1854. Student life in Edinburgh. *Tait's Edinburgh Magazine,* 21 (241), 29–33.

Matthews, P. K., Macdonald, A. A. and Warwick, C. M. 2015. The Royal (Dick) Veterinary College contingent of the Officers Training Corps. *Veterinary History,* 18 (1), 5–27. <era.ed.ac.uk/handle/1842/14176> (accessed 11 September 2022).

Mitchell, W. M. 1933. Alumnus Association annual meeting. *The Centaur,* 3 (11), 7.

Nivan, Mary, Rebecca and Ally. 2016. *Day in the life of a First Year Vet Student. Stories from the Vet School.* <facebook.com/DickVetAdmissions/videos/293864264911671 > (accessed 11 September 2022).

Olver, A. 1943. *Royal (Dick) Veterinary College. Principal's report for session 1942–1943.* CRC, University of Edinburgh.

SRC. Manuscript minute books. CRC, Edinburgh University Library.

The Centaur. The Magazine of the Royal (Dick) Veterinary College. R(D)SVS Library.

The Representative. The Magazine of the Royal (Dick) Veterinary College. R(D)SVS Library.

The Royal Dick College Magazine. R(D)SVS Library.

Tranter, N. L. 1987. The social and occupational structure of organised sport in central Scotland during the nineteenth century. *International Journal of the History of Sport,* 4 (3), 301–14.

Tranter, N. L. 1992. Organised sport and the working classes in Central Scotland, 1820–1900: the neglected sport of quoiting. In Holt, R. (ed.), *Sport and the working classes in modern Britain.* Manchester: Manchester University Press, 45–66.

Tranter, N. L. 1998. *Sport, Economy and Society in Britain 1750–1914.* Cambridge: Cambridge University Press.

VSC, 1980. Item 3 (iv) The Dick Vet News – 'Agreed it would be a very useful publication, bringing together all current aspects of activities at the Dick, including VSC developments.' *VSC Minutes,* 19 November 1980.

VSC, 1981. The Dick Vet News – An excess (500 copies) produced instead of 300. Student reaction was that it was 'too formal'. *VSC Minutes*, 23 February 1981.

Williams, W. 1875. The veterinary profession – the Scotch Colleges. *North British Agriculturist*, 26, 701, cols a–c.

Worthington, E. D. 1897. *Reminiscences of student life and practice*. Sherbrooke: Printed for Sherbrooke Protestant Hospital by Walton.

Wulfsohn, H. 2021. *Vet school?? In the pandemic???* <https://blogs.ed.ac.uk/vetstudentlife /2021/12/03/vet-school-in-the-pandemic > (accessed 11 September 2022).

Yu, V. 2020. *Changes*. <https://blogs.ed.ac.uk/vetstudentlife/2020/10/27/changes/> (accessed 11 September 2022).

Chapter 15

Summary and Conclusions

Veterinary education in Edinburgh has provided biological knowledge, understanding of veterinary ethics, knowledge of veterinary clinical diagnostics, foundational experience of veterinary medicine and surgery, technical and interpersonal skills, self-awareness and self-reliance, and much more to well over 14,000 students from at least 139 countries who have studied towards obtaining undergraduate veterinary degrees and/or postgraduate qualifications (Diplomas, Masters, Doctorates) from the Dick Vet, Gamgee's New Edinburgh Veterinary College, Williams's New Edinburgh Veterinary College, Polish Veterinary Faculty, Centre for Tropical Veterinary Medicine and the University of Edinburgh. In the process, a worldwide network of professionals trained to provide exemplary medical and surgical care to sick and injured animals of all species has been created.

The external political and social environment surrounding the provision of veterinary education has changed repeatedly over the last two centuries. Initially the drive was to supply trained practitioners of veterinary medicine to all corners of Scotland and beyond. William Dick was well qualified to do this and the young farriers who were most of his students were highly motivated to take on the task. Later there was an increased demand for more highly educated graduates and then progressively a need for research-motivated students and graduands. The upgrading, expansion and eventual replacement of ageing buildings were factors of recurring concern. Wartime and the resultant contractions and expansions in student applicants stressed the physical and staff resources available. Increased numbers of overseas students coupled with a better awareness of the need to deal with tropical and subtropical animal diseases prompted new teaching efforts to better cover these and associated topics.

The culture change of embodiment within the University of Edinburgh had to be absorbed and dealt with. The admission of women to the profession and the eventual removal of fixed-intake constrictions caused student and staff numbers to rise dramatically. External appraisal and comparative judgement of veterinary schools placed greatly increased pressure on the development of higher-quality research output and further improvements in teaching and clinical facilities. The desire to better contribute to overseas demand for veterinary surgeons stimulated further expansion in student numbers.

Progressive enlargement of teaching content from one year to five years, management of the explosion in knowledge of animal disease and treatment, shifts in the animal focus of teaching from largely domestic livestock to include cats and dogs and then exotic mammals, reptiles and birds each had an impact on the changing course content. The shift from preclinical subject teaching followed by clinical content to the integration and incorporation of clinical material throughout the course and a 'lecture-free' final year enhanced student engagement with the subjects being taught. Additional aids to student learning came with computer-assisted provision, team-working and the provision of adequate numbers of study spaces for students. Directors of studies, the Mummies and Daddies student support, VetPals and the creation of the student house scheme enhanced the interaction between students in the five different years.

By its very nature, our twenty-year-long study of this history has revealed many 'unknowns' of one sort or another. We know that students from at least 139 countries in the world have studied and obtained undergraduate veterinary degrees and postgraduate qualifications from the Dick Vet. However, it was sadly not possible in the time available to gather and survey all of the student data. The first large undergraduate data lacuna lay in the period from 1866 to 1920 and the second from 1950 to 2006. The postgraduate nationality data pertains only to the students of the Centre for Tropical Veterinary Medicine.

And, of course, a range of 'puzzles' have cropped up. These deserve and should attract research attention in the future. As an example, we draw attention to this one from about 170 years ago (Figure 15.1). We were told by a former member of staff that the well-dressed man in this photograph was William Dick's groom. Perhaps he was. One day, someone somewhere can perhaps shed further light on that assertion and tell us his name, who he was, where he was photographed and by whom. Like him, these 'unknowns' have highlighted huge gaps in our knowledge of the personalities of the individuals who taught, administered, supported, fed, housed and encouraged all the veterinary students who studied in Edinburgh. And of the students themselves, and their lives during and

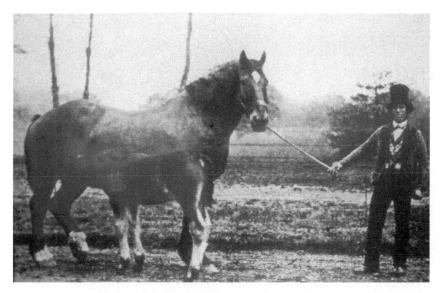

Figure 15.1 'William Dick's groom'. Photographer: unknown.

after graduation, there is much to learn, much to learn from and much to appreciate.

William Dick founded his Veterinary College two centuries ago, and Orlando Charnock Bradley published his *History of the Edinburgh Veterinary College* one hundred years ago. To mark the bicentenary in 2023, we the authors humbly submit this, our update to the Dick Vet's history, including the histories of Gamgee's New Veterinary College, Williams's New Veterinary College, the Polish Veterinary Faculty, the Centre for Tropical Veterinary Medicine and the veterinary contributions of the University of Edinburgh.

Index